The Carrier Oil Palette

Jade Shutes & Sherilyn Siegmund-Roach

Copyright
© Jade Shutes / Aromatic Studies LLC 2022

The Carrier Oil Palette book is published by the School for Aromatic Studies. No part of this publication may be reproduced in whole or in part, or stored in a retrieval system, or transmitted in any form or by any means, electronic, mechanical, photocopying, recording, or otherwise, without written permission of the School for Aromatic Studies.

Disclaimer: The information in this book is for educational purposes only. The information within is not intended as a substitute for the advice provided by your physician or other medical professional. If you have, or suspect that you, have a serious health problem, promptly contact your health care provider.

Library of Congress Cataloging-in-Publication Data has been applied for:
ISBN: 978-1-7372331-6-9

About Authors

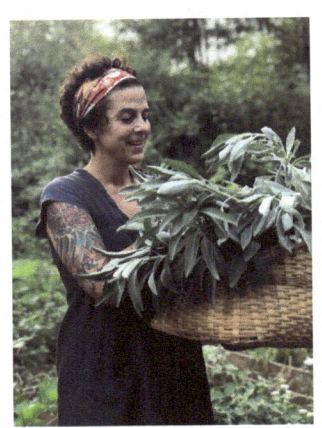

Jade Shutes, BA, Dipl. AT., Herbalist, CCA

Jade Shutes is an aromatherapist, herbalist, writer, researcher, aromatic and medicinal plants gardener, and an aromatic distiller. She holds a Diploma in Holistic Aromatherapy, Holistic Massage, Anatomy and Physiology, and Reflexology from the Raworth College of Natural Medicine in Dorking, UK, and a Diploma in Aromatherapy from the International Therapist Examining board (ITEC). She also holds certificates in herbal medicine.

Jade is the founder of the School for Aromatic Studies (aromaticstudies.com). She has also served two highly successful and rewarding terms as NAHA President (2000-2003 and 2013-2015) and was pivotal in setting educational standards for aromatherapy education. She is the author of "Aromatherapy for Bodyworkers".

Jade is currently the steward of 70 acres of land in Virginia, Yarrow Mtn. Farm, where she offers distillation, botanical body care, and aromatherapy retreats. She also offers transformational retreats for women.

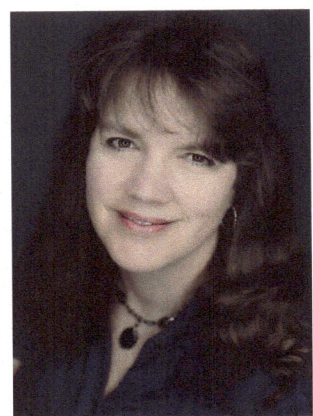

Sherilyn Siegmund-Roach, B.A., MSc., CCA

Sherilyn Siegmund-Roach has always been fascinated by the natural world and the miraculous complexities of both the human body and ecological systems. With her academic degrees in biology and science education, it was natural that phytotherapy would become a vital part of her life after she retired from a 24-year career as a K-12 public school math and science teacher. Sherilyn completed the clinical level Scholars Program at Aromahead Institute and is a professional member of both the National Association for Holistic Aromatherapy and the Alliance of International Aromatherapists.

She shares her love of herbs and essential oils with her extended family (4 generations) and friends. Her clinical aromatherapy practice, Golden Heart Essentials, has included consulting and providing education for hospice programs, as well as teaching, writing, and editing for online phytotherapy academies.

In her continuing studies, Sherilyn seeks out the best ways to combine herbs and essential oils to support a holistic approach to wellness. Sherilyn's lifelong passions for learning and sharing continue to take her down new, exciting paths every day.

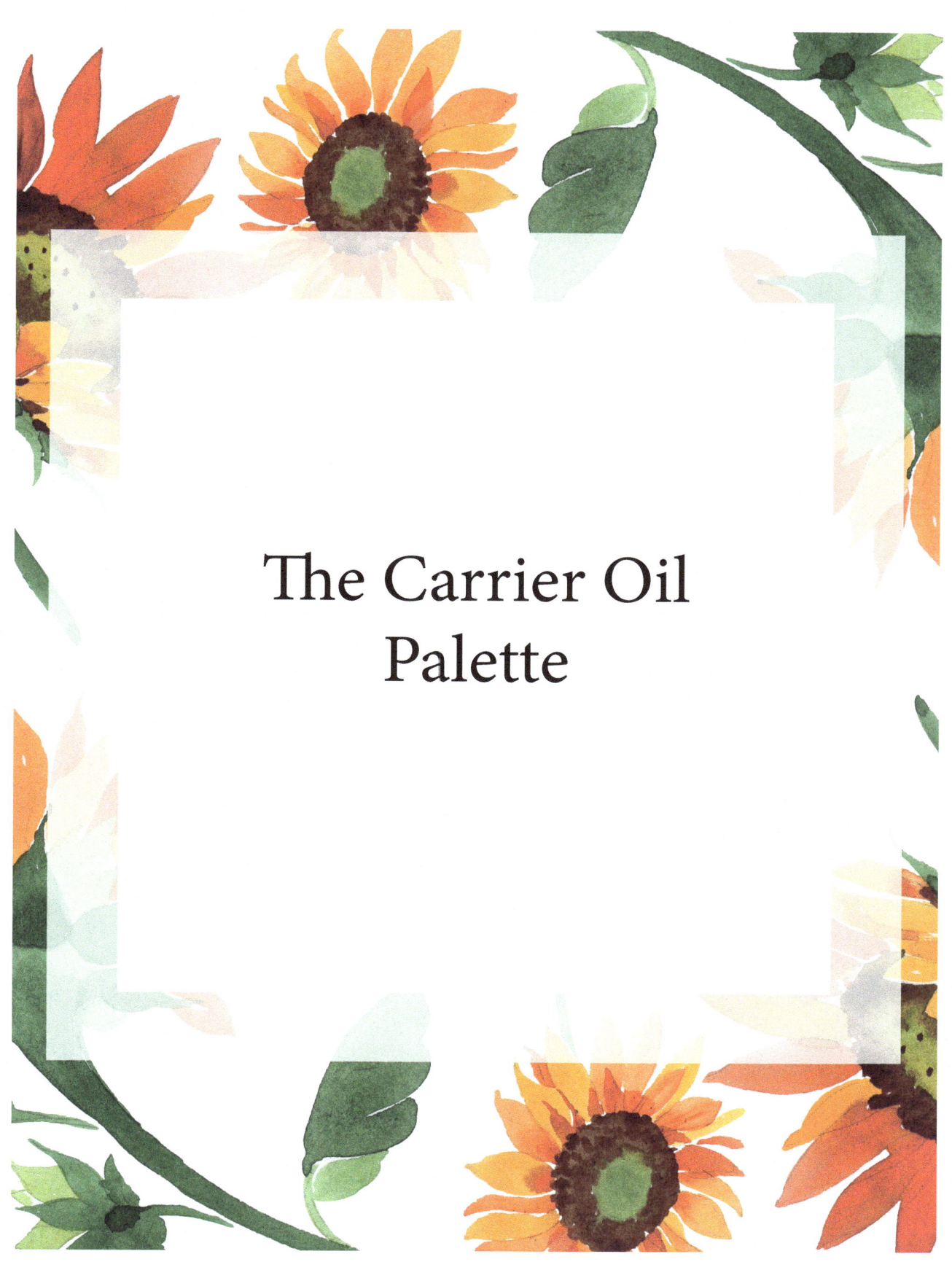

The Carrier Oil Palette

Table of Contents

Part One: About Carrier Oils

About Carrier Oils...7
Therapeutic Benefits of Oils...8
Carrier Oil Production..9
How Refining Affects Quality...9
The Chemistry of Carrier Oils...10
Major Components of Carrier Oils...12
Fatty Acid Naming Conventions..14
Fatty Acid Chart...15
Saturated Fatty Acids...16
Monounsaturated Fatty Acids..16
Polyunsaturated Fatty Acids..17
Minor Components of Carrier Oils...18
Minor Components Chart..19
Fat-soluble Vitamins and Nutrients Found in Carrier Oils...................................20
Fats vs. Oils..23

Part Two: Lipids and the Skin

Anatomy & Physiology of the Skin..25
Skin Ecology: Layers of Protection..26
The Dermal Microbiome..26
Sebaceous Glands, Sebum, and the Dermal Microbiome...................................27
The Skin's Acid Mantle..28
The Skin's Barrier Function...28
Transepidermal Water Loss and the Natural Moisturizing Factor.......................29
Fatty Acids and the Skin..29
Moisturizers and Skin Barrier Repair...30

Part Three: The Core Carrier Oils

The Core Carrier Oils...33
Carrier Oil Storage...33
Almond, Sweet...35
Apricot...37
Argan...40
Baobab...43
Camelina..47
Jojoba..50
Marula..54

Olive	56
Safflower	60
Sesame	63
Sunflower	66

PART FOUR: THE ENHANCER CARRIER OILS

The Enhancer Carrier Oils	71
About Antioxidants	71
Cold-Pressed Oils vs. CO2 Extracts	72
Avocado	73
Black Cumin	76
Borage	79
Castor	82
Evening Primrose	85
Hemp	88
Meadowfoam	92
Neem	95
Pomegranate	98
Pumpkin	101
Raspberry	104
Rose (Rosehip)	107
Sachi Inchi	111
Sea Buckthorn	114
Sea Buckthorn (seed)	116
Sea Buckthorn (pulp)	118
Tamanu	120

PART FIVE: THE HERBAL OILS

The Herbal Oils	124
How to Make an Herbal Oil	125
Arnica	127
Calendula	130
Carrot	133
Chickweed	135
Comfrey	137
Cottonwood	139
St. John's Wort	141

PART SIX: THE BUTTERS

The Butters	144
Babassu	147
Cocoa butter	150

Coconut..153
    Fractionated Coconut Oil..156
Cupuaçu...157
Kokum...160
Kombo...162
Kpangnan..164
Mango...167
Palm (kernel)..169
Shea...173

APPENDICES

Core and Enhancer Carrier Oil Charts...178
Sustainability and Zero Waste..188
Limited Glossary of Terms..190
Shelf Lives of Fixed Oils and Butters...191
Fixed Oils with >20% Essential Fatty Acids..192
Omega-3 Fatty Acids..193
Omega-6 Fatty Acids..193
Omega-9 Fatty Acids..193
Oleic Acid (Omega-9) Content >50%...193
Linoleic Acid (Omega-6) Content >50%...193
Alpha-Linolenic Acid (Omega-3) Content >25%..193
Gamma-Linolenic Acid (Omega-6) Content >10%..193
Oils with Notable Omega-6:Omega-3 ratio..193
Sources of Less Common Fatty Acids and Influential Compounds...194
Oils High in Medium Chain (C8-C12) Fatty Acids...195
Oils High in Very Long Chain (C20-C22) Fatty Acids..195
Significant Sources of Carotenoids...195
Tocopherol Content >1700mg/kg...195
Carrier Oils High in Squalene..195
Sterol Content >3000 mg/kg...196
Oils That Can Extend the Shelf Life of Other Oils...197
Top Recommended Base Oils for Herbal Infusions...197
Carrier Oils for Wound Healing or Skin Regeneration..197
Oil-Bearing Plant Botanical Families..198

REFERENCES, IMAGE CREDITS, AND INDEX

References...200
Image Credits..221
Index..223

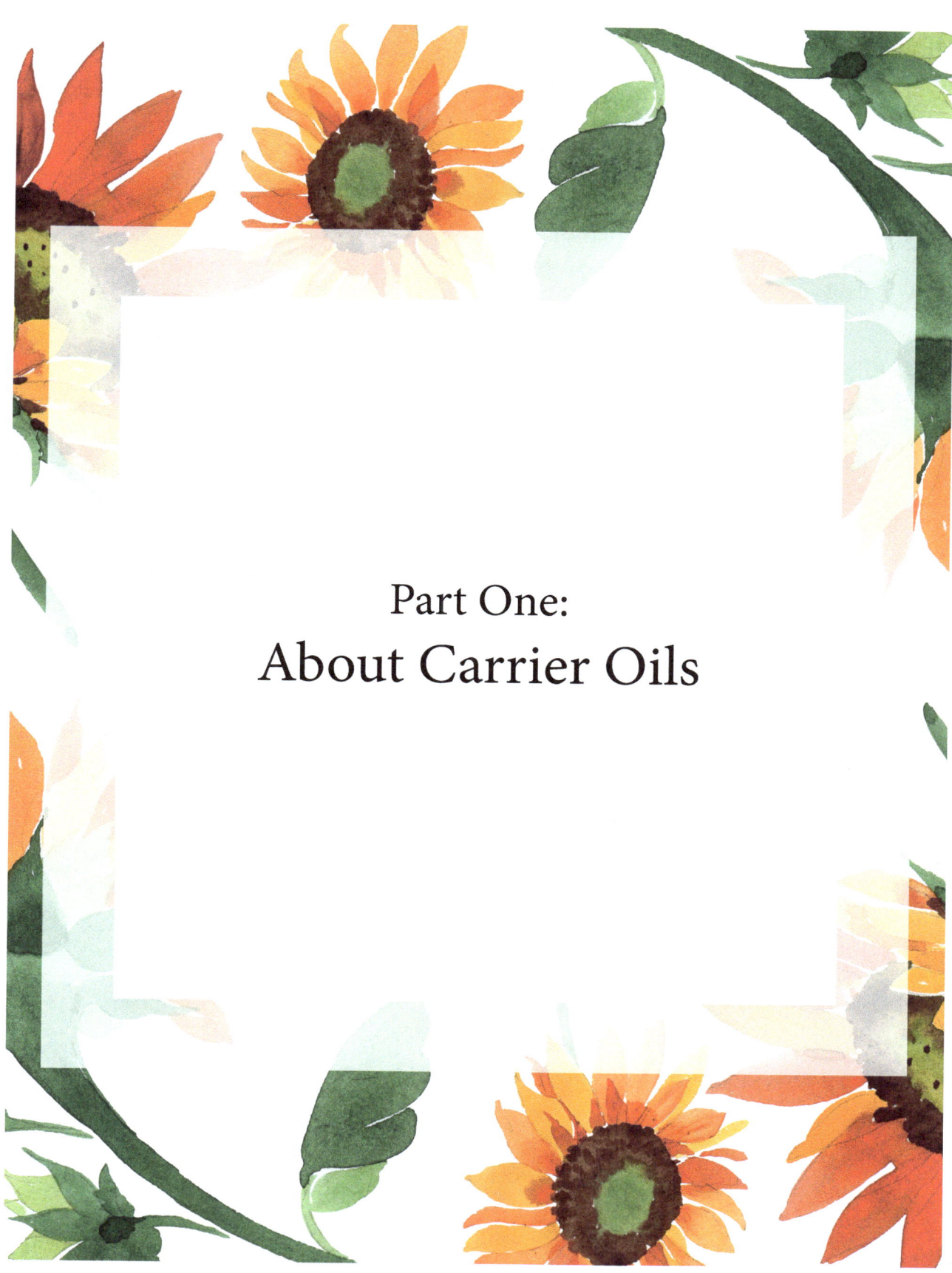

Part One:
About Carrier Oils

About Carrier Oils

Carrier oils are a vital, intrinsic part of the repertoire of aromatherapists and botanical body care product manufacturers. The term "carrier" indicates the oils' usefulness as vehicles for therapeutic plant extracts, but they are also unique, health-promoting substances with tremendous benefits for holistic skincare.[1]

Carrier oils primarily comprise two major categories, the fixed - or vegetable – oils, often called "butters" when they are solids at room temperature, and herbal oils, where herbs are infused into a fixed oil. Essential oils can then be added to any of these carrier oils, thereby increasing the therapeutic value of the overall blend. This combination of essential oils and carrier oils offers an ideal therapeutic partnership.

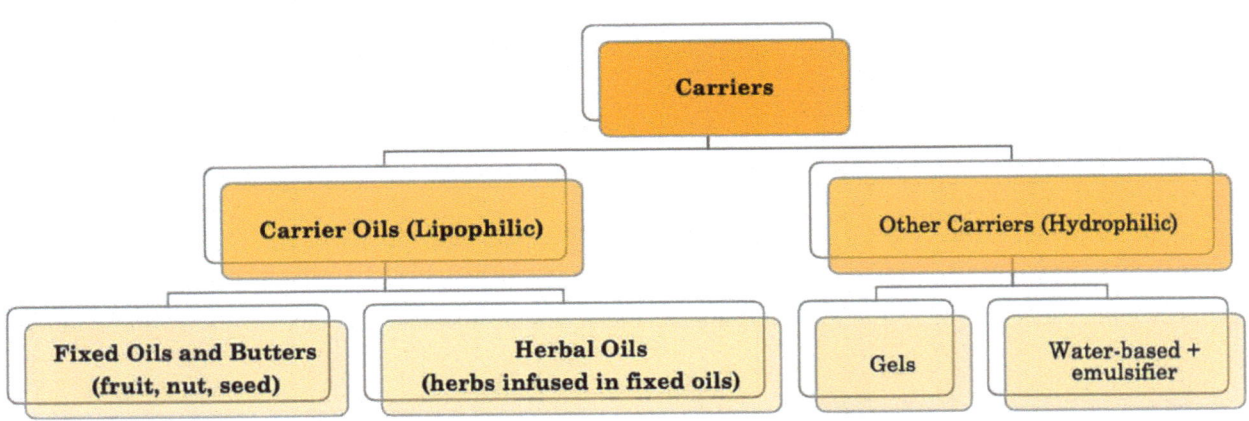

Carrier oils come from fruits (e.g., olive, sea buckthorn pulp, avocado) or seeds (e.g., pomegranate seed, apricot kernel, almond, shea nut). The main components of carrier oils are triglycerides (usually 92-98%). The rest is a complex mixture of minor compounds, including sterols, squalene, tocopherols, pigments, phospholipids, and phenolic components. The types and proportions of these components contribute to the oils' viscosity, state (solid or liquid), shelf-life, and therapeutic qualities.

Note: Mineral oil is derived from a mineral source, usually petroleum, not a plant source, so it does not contain nutrients like vitamins or fatty acids. It may even rob the body of some of its fat-soluble nutrients. Mineral oil does not penetrate healthy, intact skin and acts more as a barrier to the skin, making it an unsuitable medium for essential oils.

Examples of Carrier Oils:

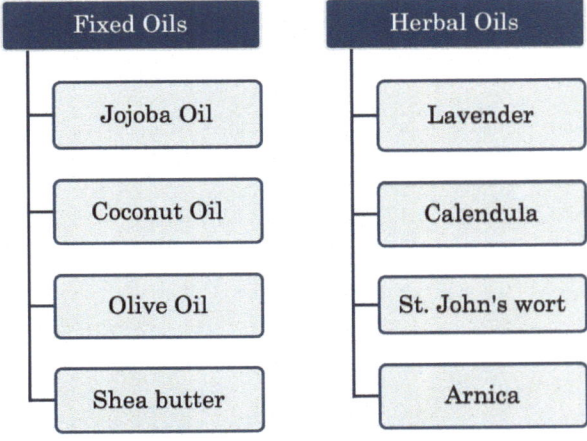

Therapeutic benefits of carrier oils

The therapeutic activities of carrier oils in this palette:
- Support and maintain the skin's intercellular lipid matrix, which in turn serves to protect the integrity of the stratum corneum and its barrier function
- Prevent transepidermal water loss (TEWL) by forming an occlusive film on the surface of the skin
- Restore barrier function, if damaged
- Provide antioxidant activity (preventative to aging)
- Provide anti-inflammatory activity

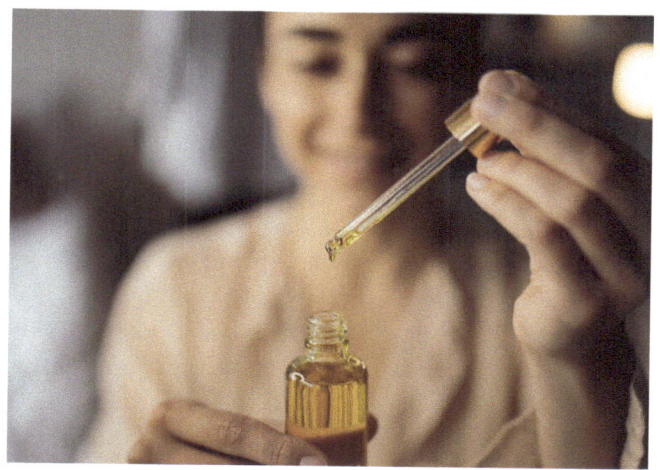

Protection	Repair	Support/Structure
• Lipid matrix integrity/barrier function • Prevent dehydration • Antioxidant • Antimicrobial • Inhibit tumor growth	• Antioxidant • Anti-inflammatory • Cell regeneration	• Cell membranes • Barrier function • Moisturize

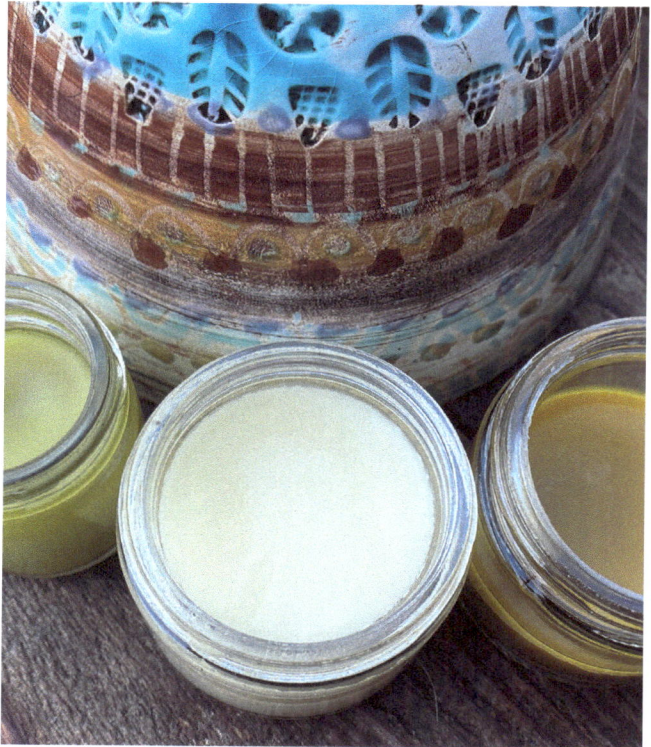

Products containing carrier oils:
- Creams
- Lotions
- Facial oils/serums
- Body/massage oils
- Salves
- Ointments
- Body butters/balms
- Lip balms
- Herbal oil infusions

Carrier Oil Production:
Methods of Extraction

There are several methods for extracting vegetable oils, from mechanical extraction to microwave-assisted extraction. In this book, we cover the most common methods, which include:

- **Cold Pressing or Expeller Pressing:** The oil is pressed using a mechanical screw press at temperatures between 45-49 degrees F. The extraction process may include enzymes to increase yield. Still, the oil yield from cold pressing tends to be lower than the yield from solvent extraction. The CODEX Alimentarius Standards define "cold-pressed oils" as "obtained, without altering the oil, by mechanical procedures only, e.g. expelling or pressing, without the application of heat. They may have been purified by washing with water, settling, filtering and centrifuging only."

The CODEX further defines "virgin" as "obtained, without altering the nature of the oil, by mechanical procedures, e.g. expelling or pressing, and the application of heat only. They may have been purified by washing with water, settling, filtering and centrifuging only."[2]

- **Solvent Extraction:** This method of oil extraction, which uses a solvent, such as benzene, to extract lipids from nuts and seeds, is a more efficient form of extraction, producing greater oil yields.

- **Supercritical Fluid CO2 Extraction:** CO2 extraction uses supercritical carbon dioxide, which has the properties of both a gas and a liquid, to extract specific compounds from a plant. Various industries have used this technique for many years (for instance, for decaffeinating coffee,) but it is relatively recently that aromatherapists have used CO2 extracts as therapeutic agents. CO2 extracts from seeds include lipids and can function as carrier oils.

The supercritical CO2 extraction process can be very precise, allowing the producer to select specific molecules to be included in the final product, potentially increasing the oil's therapeutic value. The carbon dioxide evaporates at the end of the process, leaving no residues behind in the final product. The carbon dioxide can also be fully recycled, making this extraction method relatively environmentally friendly.

How Refining Affects Quality

Refining puts the extracted fixed oil through additional processes to "purify" it. These processes remove undesirable pigments, odor, taste, and fatty acid oxidation products, such as peroxides and their degradation products. The refining process removes many of the nutritive-rich components to lengthen shelf life.

Food producers use the refining process to make oils suitable for consumption and increase their shelf lives. Unfortunately, these processes cause the loss of valuable nutrients, essential fatty acids, and natural antioxidants, producing oils with little to no therapeutic value. Many supermarket oils fall into this category.

Some companies selling carrier oils for aromatherapy and cosmetics will list the oils with RBD or RBDW after the name of the carrier oil, for example, Apricot Kernel – RBD or Black Currant Seed – RBDW. RBD stands for "Refined, Bleached, and Deodorized." RBDW stands for "Refined, Bleached, Deodorized, and Winterized." What do the terms refined, bleached, deodorized, and winterized mean?

Bleaching: The purpose of bleaching is to remove the color pigments from the oil. Bleaching also removes components of the oil that contribute to the oil's oxidation rate. The bleaching process combines the oil with a bleaching clay (a natural clay or activated with an acid wash) and heats it to high temperatures. The clay absorbs and removes undesirable components, such as the unwanted color pigments. Once the bleaching process is complete, the oil is filtered to remove the clay and other particulate matter, and the resultant oil is nearly colorless.[3]

Deodorizing: Deodorizing an oil removes the flavor and aroma of the oil by passing steam through it to remove the undesirable components, leaving an oil with no taste or smell.[3]

Winterizing: Winterization removes compounds, such as waxes, that crystallize at low temperatures and can cause an oil to become cloudy. The process occurs in three steps: heating the oil, appropriate cooling to crystallize undesirable components, and finally, filtering to remove these crystallized components. Winterization typically happens before the deodorizing.[4]

Understanding the Chemistry of Carrier Oils

Carrier oils are predominantly made up of **lipids**, which constitute a large category of molecules that are not completely soluble in water. Some lipids, like triglycerides, are hydrophobic and do not dissolve in water at all. Other lipids, like phospholipids, may have a hydrophobic section and a hydrophilic section.

The various lipids found in carrier oils interact with each other and other molecules in different ways. Based on how they interact with strong bases, lipid components in carrier oils are divided into two main categories:

1. Saponifiable fraction
2. Unsaponifiable fraction

In basic terms, a **saponifiable** lipid can be turned into soap. Saponification is the hydrolysis of the fatty acid esters in the presence of a base, a process by which sodium or potassium hydroxide (lye) reacts with triglycerides (fat) to produce glycerol molecules soap.[5]

The saponifiable part of lipids includes waxes, triglycerides, and phospholipids (phosphoglycerides and sphingolipids).

Lipids that do not contain an ester group and cannot be saponified, i.e., they do not react with bases to form soap, comprise the **unsaponifiable** fraction. These compounds play crucial supporting roles in carrier oils, including acting as oxidation inhibitors (antioxidants). This fraction constitutes on average 0.3 to 2% of the carrier oil, but it can reach more than 10% in certain plants such as *Amaranthus* or *Butyrospermum parkii*.[6]

Nonsaponifiable lipid constituents of carrier oils include hydrocarbons, terpene alcohols, sterols, tocopherols, pigments, and other phenolic compounds.

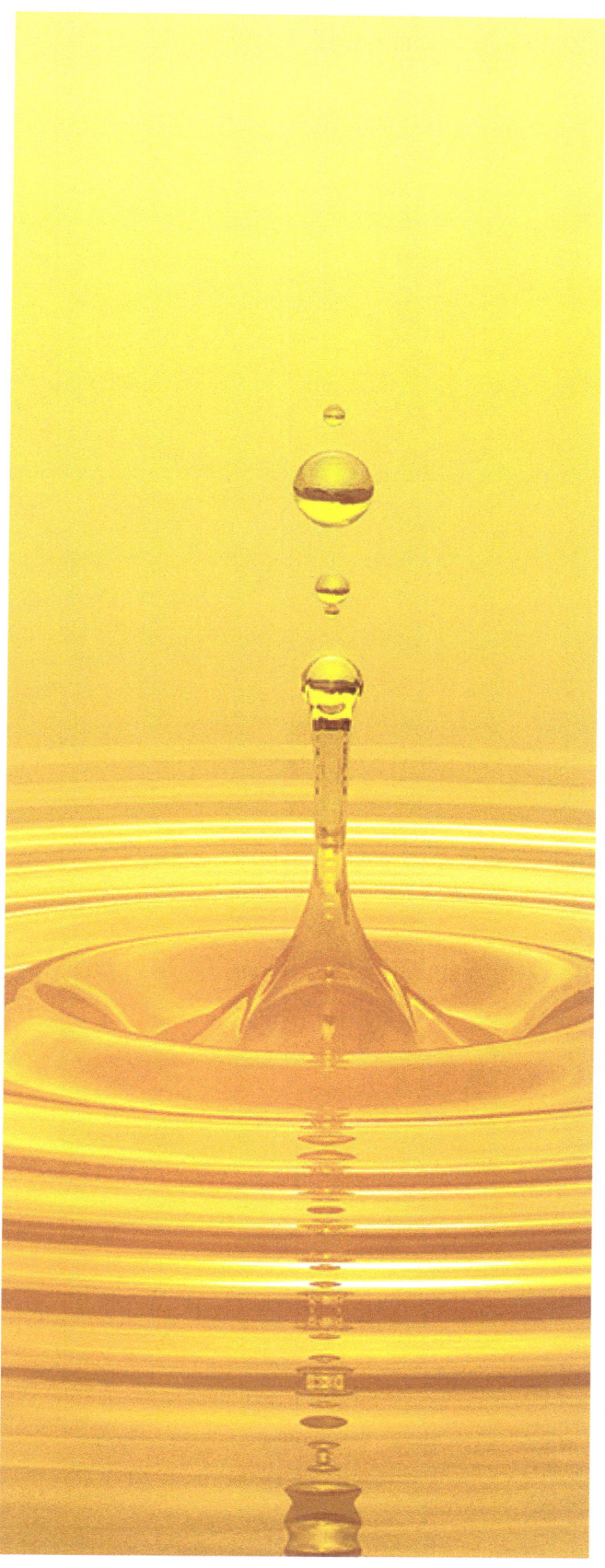

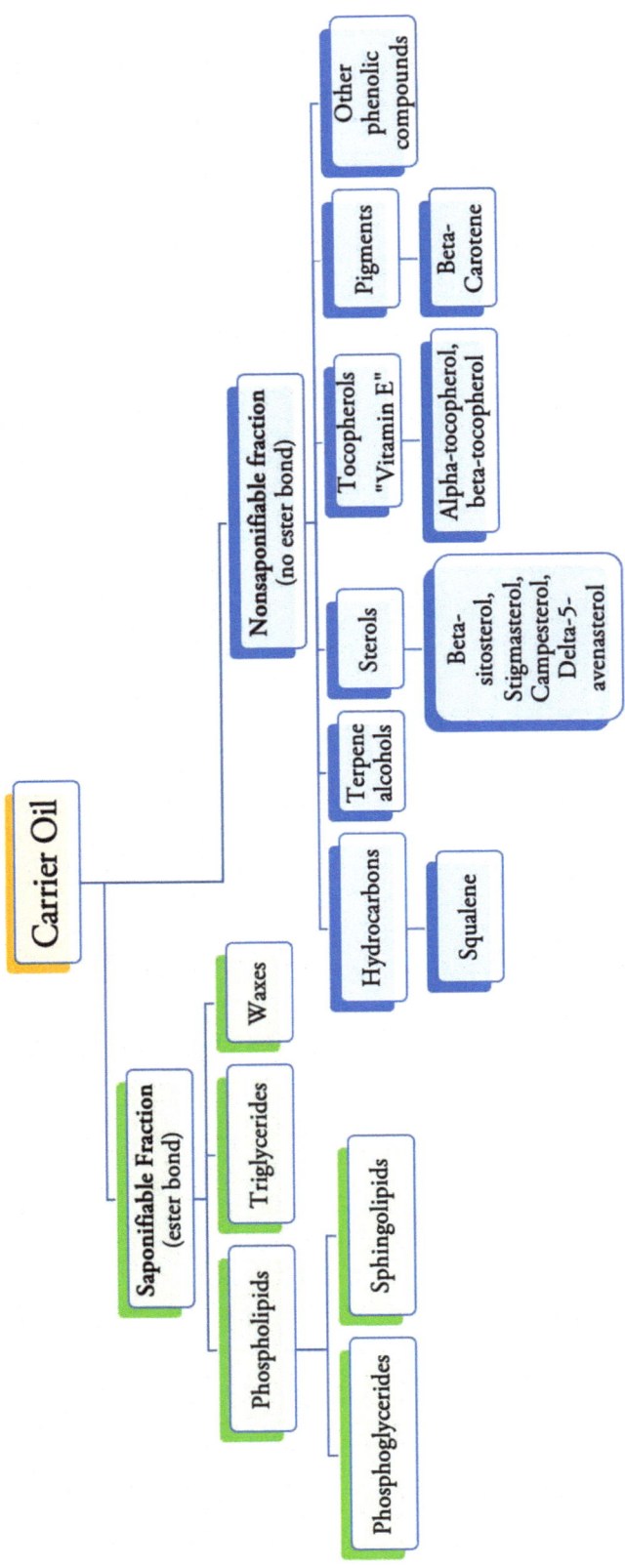

Major Components of Carrier Oils
(Saponifiable Fraction)

Fatty Acids

Fats and oils consist of approximately 95% fatty acids, often bonded to glycerol molecules to form triglycerides. Fatty acids are hydrocarbons and consist of the elements carbon (C), hydrogen (H), and oxygen (O) arranged as a carbon chain skeleton with a carboxyl group (-COOH) at one end and a methyl group (-CH3) at the other.

These molecules play essential roles in cell membrane function and metabolic processes.

Applied to the skin, triglycerides and fatty acids help protect the skin from moisture loss (known as transepidermal water loss or TEWL), soften the stratum corneum, reduce inflammation, reduce oxidative stress, improve cell proliferation, and provide a host of other benefits.

There are three types of fatty acids:

- **Saturated fatty acids (SFAs)** contain the maximum possible number of hydrogen atoms attached to every carbon atom, and the molecule is said to be "saturated" with hydrogen atoms. Saturated fatty acid oils are solid at room temperature. Oils rich in saturated fatty acids include coconut oil and palm kernel oil.

Saturated Fatty Acid (Stearic Acid)

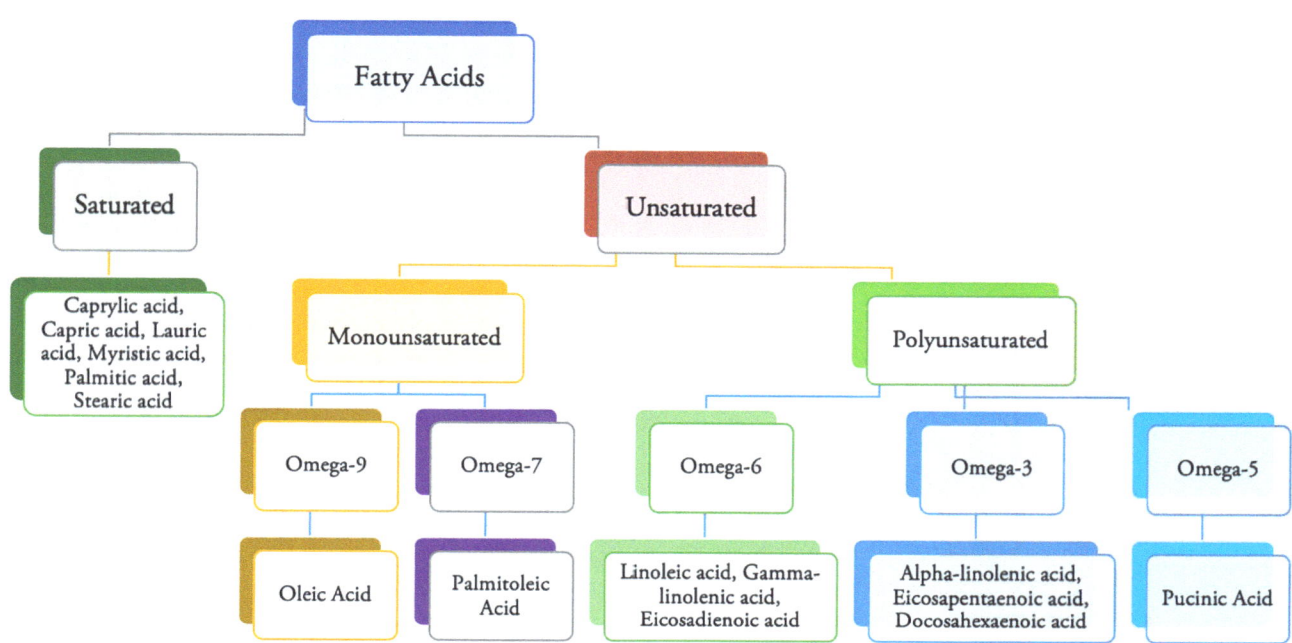

- **Monounsaturated fatty acids (MUFAs)** are fatty acids that are missing two neighboring hydrogen atoms somewhere in the chain, resulting in one double bond between two carbon atoms. One of the most common monounsaturated fatty acids is oleic acid, which is relatively abundant in olive, canola, sunflower (high oleic acid version), and safflower oils.

Monounsaturated Fatty Acid (Oleic Acid)

- **Polyunsaturated fatty acids (PUFAs)** have two or more carbon double bonds. The most important polyunsaturated fatty acids in carrier oils are alpha-linolenic acid and linoleic acid. These two fatty acids are called essential fatty acids (EFAs). They are necessary for human health, but the human body cannot synthesize them; we must either consume them in our diets or apply them to our skin.[7]

Polyunsaturated fatty acids are highly unstable and oxidize easily if exposed to oxygen and light. The presence of tocopherols in oils rich in PUFAs may contribute to their lipid stability.

Polyunsaturated Fatty Acid (Linoleic Acid)

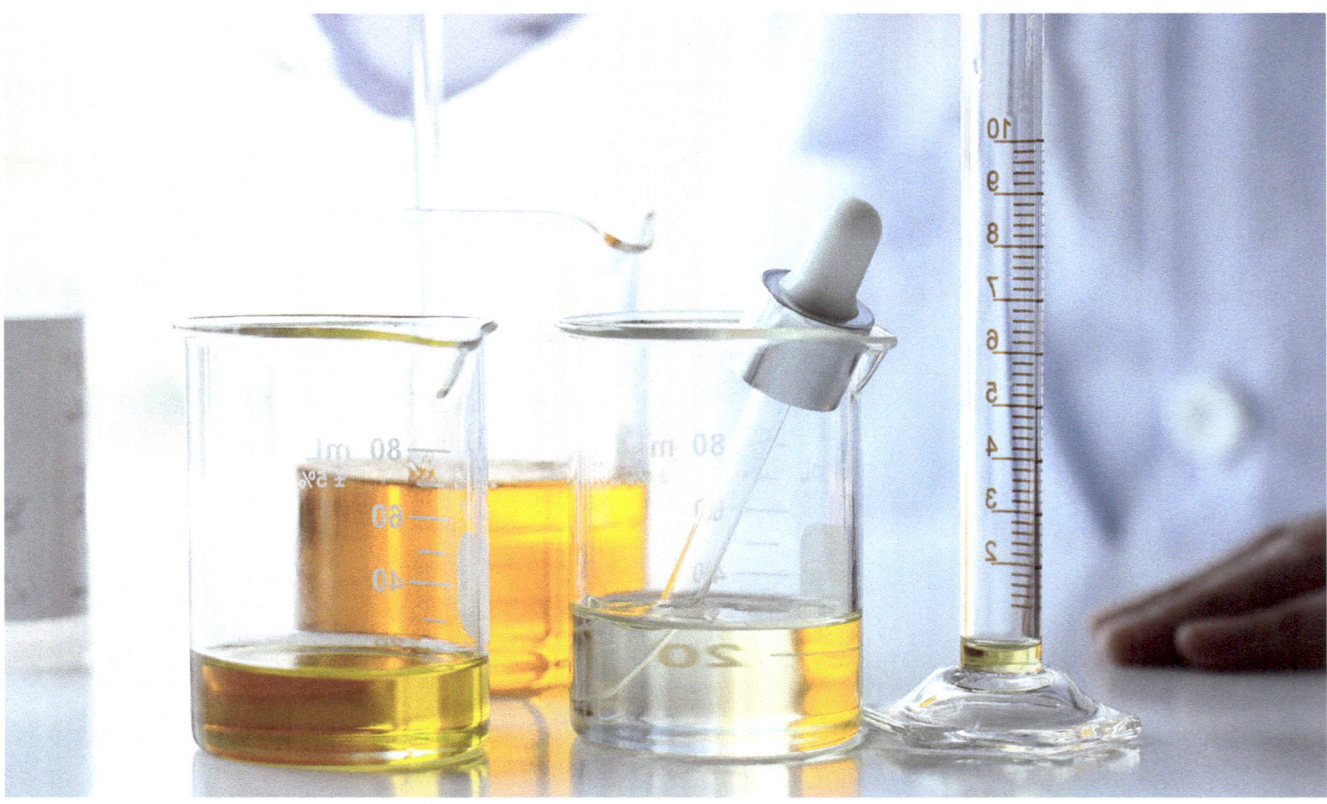

Fatty Acid Naming Conventions[8, 9, 10]

Although there are several naming conventions for organic chemicals, these monographs use two standard conventions to identify fatty acids - common or "trivial" names and shorthand nomenclature. The monographs will use the International Union of Pure and Applied Chemistry (IUPAC) or "systematic" names in those few cases where there is no trivial name for a fatty acid.

Fatty acid common names are the most familiar, e.g., oleic acid and linoleic acid. Systematic names are long and descriptive but cumbersome, e.g., (Z,Z)-5,13-docosadienoic acid.

The scientific literature most frequently uses either shorthand nomenclature or a combination of common names and shorthand. The shorthand combines the number of carbon atoms with the number of double bonds, including the position of the first double bond in unsaturated fatty acids. The shorthand format is (Cx:D ny), or (Cx:D n-y), where x indicates the number of carbon atoms and D designates the number of double bonds. The y in the ny or n-y indicates the position of the double bond along the carbon backbone.

There are two naming conventions, Delta and Omega Nomenclature, for unsaturated fatty acids. Chemists may use the Delta Nomenclature, which indicates where the first double bond is relative to the carboxylic, or acid (delta), end of the fatty acid molecule. An example would be palmitoleic acid, which is 16:1Δ9 or C16:1 cis-9, which shows that the fatty acid has 16 carbons and 1 double bond (cis configuration) found 9 carbons from the carboxylic end of the chain.

Nutritionists use the Omega Nomenclature, the naming convention we encounter more often. The omega format describes how far the first double bond is from the chain's methyl (omega) end. Palmitoleic acid is also known as 16:1 n-7 or 16:1 ω-7 because the first double bond is 7 carbons away from the methyl end of the molecule; hence it is classified as an omega-7 fatty acid. These monographs will use the Omega Nomenclature.

A few examples:

Common name	IUPAC name	Shorthand Nomenclature	
		Delta	Omega
Butyric acid	Butanoic acid	C20:0	C20:0
Arachidic acid	Eicosenoic/Icosenoic acid	C20:0	C20:0
Oleic acid	(9Z)-octadec-9-enoic acid	C18:1 cis-9	C18:1 n-9
Linoleic acid	(gZ,12Z)-octadeca-9,12-dienoic acid	C18:2 cis-9,12	C18:2 n-6

Fatty Acid Chart		
Type of Fatty Acids	**Important examples**	**Found in**
Saturated fatty acids	Caprylic acid (C8:0)	Coconut <10%
	Capric acid (C10:0)	Coconut <8%
	Lauric acid (C12:0)	Babassu, Coconut, Palm kernel
	Myristic acid (C14:0)	Babassu, Coconut, Kombo butter, Palm kernel
	Palmitic acid (C16:0)	Cocoa butter, Sea buckthorn pulp
	Stearic acid (C18:0)	Cocoa butter, Cupuaçu butter, Kokum butter, Kpangnan butter, Mango butter, Marula, Neem, Shea butter, Tamanu
	Arachidic acid (C20:0)	Cupuaçu butter and small amounts are found in various fixed oils and butters
	Behenic acid (C22:0)	Small amounts are found in various fixed oils and butters
Monounsaturated fatty acids	Palmitoleic acid (C16:1 n-7)	Sea buckthorn pulp
	Oleic acid (C18:1 n-9)	Sweet almond, Apricot kernel, Argan, Avocado, Baobab, Cocoa butter, Cupuaçu butter, Kokum butter, Kpangnan butter, Mango butter, Marula, Neem, Olive, Safflower and Sunflower (oleic acid-rich), Sesame seed, Shea butter
	Ricinoleic acid (C18:1 -OH)	Castor
	Gondoic acid (C20:1 n-9)	Jojoba, Meadowfoam
Polyunsaturated fatty acids	Linoleic acid (C18:2 n-6)	Black cumin seed, Evening primrose, Hemp seed, Pumpkin seed, Rosehip seed, Safflower and Sunflower (linoleic acid-rich oils), Sea buckthorn seed, Sesame seed Sweet almond, Apricot kernel, Argan, Baobab, Borage, Sacha inchi, and Tamanu contain appreciable amounts.
	Alpha-linolenic acid (C18:3 n-3)	Camelina, Hemp seed, Rosehip seed, Sacha inchi, Sea buckthorn seed
	Punicic acid (C18:3 n-5)	Pomegranate seed
	Gamma-linolenic acid (C18:3 n-6)	Borage seed, Evening primrose, Hemp seed

Saturated fatty acids
- Caprylic acid (C6:0)
- Capric acid (C10:0)
- Lauric acid (C12:0)
- Myristic acid (C14:0)
- Palmitic acid (C16:0)
- Stearic acid (C18:0)

→ Caprylic acid
Caprylic acid, a minor component of coconut oil and palm kernel oils, exhibits antibacterial activity.[11]

→ Capric acid
Capric acid, a minor component of coconut and palm kernel oils, exhibits antibacterial and anti-inflammatory activity.[12]

→ Lauric acid
Lauric acid is a major component of babassu, coconut, and palm kernel oils. An *in vivo* study showed the antimicrobial properties of lauric acid against *Cutibacterium acnes* (syn. *Propionibacterium acnes*), indicating its potential use in cases of acne vulgaris.[13,14]

→ Myristic acid
Myristic acid is a minor component of coconut and palm kernel oils and a major component in babassu oil and kombo butter. Myristic acid has demonstrated anti-inflammatory and antinociceptive activity in animal studies.[15]

→ Palmitic acid
Palmitic acid is the most common saturated fatty acid in the human body, accounting for 20–30% of the total fatty acids. One of its key roles is to create a protective coating on the skin's surface.[16] It is also found in sea buckthorn pulp oil (34-35%), cocoa butter (23-33%), olive oil (7-20%), and meat and dairy products (50-60%). (Percentages are based on total fat content.)

→ Stearic acid
Stearic acid, one of the most commonly occurring fatty acids, is a saturated fatty acid found in both animal and vegetable fats, including beef fat and cocoa butter. It is abundant in tallow (38%),[17] cocoa butter (33-40%),[18] and shea nut butter (25-50%).[19] It is a minor component in coconut and palm kernel oils.

Stearic acid is used in pharmaceutical product delivery systems and to mask pharmaceutical compounds' bitter taste. Isolated stearic acid acts as a thickening and emollient agent in creams. If you are purchasing isolated stearic acid to use in emulsion formulation, be sure to buy either organic stearic acid or regular stearic acid that is plant-derived, not animal fat-derived.

Monounsaturated fatty acids
- Palmitoleic acid (C16:1 n-7)
- Oleic acid (C18:1 n-9)

→ Palmitoleic acid
Palmitoleic acid, an omega-7 fatty acid, is a promising anti-inflammatory MUFA that may help to ameliorate metabolic disorders when used as a dietary supplement. Although it is uncommon in plants, it is a component of skin lipids and supports the regeneration processes required for wound healing in the epidermis. *In vivo* and *in vitro* trials support palmitoleic acid in treating vaginal atrophy, skin hyperpigmentation, wound infections, diabetes, and liver dysfunctions.[20]

Sea buckthorn pulp oil contains significant amounts (34-36%) of palmitoleic acid.

→ Oleic acid (Omega-9)
Oleic acid is probably the most prevalent fatty acid in vegetable oils. The most common human food sources are almond, olive, macadamia, high oleic sunflower and safflower, grapeseed, sesame, palm, canola, soybean, butter, lard, and tallow. Carrier oils with a high oleic acid content, such as olive oil (60-70%), are more resistant to the damaging effects of heat and light than those containing mostly SFAs. Cocoa, cupuaçu, kokum, kpangnan, mango, and shea butters are all rich in oleic acid.

Studies have found oleic acid to be fungistatic against a broad spectrum of saprophytic molds and yeasts.[21] Oleic acid has also demonstrated the ability to penetrate the dermal-epidermal junction in a dose-dependent fashion, which can result in increased TEWL, as well as increased skin penetration of other oil constituents.[22] Balancing oleic acid content with other fatty acids can mitigate concerns associated with this increase in TEWL.

Studies have shown oleic acid and lauric acid to be effective skin penetration enhancers by disrupting the lipid structure of the stratum corneum.[23] One study showed that oleic acid optimized the cutaneous delivery of Lumiracoxib, a non-steroidal COX-2 selective inhibitor anti-inflammatory drug, by significantly increasing drug retention in both the epidermis and the dermis.[24] This activity ensures the drug moves continuously and consistently through the skin.

Another *in vivo* study showed that unsaturated fatty acids, specifically omega-9 fatty acids (oleic acid), modulate the inflammation in wounds and enhance the reparative response. Therefore, oleic acid-containing carrier oils may be useful in treating cutaneous wounds.[25, 26, 27, 28]

Polyunsaturated fatty acids

- Linoleic acid* (C18:2 n-6)
- Alpha-linolenic acid* (C18:3 n-3)
- Punicic acid (C18:3 n-5)
- Gamma-linolenic acid (C18:3 n-6)
- Eicosapentaenoic acid (C20:5 n-3)
- Docosahexaenoic acid (C22:6 n-3)

Polyunsaturated oils are highly susceptible to oxidation, often resulting in shortened product shelf lives. Dietary consumption of PUFAs can be used in the prevention of several human diseases, many of which are associated with excess inflammation.[29]

* The polyunsaturated fatty acids linoleic acid and alpha-linolenic acid are considered **essential fatty acids** making them especially important. These fatty acids are necessary for human health, but our bodies cannot synthesize them. Therefore, we must consume them in our diets and apply them to our skin.

→ Linoleic acid (Omega-6) (LA)

Linoleic acid is a polyunsaturated essential fatty acid (PUFA) of the omega-6 series that is important in building the membranes surrounding every skin cell. It is necessary for the proper growth and development of the epidermis and the synthesis of the critical long-chain ceramides required to protect against dry skin. Within the lipid matrix of the stratum corneum, linoleic acid plays a homeostatic role in the water permeability barrier of the skin,[25] prevents the skin from peeling, prevents TEWL,[30] improves the skin's softness and elasticity, and regulates the process of epidermal keratinization.[31]

Linoleic acid also displays antibacterial activity[32] and improves the functioning of sebaceous glands in oily or problematic skin types, thereby unblocking pores and reducing the formation or number of blackheads.[33] It can also play a role in cellular regeneration and moderating inflammation.[34] Both linoleic and alpha-linolenic acid may reduce UV-associated damage and hyperpigmentation of the skin.[35]

A deficiency of linoleic acid in the skin can lead to its replacement by oleic acid, negatively impacting the skin's barrier function and increasing TEWL.[36] This lack can further lead to other serious skin problems, such as premature skin aging with a reduction in the integrity of the collagen fibers supporting the skin, which may also slow wound healing. Dietary deficiency of linoleic acid results in a characteristic scaly skin disorder and excessive epidermal water loss. A linoleic acid deficiency may also trigger hair loss.[37]

Carrier oils rich in linoleic acid include black cumin seed, evening primrose, hemp seed, pumpkin seed, rosehip seed, and sesame seed. Sunflower and safflower oil can also be found as linoleic acid-rich, although the oleic acid-rich version of each of these two oils is more readily and commonly available.

→ Alpha-linolenic acid (Omega-3) (ALA)

Alpha-linolenic acid, another essential fatty acid, is highly concentrated in flaxseed oil and to a lesser extent in canola, soy, perilla, and walnut oils. When ingested, the body converts ALA to eicosapentaenoic acid and docosahexaenoic acid, both of which are also omega-3 fatty acids. Omega-3 fatty acids help to reduce inflammation. When applied topically, alpha-linolenic acid reduces inflammation[38] and may be beneficial for chronic inflammatory skin conditions. Alpha-linolenic acid-rich carrier oils include camelina, hemp seed, rosehip seed, sacha inchi, and sea buckthorn seed oil.

→ Gamma-linolenic acid (Omega-6) (GLA)
One of the fatty acids derived from linoleic acid is gamma-linolenic acid (GLA). GLA plays an important role in the formation of prostaglandins, which, in turn, play an important role in the inflammatory process, blood clotting, stimulating smooth muscle in the uterus, inhibiting the secretion of gastrointestinal acid, and increasing the secretion of a protective mucous layer in the stomach. GLA deficiency can lead to various inflammatory, autoimmune, and other disorders.[39]

Carrier oils rich in gamma-linolenic acid may help with inflammatory conditions, including eczema, atopic dermatitis, acne, psoriasis, and rheumatoid arthritis. Hemp seed oil and GLA appear to alleviate symptoms of atopic dermatitis and other skin diseases. GLA also serves as an emollient for the skin and mucous membranes both internally and externally.[40] Apart from human breast milk, evening primrose oil, black currant seed oil, hemp seed, and borage seed oil are the primary sources of GLA, although there are also trace amounts in green leafy vegetables.

→ Eicosapentaenoic acid (Omega-3) (EHA)
Found in high concentrations in fish oil, this omega-3 oil is an important food supplement. It is also a metabolite of alpha-linolenic acid.

→ Docosahexaenoic acid (Omega-3) (DHA)
Found in high concentrations in fish oil, this omega-3 oil is an important food supplement. It is also a metabolite of alpha-linolenic acid. Both DHA and EHA has been found to reduce UVB-induced skin inflammation and damage.[41]

Minor Components of Carrier Oils
(Mostly unsaponifiable fraction)

The main groups of minor components present in carrier oils are:
- Sterols
- Tocopherols
- Wax esters*
- Hydrocarbons (e.g., squalene)
- Phenolic compounds
- Volatiles
- Pigments
- Minor glyceridic compounds*
- and Phospholipids*[42]

*Wax esters, minor glyceridic compounds, and phospholipids are part of the saponifiable fraction. The other minor components are nonsaponifiable.

Although these components constitute a small portion of the carrier oils, they still play critical roles. The primary nonsaponifiable contents in carrier oils, including sterols, tocopherols, and squalene, contribute significantly toward the stability of the oils, protecting the oils from oxidative changes. These components also exhibit anti-inflammatory activity and perform other desirable functions in the skin. In many cases, selecting a specific carrier oil for therapeutic purposes can depend on its minor components.

Minor Components Chart		
Component	**Examples**	**Activity**
Sterols/ Phytosterols	Beta-sitosterol, Campesterol, Stigmasterol, and Delta-5-avenasterol Plant sterols play a role in lowering cholesterol levels in the human body.[43]	• May play a role in supporting the antioxidant activity of tocopherols and supporting a carrier oil's shelf-life stability[44] • Strengthen the lipid barrier and protect skin from external noxious substances[45] • Decrease water loss and improves skin elasticity and firmness • Exhibit anti-inflammatory, antibacterial, and anticarcinogenic activity[46]
Wax esters*	Jojoba oil, Meadowfoam seed oil, Carnauba wax, Candelilla wax, and Beeswax	Emollient and prevents TEWL
Hydrocarbons	Squalene	Squalene appears to function in the skin as an antioxidant, protecting the human skin surface from lipid peroxidation due to exposure to UV radiation.[47]
Tocopherols	Includes alpha (α), beta (β), gamma (γ), and delta (δ) tocopherols	Antioxidant and free radical scavenging
Phenolic compounds	3-Hydroxybenzoic acid; p- Hydroxybenzoic acid; 3,4-Dihydroxybenzoic acid; Gentisic acid	Antioxidant and free radical scavenging
Volatiles (found in extremely low concentrations)	Calarene, Kaurene	Flavor and aroma of carrier oils
Pigments	Carotenes are responsible for some oils' yellow, orange, and red color. Chlorophyll is often responsible for the green color.	The core pigments found in fixed oils are the carotenes, specifically alpha and beta-carotene, which give palm fruit and sea buckthorn pulp their rich orange-red color. Beta-carotene is a powerful antioxidant and exhibits photoprotective (prevents damage from sun) activity.[48]

Minor Components Chart		
Component	**Examples**	**Activity**
Phospholipids* Phospholipids are natural surfactants and emulsifiers consisting of an alcohol, such as glycerol, one or two molecules of fatty acids, and a phosphoric acid compound. They are found in all plants and animals.[51]		**In animals and plants:** Phospholipids are the primary components of cell and organelle membranes, which surround the cells or organelles with a semi-permeable barrier separating them from their outside environment. **In carrier oils:** Phospholipids contribute to the stability and quality of edible oils, fats, and fatty foods through their antioxidative activity. They may also contribute to the texture of the oil.[49] Applied phospholipids mainly fuse with the outer lipid layer of the stratum corneum, potentially acting as chemical permeability enhancers.[25] They also moisturize and soften skin, improve elasticity, and delay aging.[50]
*Wax esters and phospholipids are part of the saponifiable fraction.		

Fat-soluble Vitamins and Nutrients Found in Carrier Oils
(Mostly unsaponifiable fraction)

→ Phytosterols

Sterols, natural components present in many plants and animal species, are also essential for human and animal health.[51] The richest natural sources of plant sterols in the human diet are unrefined vegetable oils, seeds, nuts, and legumes. Phytosterols are similar in structure and function to cholesterol, a lipid naturally found in human skin where it has a water-binding capacity and is very important in repairing damaged skin barrier function.[52] Sterols in carrier oils may play similar roles when applied to human skin. Carrier oil phytosterols are also useful in reducing inflammation for such skin conditions as skin eruptions, eczema, and itchy skin.[53]

In plant oils, the composition of phytosterols may vary due to plant species, agronomic and climatic conditions, extraction and refining procedures, and the quality of the fruits or seeds.[54] Although phytosterols are minor components of carrier oils, they comprise the major portion of the unsaponifiable fraction and generally account for about 1% of the oil.[55] One study found the mean content of sterols for a selection of vegetable oils to be 4866.6 mg/kg oil.[56]

Phytosterols possess a variety of bio-actions that have been implicated in slowing the pathogenesis of chronic disease, demonstrating antioxidant and anti-inflammatory activity as well as the capacity to promote detoxification, reduce cell proliferation, and/or lower serum low-density lipoprotein (LDL) cholesterol.[57] Sterols are generally considered to be heat-stable, odorless, and tasteless.

The main phytosterols found in carrier oils are:
- Beta-sitosterol
- Stigmasterol
- Campesterol
- Delta-5-avenasterol

Beta-sitosterol is the major phytosterol found in higher plants. In animals, beta-sitosterol exhibited anti-inflammatory, anti-pyretic,[58] anti-neoplastic, and immune-modulating activity.[59] It is also a known antioxidant. Along with reducing DNA damage caused by free radicals, it also may increase the level of antioxidant enzymes in the cells.[60]

→ Squalene

Squalene, a triterpene, polyunsaturated hydrocarbon, derives its name from the shark, whose liver oil contains the richest source of squalene. In humans, squalene makes up approximately 13% of sebum.[47]

Squalene shows some advantages for the skin as an emollient, antioxidant, and for its antitumor activities.[47] Squalene appears to be highly effective for reducing free radical oxidative damage to the skin and inhibiting chemically induced skin, colon, and lung tumorigenesis in rodents.[57] Squalene protects the skin surface lipids by inhibiting lipid peroxidation, acting as a quencher of singlet oxygen.[61] Truly one of nature's great emollients, squalene is quickly and efficiently absorbed deep into the skin, restoring healthy suppleness and flexibility without leaving an oily residue.[47]

Squalene can be a material (in carrier oils) or additive (isolated ingredient) in topically applied vehicles such as lipid emulsions, creams, and lotions.

→ Vitamin E and the Tocopherols

The vitamin E family comprises several molecules, one group of which, called the tocopherols, includes alpha (α), beta (β), gamma (γ), and delta (δ) tocopherols, named here in order of their biological importance.[62] Some consider alpha-tocopherol to be the most biologically active. However, gamma- and delta-tocopherol are the most active within the carrier oils, followed by alpha- and beta-.[63] Carrier oils often contain between 200-800 mg/kg of tocopherols.

Vitamin E is yet another nutrient that humans cannot synthesize and must acquire from plants.[64] It is one of the most important and potent antioxidants, able to prevent cell damage from free radicals found in carrier oils. Excess free radicals destroy the collagen and elastin fibers that support the skin and interfere with the formation of new, healthy skin cells, resulting in aging of the skin and making complexions blotchy and dull.

Vitamin E protects the skin against environmental pollutants and has excellent repairing and regenerating properties. It is used topically to treat burns, including radiation burns, and can assist in wound healing and reducing scar formation. In conjunction with beta-carotene, vitamin E decreases the harmful effects of the sun and photoaging.

One research study showed that vitamin E levels in the upper layers of the stratum corneum drop

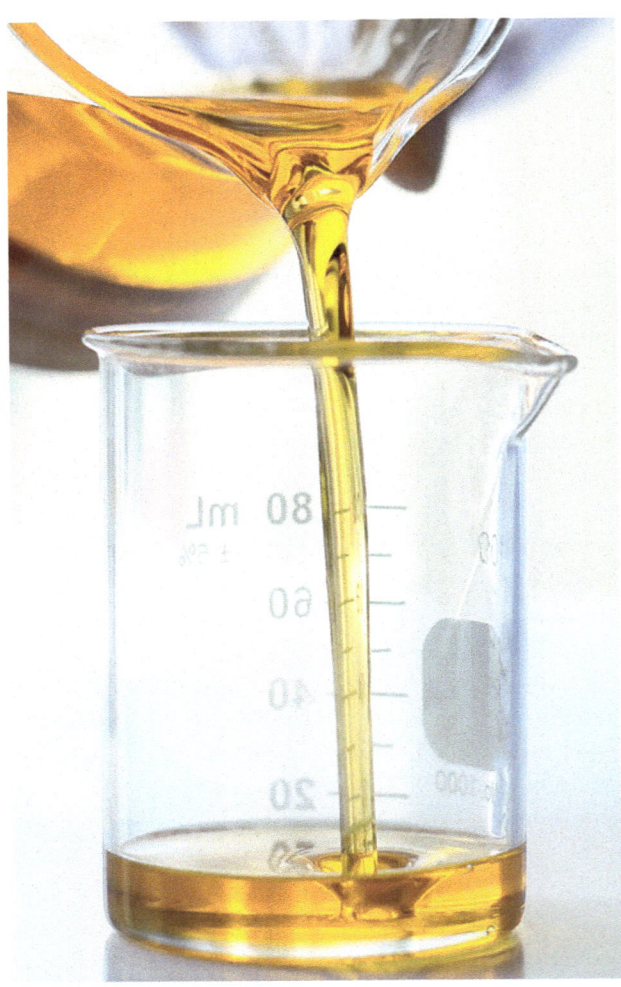

significantly after even brief exposure to sunlight, but a topical application of vitamin E (the study applied vitamin E in a body wash) can reverse this loss. This topical application was also more effective at replacing the vitamin E in the skin than the use of a dietary supplement.[65]

Studies have shown that alpha-tocopherol provides a highly protective antioxidant activity in the skin, and concentrations ranging from 0.1 to 1% are likely to be adequate to provide effective skin barrier protection.[47] Vitamin E can be added to carrier oils as an isolated component to prevent the oxidation of beta-carotene and vitamin A.

→ Vitamin A and the Carotenoids

Vitamin A is the collective name of a group of fat-soluble retinoid molecules, including retinol, retinal, retinoic acid, and retinyl esters. Human immune function, vision, reproduction, and cellular communication all require this vitamin to function properly. Animals provide most of the preformed vitamin A in the human diet, but provitamin A, which we metabolize to create the other retinoids, comes from plants. Beta-carotene is the most important provitamin A carotenoid.[66]

One study found that naturally aged, sun-protected skin and photoaged skin have important molecular features in common, including connective tissue damage, elevated matrix metalloproteinase levels, and reduced collagen production. Topical application of a 1% vitamin A solution for seven days improved all of these indicators in both naturally aged and photoaged skin.[67]

Some symptoms of vitamin A deficiency include rough, dry, scaly skin; problems with gums and teeth; loss of smell and appetite; and night blindness.

Toxicity: Large dietary intake of vitamin A for long periods can lead to hypervitaminosis (excessive vitamin intake) with symptoms such as nausea, headache, vomiting, skin discoloration, and excessive skin drying.[68]

→ β-carotene (Beta-carotene, B-carotene)

Over five hundred carotenes occur in nature. Beta-carotene, one of the most active carotenes, is a precursor to vitamin A. It is a potent scavenger of toxic oxygen radicals, especially those produced by chemicals in the air and those generated by our metabolism. It has stronger immune-stimulating and thymic supportive activity than vitamin A.[69]

Oils rich in beta-carotene, such as carrot herbal oil, palm fruit oil, and sea buckthorn oil, tend to be a rich orange color. Palm fruit oil also contains lycopene, a carotene, which, like beta-carotene, exhibits anticancer abilities.[70]

Beta-carotene can accumulate in the skin as a result of dietary supplementation. It acts as a photoprotective agent in the skin,[47] as it functions as a cellular screen against sunlight-induced free radical change.[71] However, as with vitamin A, higher doses (15 mg/day) and long-term usage (8 weeks) can be harmful.[47]

→ Vitamin D

Vitamin D, sometimes called "the sunshine vitamin," works with calcium to build strong, healthy bones and teeth. Studies suggest that vitamin D also plays a role in cell proliferation and maturation.[1]

→ *Lecithin

*As a phospholipid, lecithin is part of the saponifiable fraction.

Lecithin is a phospholipid commonly derived from egg yolk or soy oil. The name "lecithin" is derived from the Greek word *likithos*, meaning egg yolk.

In the human body, lecithin is an integral component of cellular membranes, particularly those found in the nervous system. It is also an effective, natural emulsifying agent often used in food products, cosmetics like creams and lotions, and many transdermal drug delivery systems.[72] Since lecithin is an integral part of cell membranes, it is considered highly biocompatible and is indicated for psoriasis and eczema.

Lecithin is removed from some carrier oils by a process called "degumming." Lecithin is usually extracted from soybean oil, rapeseed oil, and sunflower seed oil.

Note: Because lecithin is usually produced from soy (a heavily genetically modified crop), it is better to purchase only organic or sunflower lecithin when using it as an individual ingredient.

Fats vs. Oils

Some generalities comparing fats and oils, which are both lipids. Many of these statements demonstrate broad patterns but may include individual exceptions.

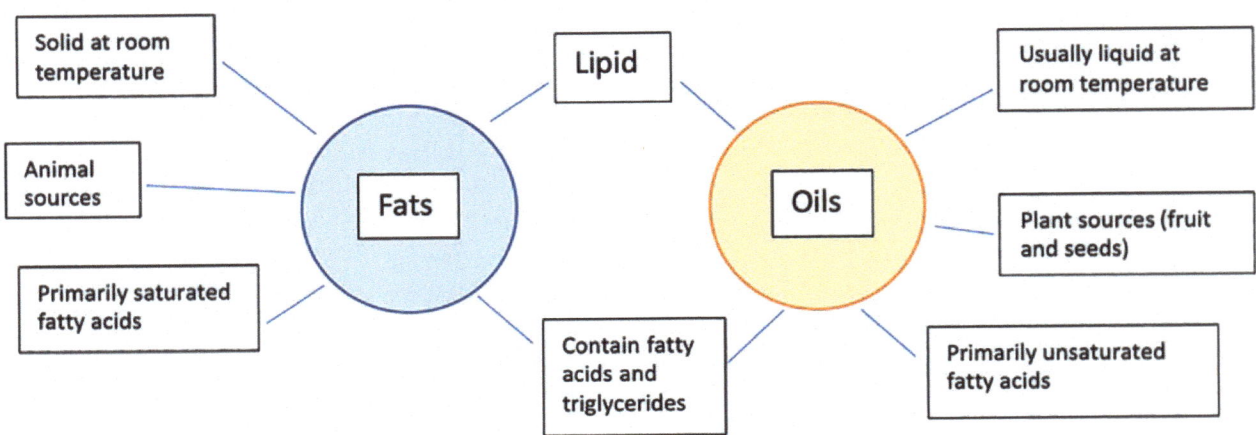

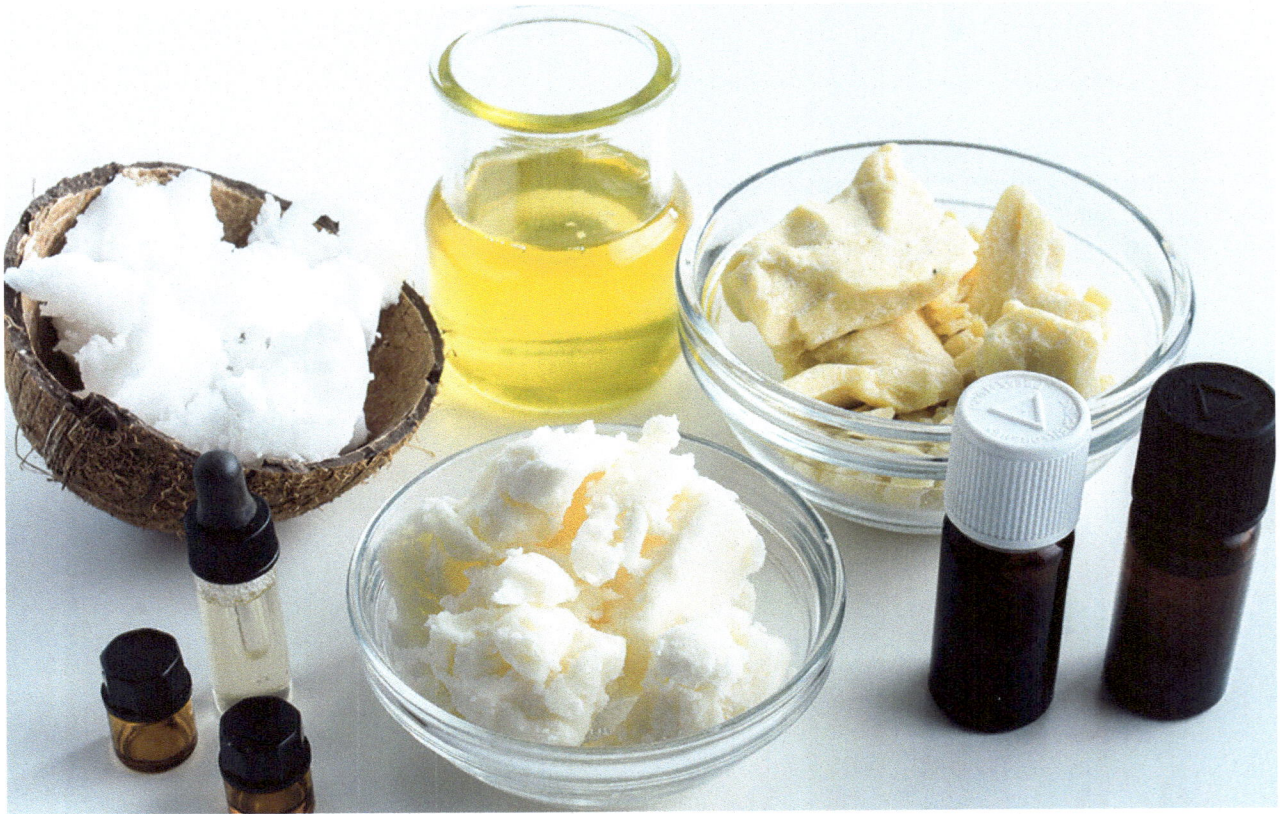

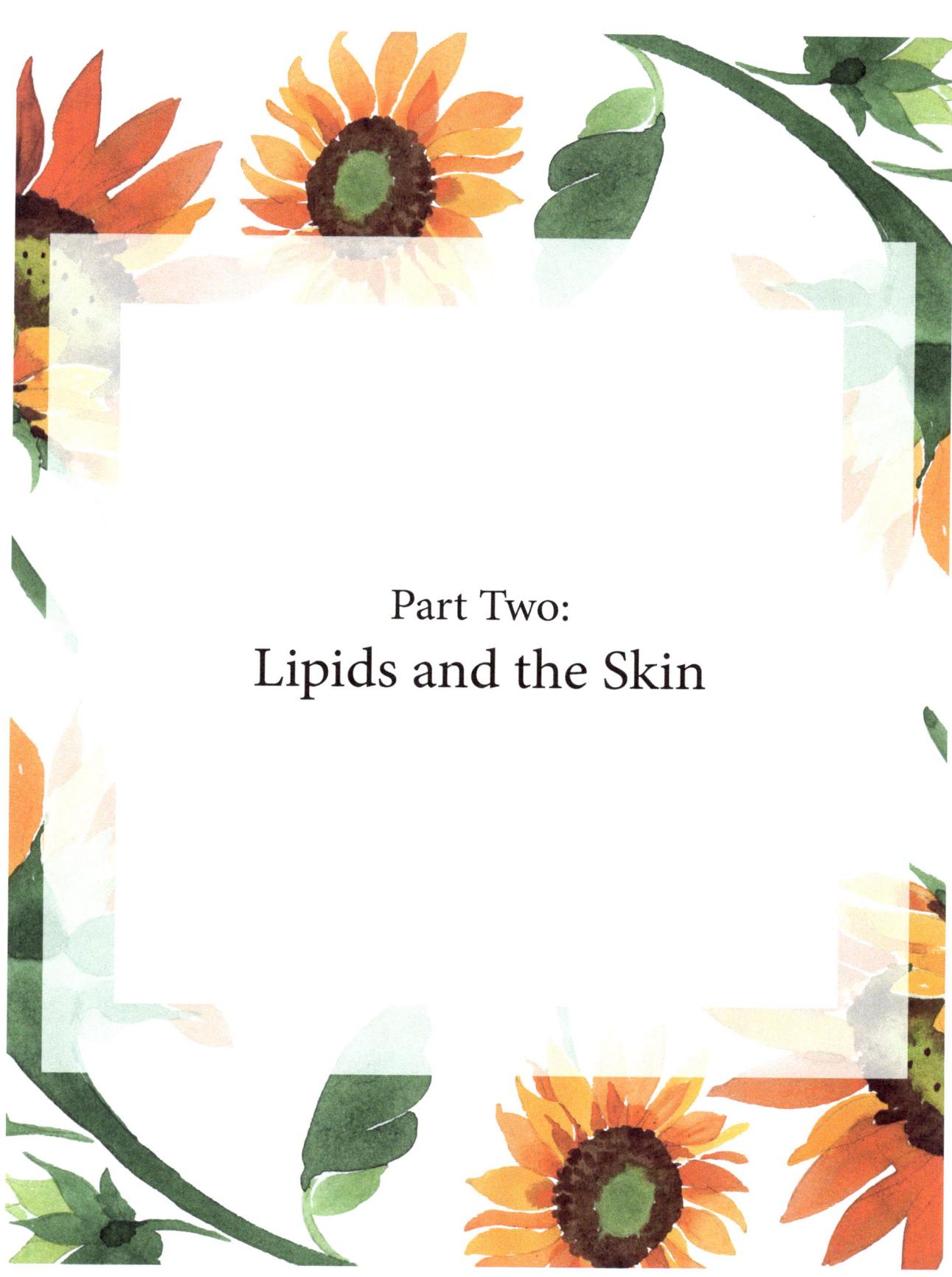

Part Two:
Lipids and the Skin

Anatomy & Physiology of the Skin

The skin is the most voluminous organ in the human body, comprising 15-16% of the total adult body weight. It is the principal barrier between the internal body and the external world. A deeply sensitive and resilient organ, the skin protects the body against biological, chemical, mechanical, and ultraviolet threats. As a significant player in systemic homeostasis, the skin is responsible for thermoregulation, water balance, absorption and elimination, vitamin D synthesis, and mediating the interrelationships among the immune, neurologic, and endocrine systems.

The skin consists of three primary layers: **the epidermis**, **the dermis**, and the **hypodermis**. The outermost layer of the epidermis, **the stratum corneum**, is characterized by a constellation of tough cells known as **keratinocytes**. These cells synthesize the protective protein **keratin**, a fibrous alpha-helical filament that renders the epidermis strong and flexible while waterproofing the skin surface.

Other cells of the epidermis include the **melanocytes** (that generate the ultraviolet radiation-protective pigment melanin), the **Langerhans cells** (involved in immune response), and **Merkel cells** (mechanoreceptors involved in light touch sensations). This skin layer perpetually renews itself and gives rise to the cutaneous **adnexa** — the skin appendages that play functional roles in sensation, contractility, lubrication, and homeostatic heat loss. The adnexa include hair, hair follicles, sebaceous glands, sweat glands, and nails.

Below the epidermis lies the **dermis**. The primary function of the dermis is to sustain and support the epidermis by providing physical and nutritional support. The dermis is the thickest layer of the skin, accounting for over 90% of the skin's mass. The two layers of the dermis are the **papillary layer**, the outermost layer in direct contact with the epidermis, and the **reticular layer**.

The papillary layer is thinner, consisting of loose connective tissue containing capillaries, lymphatics, sensory neurons, elastic fibers, reticular fibers, and collagen. It accounts for about 1/5th of the dermis and lies just under the basement membrane. This layer's papillae (projections) form the base for the friction ridges on the fingers and toes.

On the other hand, the reticular layer, which carries most of the physical stress of the skin, is thicker and has dense collagen bundles and coarse elastin fibers. The reticular layer also contains fibroblasts, mast cells, nerve fibers, lymph vessels, and epidermal appendages (hair follicles, sebaceous and sweat glands). This layer can stretch (e.g., during pregnancy or obesity), yet it tears when the dermis stretches too far. The repair of this tearing is what leaves stretch marks on the skin.

The innermost layer is the **hypodermis**, composed of fat and connective tissues that house larger blood vessels and nerves. Subcutaneous tissue insulates the body and helps to regulate body temperature. The hypodermis is classified as an endocrine organ and is involved in the immune response.[1]

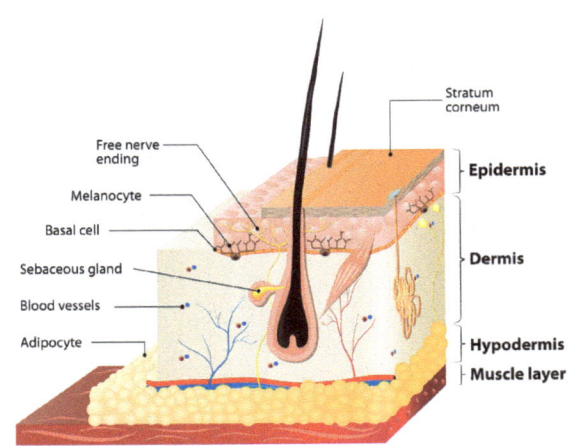

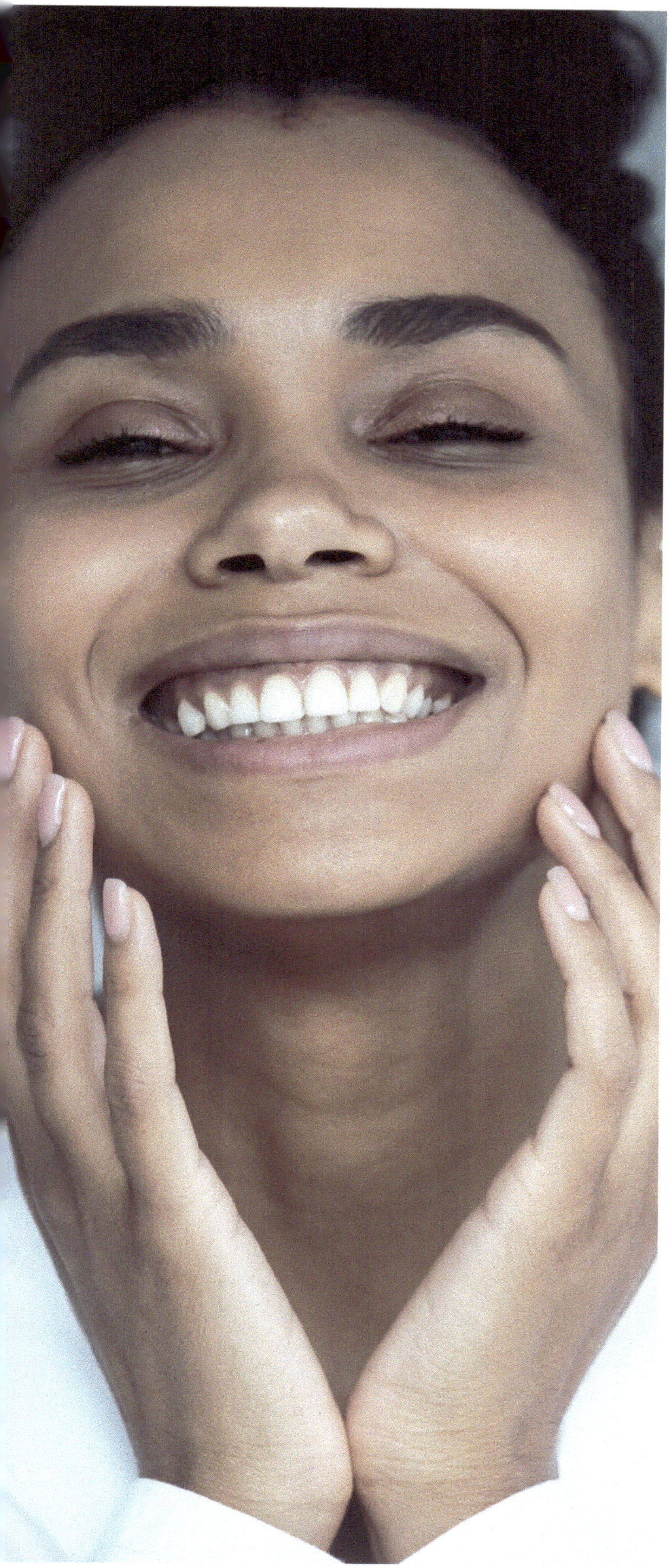

Skin Ecology: Layers of Protection

As the principal barrier between the internal body and the external world, the skin maintains three interdependent layers of protection, collectively called the skin's barrier. These protective layers include the **dermal microbiome**, the **acid mantle**, and the **barrier function** of the stratum corneum. Dysbiosis of the skin's microbiome, disruption of the acid mantle, or any dysfunction within the skin's physical barrier have all been implicated in inflammatory skin diseases, including acne, rosacea, eczema, psoriasis, and atopic dermatitis. To understand their interconnectedness, we will explore each layer and how each may contribute to the expression of inflammatory skin diseases. These layers work together to prevent infection and the entry of harmful substances, prevent water and nutrient loss, and support the skin's overall health.[2]

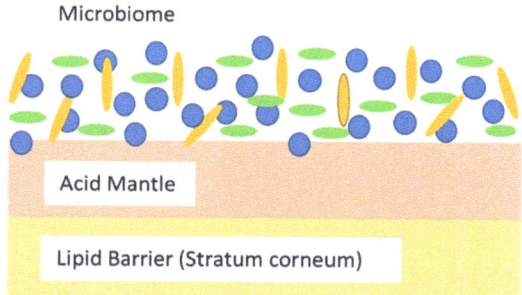

The Dermal Microbiome

The **microbiome of human skin** is composed of bacteria, fungi, and viruses. Like the gut microbiome, the dermal microbiome plays a significant role in health and pathogenesis. Scientists have found that not only do diverse microbial populations colonize the epidermis and dermis, but they also modulate and inform the development of the human immune system. The skin forms an immense interface between the body and its environment, thus serving as a crucial site of convergence between the inside and outside of the body.

A vital feature of the human dermal microbiome is site-specific colonization — unique microbial communities reside in distinct epidermal topographical niches. These niches are determined by moisture content, anatomical location, and the prevalence of sebaceous (oil) glands. Researchers explain that moist and dry sites in human skin are "as ecologically dissimilar as rain forests are to deserts."[3] Body sites loaded with sebaceous glands, like the back, face, and chest, are dominated by several species of *Cutibacterium* (formerly *Propionibacterium*) bacteria and *Malassezia* yeasts. "Dry" sites like the buttocks, arms, and legs exhibit the highest microbial diversity and variability, mostly *Cutibacterium acnes* and *Staphylococcus* species. These microbes, along with *Corynebacterium*, are the predominant commensal organisms found on the skin.[4]

In addition to the differences found across body sites, microbial signatures vary with changes in the local microenvironment, between individuals and age groups, and with health, behavior, and environmental contacts. Most microbiota colonizing the skin are harmless or beneficial and essential for host defense. Despite the popular belief that certain microbes are inherently dangerous, pathogenicity only occurs during dysbiosis - when the microbial ecosystem balance is disturbed or when diversity diminishes - or when opportunistic bacteria breach the skin surface.

Microbes living on and in the skin play key roles in host defense and tissue repair. Disturbances of the microbiome of the stratum corneum, such as from antibiotic use, hygiene practices, lifestyle factors (stress),[3] and even gut dysbiosis[5] can result in skin barrier dysfunction and transepidermal water loss (TEWL). Dysbiosis and loss of dermal biodiversity have been linked to numerous skin diseases, including atopic eczema,[6] atopic dermatitis,[7] acne,[8] rosacea,[9] psoriasis,[10] slow wound healing,[11] inflammation,[12] and skin cancer.[13]

Sebaceous Glands, Sebum, and the Dermal Microbiome

Sebaceous glands, microscopic exocrine glands in the skin that secrete an oily substance known as sebum, are crucial regulators of skin homeostasis. They play an important role in supporting the skin's barrier functions, promoting skin integrity, mediating inflammatory processes, delivering antioxidants, and managing microbial populations. They also participate in the cutaneous endocrine and immune systems and serve as stem cell reservoirs.[14] Sebaceous glands are distributed over the entire body - except for the palms of the hands and the soles of the feet - and are most plentiful on the scalp and face.

Sebum is a mixture of fats (triglycerides, wax esters, squalene, and cholesterol) and cellular debris discharged via the sebaceous duct, a structure that connects the sebaceous gland to the hair follicle. Sebum forms a protective film on the skin, maintaining the skin's pliability and helping to regulate fluid loss and absorption. Sebaceous glands produce lipids that are different from most lipids produced by other human body organs. The main sebaceous lipid components

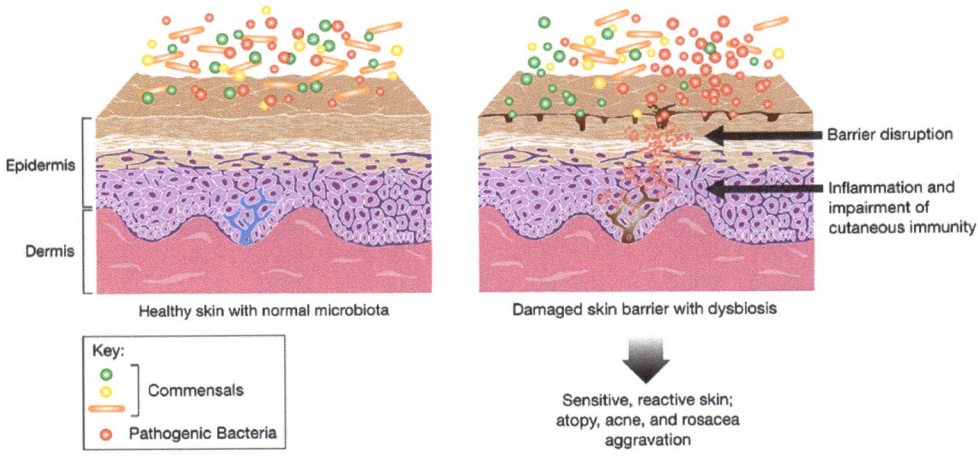

Relationship Between Skin Barrier and Dermal Microbiota

include sapienic acid (only found in sebum), squalene, wax esters, triglycerides (triaglycerols), and smaller amounts of cholesterol, cholesterol esters, and diglycerides.[15]

Sebaceous glands facilitate healthy skin homeostasis through the maintenance of a healthy microbiome. As the cutaneous microbiota play a crucial role in skin health, the sebum composition plays a major role in regulating the cutaneous microbiota. Depending on the molecular makeup of sebum, it can restrict undesired microbes while promoting preferred populations. Sapienic acid (C16:1 n-10), in particular, has demonstrated antibacterial properties.[16]

Dysfunction of the sebaceous gland contributes to skin pathologies such as acne and dry skin. Sebum overproduction, or pathological alterations of its chemical composition, can cause acne, while insufficient sebum production may lead to **xerosis** (abnormal dryness of the skin or mucus membranes), skin aging, and atopic dermatitis.

The Skin's Acid Mantle

The epidermis is covered with a thin layer of natural lipids and perspiration called the **acid mantle**. The lipids are derived from sebum and stratum corneum lipids. Perspiration is produced via the sweat glands. The acid mantle's main functions are to protect the skin against microbial infections and support the barrier function and integrity of the stratum corneum. The acid mantle has an average pH of 4 to 6, depending on gender, age, and anatomical site.[17] Other factors that may influence the skin's pH include sebum, skin moisture, sweat, genetics, detergents, topical antibacterial products, occlusive dressings, and skin irritants.[18,19]

If the acid mantle loses its acidity, the skin becomes more prone to damage and infection as well as irritation and sensitivity. Kusmirek points out that the skin's acid mantle is vital to the skin's health as it is our first line of defense against germs and contains elements that maintain crucial moisture. Carrier oils support this valuable system.[20]

The Skin's Barrier Function

The skin's barrier function is essential to human health. Under normal conditions, the stratum corneum maintains an ideal level of skin hydration, supports the innate antioxidant system, produces microbe-regulating peptides, activates innate immune responses, and serves as a line of defense against external threats, such as ultraviolet radiation, environmental toxins, allergens, and pathogens. "The skin," Belkaid and Tamoutounour write in *The Influence of Skin Microorganisms on Cutaneous Immunity*, "is therefore charged with the formidable task of protecting the host from microbial invasion while maintaining a peaceful coexistence with its resident microbiota."[21]

The outermost layer of the epidermis, the stratum corneum, prevents the absorption of noxious substances and the entry of pathogens while preventing excessive water loss by providing a physical barrier between our bodies and the outside environment. The stratum corneum is comprised of **corneocytes**, terminally differentiated keratinocytes encased in an extracellular protein and lipid matrix. The stratum corneum has

About pH

The abbreviation pH stands for "power of hydrogen" or "potential of hydrogen" and measures a substance's acidity or alkalinity. pH is measured on a scale of 1 to 14, going from acid (1) to alkaline (14). Water has a neutral pH of 7. Skin pH is slightly acidic, ranging from 4 to 6. Therefore, the skin needs more neutral to slightly acidic pH products to support overall skin health.

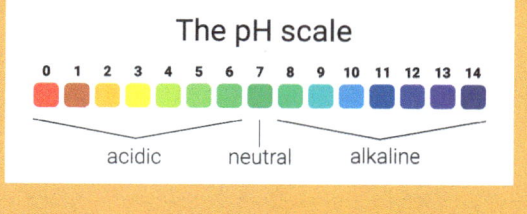
The pH scale

what is known as a "brick and mortar" design. The bricks are the cells (corneocytes) that make up this layer, while the mortar is the complex of intercellular lipids that hold or bind moisture between the "bricks."

The process of keratinocyte differentiation is closely linked with the development of the extracellular matrix. Lipids are produced during the process of epidermal differentiation. They originate from lamellar bodies (small secretory cells in the keratinocytes) that are expelled from keratinocytes in the stratum granulosum. As the differentiation process nears its end, the lamellar granules discharge their contents, both lipids and hydrolytic enzymes, into the intercellular space. The hydrolytic enzymes act on phospholipids in the vicinity of the stratum granulosum - stratum corneum interface resulting in the production of the principal lipids of the stratum corneum.

This extracellular lipid matrix provides the mechanical barrier functions of the skin, protecting the underlying epidermis and acting as a barrier to water loss (outward) and invasion by exogenous particles and pathogens (inward). This bi-directional protective barrier function is the principal role of the epidermis and specifically that of the stratum corneum.

Lipids of the Stratum Corneum

The principal lipids found in the stratum corneum include ceramides (approx. 50%), cholesterol (27%) and its esters (10%), and fatty acids (10-15%).[22,23] This mortar of lipids prevents water loss through the stratum corneum.

Ceramides, members of a class of lipids called sphingolipids, trap water molecules in their hydrophilic region. These lipids form a stacked bilayer, where their hydrophobic "heads" are to the outside and their hydrophilic "tails" point toward the other layer, which surrounds the corneocytes. This bilayer is impermeable to water, preventing the loss of water and natural moisturizing factor (NMF) through the skin.[24]

Cholesterol is the most common lipid in the stratum corneum. It lubricates these multiple layers of dry, dead cells, making the stratum corneum more flexible.[26] The precursor of cholesterol is **squalene**, which the sebaceous glands secrete onto the skin.[22]

Fatty acids in the skin provide lubrication, play an important role in barrier function, prevent moisture loss, maintain the skin's acid pH, and support innate immunity by exerting antimicrobial activity.[23,26] Some of the fatty acids found in the skin include palmitic acid (C16:0), palmitoleic acid (C16:1 n-7), myristic acid (C14:0), stearic acid (C18:0), and linoleic acid (C18:2 n-6), which is the most abundant polyunsaturated fatty acid (PUFA) present in the epidermis.[27]

Transepidermal Water Loss (TEWL) and the Natural Moisturizing Factor (NMF)

The stratum corneum plays a key role in maintaining the water level of the skin below it and in regulating the natural moisture flow out from the deeper layers, to be lost eventually by evaporation from the skin surface. This flow is known as **transepidermal water loss** (TEWL). Moisture homeostasis is crucial in maintaining the skin's barrier function and overall health.

The lipids and the **natural moisturizing factor (NMF)** of the stratum corneum play a crucial role in maintaining the water level of the skin as well as reducing TEWL. The NMF, found within the corneocytes, is a collection of water-soluble compounds, including amino acids (which make up approximately 50% of the NMF), urea, lactic acid, inorganic salts, sugars, and electrolytes. These compounds, derived from the breakdown of filaggrin proteins, are responsible for keeping the skin moist and pliable by attracting and holding water, supporting the process of desquamation (the shedding of corneocytes), and supporting the health of the stratum corneum barrier function.[28] NMF components act as humectants, attracting and absorbing water from the atmosphere and drawing the moisture into the corneocytes.[29] When NMF levels are low, skin aging, skin disorders, ichthyosis, and general xerosis may arise.[28]

Fatty Acids and the Skin

Lipids are a fundamental component of the membranes of every cell in our body, influencing the permeability of substances into and out of cells. Triglycerides, phospholipids, sphingolipids (syn. glycosylceramides), and ceramides all play a vital role in forming the epidermal barrier function. Fatty acids, which make up these cellular lipids, are crucial in maintaining the structure and function of the stratum corneum, where they provide a moisture and insulation barrier. They improve skin barrier function, provide anti-inflammatory activity, are natural penetration enhancers, and support healthy skin activities.

Essential fatty acids (EFAs), in particular, are integral for normal stratum corneum structure and function.[30] EFAs, specifically linoleic acid (LA), an essential fatty acid component of ceramides, are important to the formation of the intercellular lipid complex.[31] EFA deficiency alters the skin's barrier function, disrupts epidermic homeostasis, and can lead to marked skin abnormalities, including excessive TEWL, dryness, scaliness, redness, dermatitis, and other signs of inflammation.[32]

Other factors such as cold or heat exposure (sunburn, windburn, frostbite), low ambient humidity, home heating during the winter months, age, genetics, seasonal influences, and diet also affect the stratum corneum lipids. Using solvents, detergents, and other irritating chemicals, even the excessive use of water and soap, can break down the protective lipid layer and increase TEWL by altering the skin's natural water-holding capacity. A deficiency in these lipids can result in dehydrated skin or xerosis. Even acute psychological stress can negatively impact the skin barrier function.[33]

Moisturizers and Skin Barrier Repair

Maintaining a healthy skin barrier is essential, especially for those individuals who suffer from common skin disorders that can be exacerbated by dry skin, e.g., psoriasis, atopic dermatitis, and photodamage. All these disorders can be linked to fundamental barrier dysfunction, which makes the skin even more vulnerable to environmental insults that cause dryness and irritation. Maintaining healthy skin on a daily basis is crucial for adults and children, even in the absence of such disorders.[32]

Topical products that come under the heading of **moisturizers** include emollients, humectants, and occlusives. When applied to the skin, moisturizers can improve, maintain, and support the skin barrier function and improve skin hydration by preventing or reducing TEWL.[29] The term **emollient** is derived from the Latin - meaning "to soften" - and implies a substance that acts to smooth the skin surface. Emollients soften

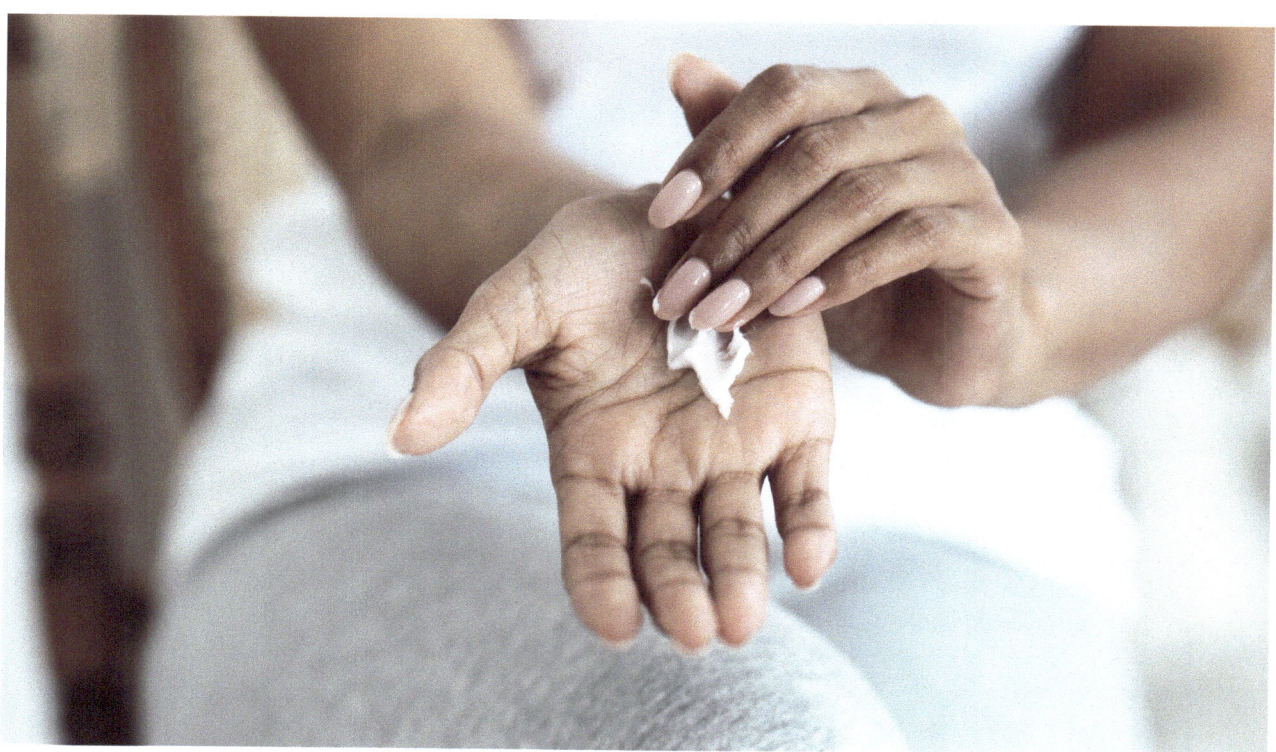

the skin, prevent TEWL, reduce inflammation, and support the lipid matrix.[34] Emollient cosmetics include carrier oils, creams, lotions, ointments, butters, and balms. **Humectants** (honey, glycerine) are substances that attract water. **Occlusive substances** (waxes, lecithin) provide a hydrophobic layer on top of the skin, preventing TEWL.[35]

The topical application of carrier oils is a successful route of both fatty acid and essential fatty acid delivery to the skin. It can play a role in the prevention and treatment of skin pathologies. In general, fatty acids applied to the skin can support the structure of the stratum corneum and its barrier function. Both topical application and ingestion of linoleic acid-rich fatty oils can reverse symptoms of EFA deficiency in both animals and humans.[36] The topical application of carrier oils, especially those rich in essential fatty acids, can be of great benefit in restoring the skin barrier, healing wounds, preventing wrinkles, and treating inflammatory disorders including eczema, dermatitis, and psoriasis.

The name "carrier oil" implies that these oils are merely vehicles for distributing other substances onto our skin. However, they are valuable therapeutic substances in their own rights. Knowing how to select appropriate carrier oils for a particular application is a key skill for any aromatherapist or botanical skincare product manufacturer. When topically applied, fixed oils, and their various components, can:

- Support and maintain the intercellular lipid matrix (the mortar), which in turn serves to protect the integrity of the stratum corneum and its barrier function.
- Restore barrier function, if damaged, and support cell proliferation.
- Prevent transepidermal water loss (TEWL) by forming an occlusive film on the skin's surface.
- Provide antioxidant activity.
- Provide anti-inflammatory activity.

It is important to cultivate a relationship with carrier oils, as with essential oils. Getting to know a few carrier oils well can be of greater benefit than knowing only very little about many oils. As your relationship with these important oils develops, your knowledge will enhance the therapeutic value of the blends you create.

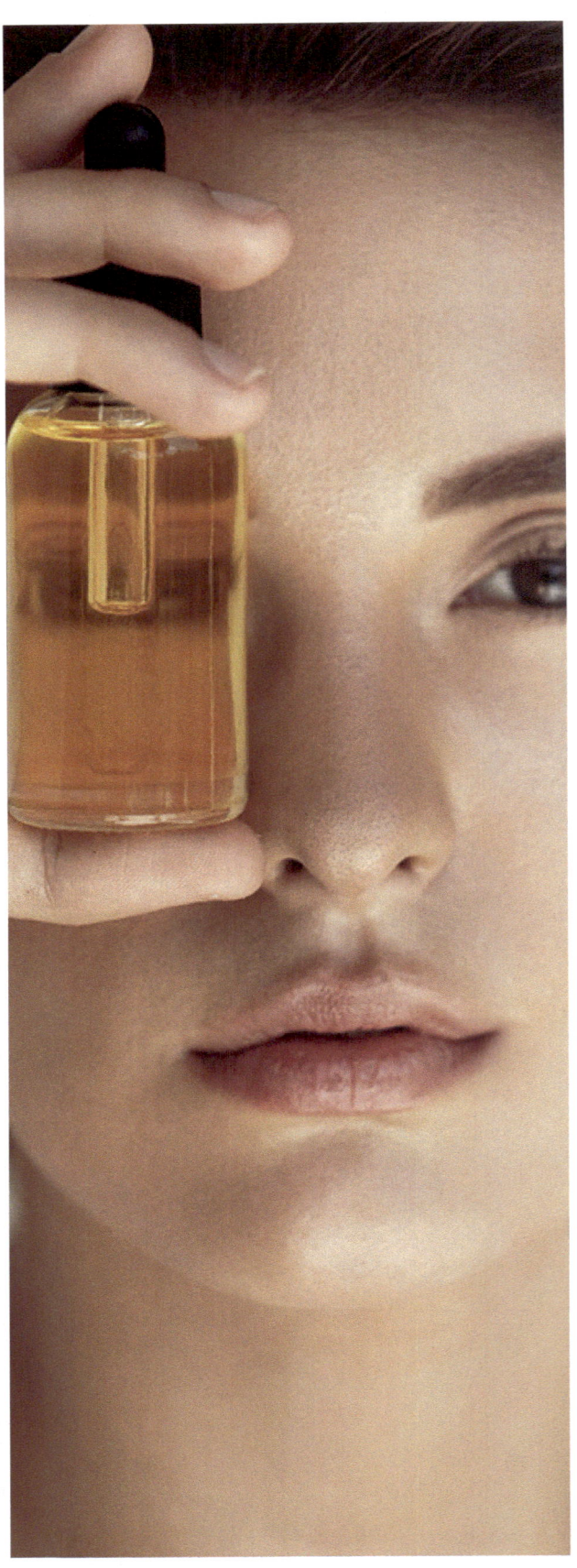

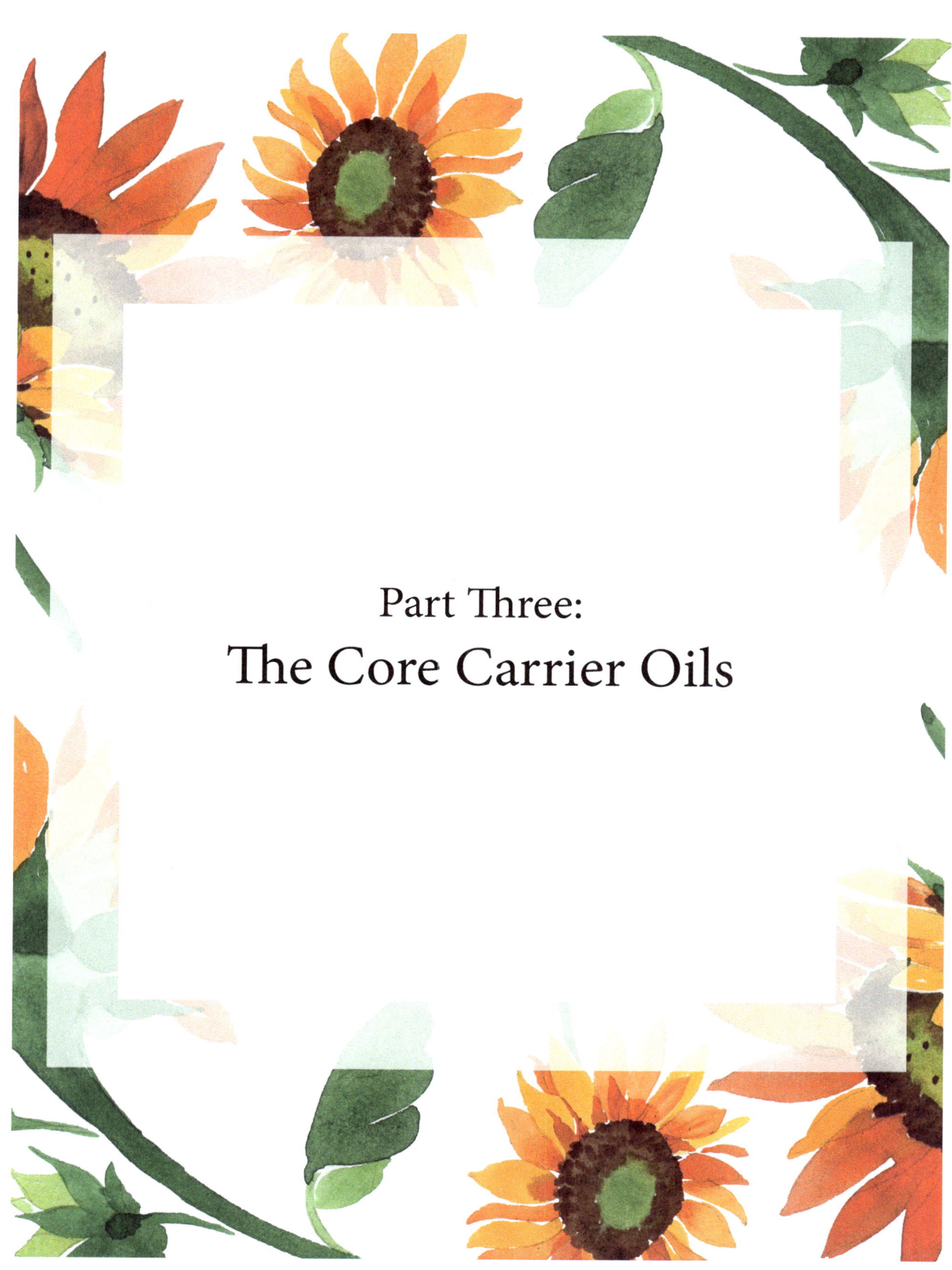

Part Three:
The Core Carrier Oils

The Core Carrier Oils

Core carrier oils are the oils that will make up 50-100% of oil-based formulations. They have a stable shelf life of at least 12 to 24 months, depending on storage.

Carrier Oil Storage

Carrier oils deteriorate via two separate processes: oxidation and spoilage. To prevent such deterioration, you must protect carrier oils from light, air, heat (oxidation), and microbes (spoilage). Storing them in tightly sealed containers in cool, dark locations protects them from both forms of deterioration and maximizes their shelf lives.

Oxidation

Light and oxygen can cause lipid peroxidation processes where fatty acids undergo reactions that produce peroxides and hydroperoxides, causing the oil to become rancid.[1] Rancid oils may be tacky or sticky and will smell "off." If the oil has a color, that color may change or disappear altogether. Carrier oils can experience significant oxidation before we detect these changes, so do not wait for your oil to smell bad before you stop using it.

There are several problems with rancid oils. First, the fatty acids we value are no longer in the carrier oil. Second, the peroxides and hydroperoxides are highly irritating to the skin, and eating rancid oils can cause or exacerbate various diseases. Third, the smell and change in the texture of a rancid carrier oil are unpleasant. Finally, once an oil is rancid, it cannot become fresh again and must be thrown out.

Antioxidant substances will oxidize more readily than fatty acids, which is how they "protect" the carrier oils and maximize their shelf lives. Many carrier oils contain naturally-occurring antioxidant ingredients, which, in effect, sacrifice themselves by reacting with unstable molecules called free radicals. Eventually, these antioxidant molecules and any additional antioxidant ingredients in your product will have reacted, leaving only the other chemicals in the carrier oil to oxidize. As you increase temperature, you increase the rate of these oxidation reactions.[2]

Spoilage and decomposing

Carrier oil spoilage requires the growth of microorganisms, such as bacteria or fungi. Once microbes in the environment infect an open container through the air or direct transfer, such as on a tool or finger, moisture and warmer temperatures support and encourage the microbes' multiplication and growth. Careful storage (cool, sealed) can prevent or minimize such growth in carrier oils and their products.

Fungal growth on a carrier oil is easiest to see, and it may appear as cloudiness or fogginess within the oil or as a fuzzy growth. The part of a fungal growth you might see, such as the fuzzy spot at the top of an oil, is only a tiny part of the fungal organism, which grows in long threads, called mycelium. If you spot any fungal growth, you can be confident that it has spread through much more of the product.

Bacterial growth is similar in that bacteria are so small that a spot of bacterial growth represents thousands of individuals. Bacterial growth is more challenging to identify or see but is just as insidious and destructive as fungal growth.

Often, a key indicator of spoiled or decomposing carrier oils is a softening, thinning, or liquifying of the oil or butter that does not result from an increase in temperature (melting.) If this occurs, the bacterial or fungal growth will be beyond what you can identify visually, possibly affecting the whole container.

Refrigeration v. shelf storage

Some carrier oils, especially those high in PUFAs, may benefit from refrigeration, as identified in their monographs. However, others, often those with more SFAs, may separate, become solid, or become more difficult to use under refrigeration. Refrigeration is not necessary or recommended for most carrier oils.

Some butters, such as coconut oil, have melting points close to room temperature. Depending on their surrounding temperature, they may become harder, softer, or melt into a liquid. These changes will not usually affect quality, other than the oxidation rate, but they may affect how you store these butters or products that contain them.

Antioxidants and preservatives in end products

If your final products contain only carrier oils and waxes, the addition of an antioxidant ingredient is helpful to maximize the product's shelf life, but a preservative is not necessary. Products that include water require a preservative to maximize product shelf life. For personal product use, only making up as much product as can be used within a reasonable period is the best way to avoid the problems associated with lipid peroxidation and microbial growth.

Adding antioxidant and preservative ingredients to your pure carrier oils is not always practical, especially with butters, so proper storage conditions are critical to making your carrier oils last as long as possible. Eventually, often within 12-24 months of opening, carrier oils will oxidize, even if they do not spoil, so it is best that you only purchase as much as you can use within a year or so.

Proper storage

Therefore, proper storage for all carrier oils and butters requires they be kept away from light, particularly UV light, sealed to prevent contact with oxygen and water, and in cool temperatures to avoid melting and minimize the rate of oxidation reactions.

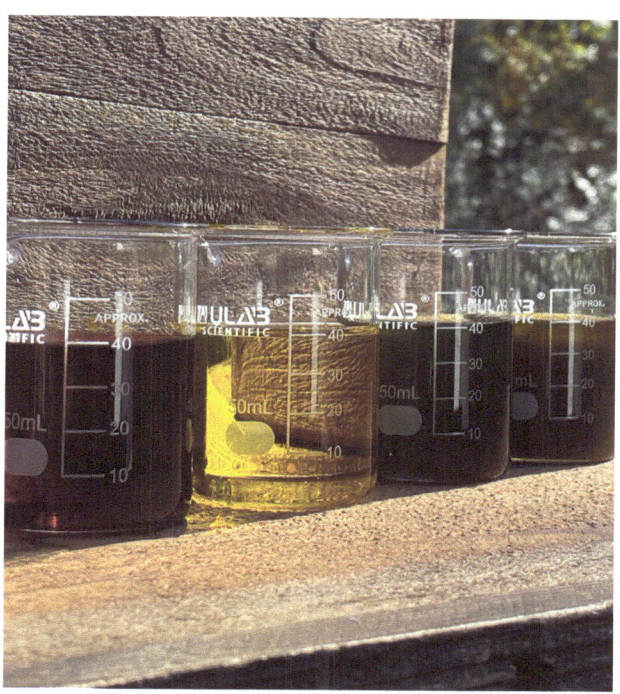

Are Essential Oils Antioxidants?

Do not consider essential oils as antioxidant ingredients. If an essential oil operates as an antioxidant within a product, they will also sacrifice themselves, reacting with free radicals, thereby losing their therapeutic value. Protect both the essential oils and carrier oils in your products by adding an appropriate antioxidant ingredient.

Sweet Almond
Prunus amygdalis var. *dulcis*

Common names: Sweet Almond
Scientific name: *Prunus amygdalis* var. *dulcis* (Mill.) D.A. Webb
Botanical family: Rosaceae
Conservation status: Not yet assessed

Description: Almond is a deciduous large, many-stemmed shrub or tree in the Rosaceae family native to Western Asia and Northern Africa. The tree grows 10-15 feet tall (sometimes up to 30 feet) and is equally wide. Flowers, borne laterally on spurs or short branches, are fragrant, five-petaled, light pink to white, and grow singly or in pairs in early spring before leaves emerge. Leaves are lanceolate to oblong-lanceolate, serrate, green, and grow to 5 inches in length. The fruit, an oblong drupe, matures 7-8 months after the flowers appear and splits open to disclose the stone inside. *P. dulcis* grows best in deep, fertile, well-drained loamy soil in full sun.

The genus name *Prunus* refers to the Latin for "plum" or "cherry tree;" the specific epithet *dulcis* means "sweet."[3]

Ethnobotany: Ayurvedic, Chinese, and Greco-Persian schools of medicine used almond oil to treat dry skin conditions, including psoriasis and eczema. These and other ancient civilizations also valued its emollient and scar-healing properties. Almond oil has been used to improve complexion and promote soft, healthy skin.

Prior to 3,000 BC, before almonds were cultivated, wild almonds were harvested as a rich nutritional source. These contained high concentrations of a constituent that, when crushed or chewed, is converted to hydrogen cyanide. Wild almonds were thus first roasted or leached to purge the toxins.[4]

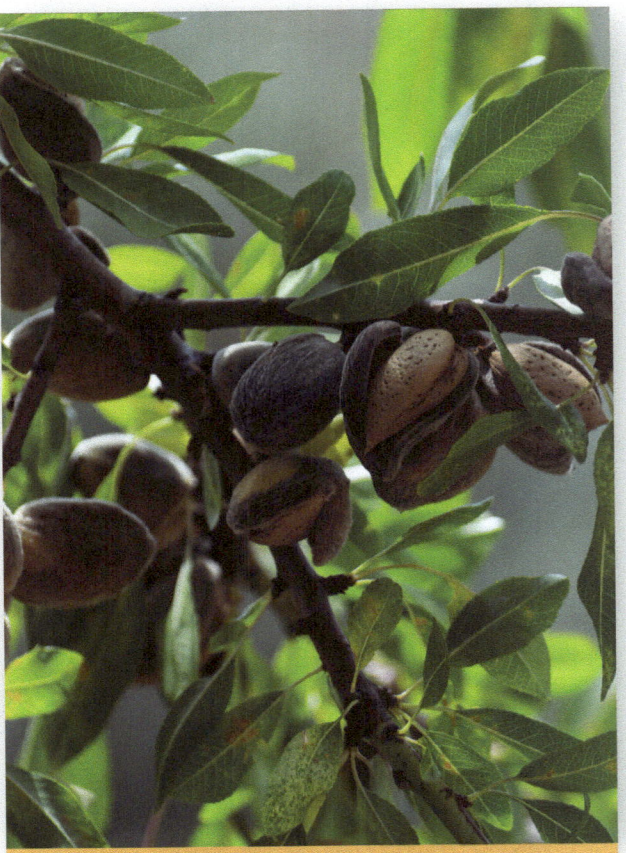

EXTRACTION INFORMATION

Country of origin: Italy, Spain, USA
Part of plant: Seed
Oil content: 18-25%
Extraction method: Cold pressing

MANUFACTURING INFORMATION

CAS number: 8007-69-0 / 90320-37-9
EC number: 291-063-5
INCI name: Prunus Amygdalis Dulcis (Sweet Almond Oil) or Prunus Dulcis
CosIng (functions): Fragrance, Hair conditioning, Perfuming, Skin conditioning

SHELF LIFE

12-24 months

NUTRIENT PROFILE

Rich in the monounsaturated fatty acid, oleic acid, with a strong presence of linoleic acid, sweet almond oil is widely used for its emollient properties and massage due to its slow absorption into the skin.

Sweet Almond Oil[5, 6, 7]	
SATURATED FATTY ACIDS	
Palmitic acid (C16:0)	3 - 9%
Stearic acid (C18:0)	0.3 - 5%
MONOUNSATURATED FATTY ACIDS	
Oleic acid (C18:1 n-9)	60.0 - 86.0%
POLYUNSATURATED FATTY ACIDS	
Linoleic acid (C18:2 n-6)	15 - 30%
UNSAPONIFIABLE FRACTION 1.5%	
Sterols 1281.3 mg/kg	Beta-sitosterol (820.7 mg/kg), stigmasterol (310 mg/kg), brassicasterol (99.1 mg/kg), campesterol (51.2 mg/kg)
Tocopherols 45-50+ mg/kg	Alpha-tocopherol (30.9-50+ mg/kg), beta-tocopherol (0.18-3.1 mg/kg), gamma-tocopherol (0.54-5.7 mg/kg), delta-tocopherol (n.d.-1.7 mg/kg)
Squalene	96-113 mg/kg

Formulating with Sweet Almond Oil

Sensory info: Light yellow, oily liquid; generally clear. Has a very light almond aroma.
Absorption rate: Wet – absorbs slowly
Dilution: Can be used 100% or in a blend of other oils.

Therapeutic applications:
A good emollient, it protects and nourishes the skin. It helps relieve skin itching, soreness, dryness, and inflammation, making it a good choice for inflammatory concerns such as eczema. Suitable for all skin types, especially dry skin.

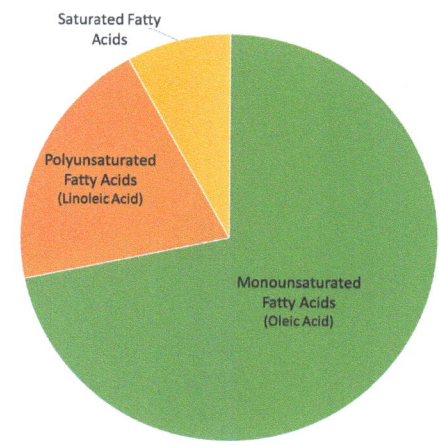

Apricot
Prunus armeniaca

Common name: Apricot kernel
Scientific name: *Prunus armeniaca* L.
Botanical family: Rosaceae
Conservation status: Not yet assessed

Description: Apricots are small-to-medium-sized deciduous trees in the Rosaceae family, which likely originated in China. *P. armeniaca* grows 10-15 meters high under natural conditions and around 4 meters when cultivated, with a spreading or upright habit. The bark is reddish to grey-brown, with reddish leaves and young twigs. Leaves are simple, alternate, ovate to round-ovate, pointed, and glabrous with serrated margins and red-purple petioles. Solitary flowers, which bloom in the early spring, are pink to white with dark red sepals. The fruit is a somewhat flattened drupe 3.5-8 cm wide, with a distinct furrow. The skin color ranges from yellow to deep orange, with a marked red blush in many modern cultivars. The apricot kernel is the seed contained within a hard endocarp, together with which it forms the stone or pit of the fruit.

Apricot trees thrive in deep, fertile, well-drained soils. They grow best in Mediterranean climates, where frosts in late winter or early spring are unlikely.

Many historians agree that the cultivation of apricots dates back 3,000 - 4000 years. *Prunus armeniaca* was thought to spread originate in China, then spread throughout Central Asia, Armenia, Anatolia, and then to Europe, likely via the Romans. Apricots arrived in Greece by way of the Romans around 70-60 BC and became an important crop in the 17th century. Spaniards and English colonists likely exported the tree to the New World.

Like many other stone fruit trees, apricot flowers, leaves, kernels, and bark contain the toxic, cyanide-generating amygdalin that can be lethal at high doses. Amygdalin is a bitter cyanogenic glycoside that the human body converts to hydrogen cyanide. The apricot kernel contains the highest levels of amygdalin of any stone fruit.[8]

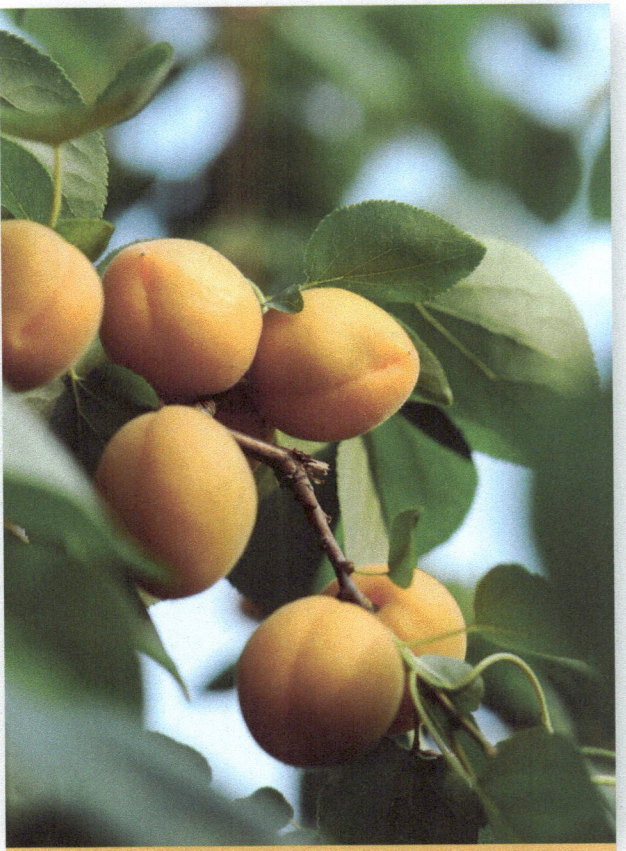

EXTRACTION INFORMATION

Country of origin: Turkey, Uzbekistan, Italy, Algeria
Part of plant: Kernel or seed
Oil content: 37-44%
Extraction method: Cold pressing

MANUFACTURING INFORMATION

CAS number: 72869-69-3
EC number: 272-046-1
INCI name: Prunus Armeniaca (Apricot) Kernel Oil
CosIng (functions): Fragrance, Skin conditioning

SHELF LIFE

12 months

Ethnobotany: The whole apricot tree is used as food and medicine. The fruits are nutritive and mildly laxative; they have been used in Vietnam to treat digestive and respiratory disorders. The flowers are considered to be tonic and to promote fertility. The seed has been used to treat asthma, coughs, acute or chronic bronchitis, and constipation.[9]

NUTRIENT PROFILE

Rich in the monounsaturated fatty acid oleic acid, with a strong presence of linoleic acid (20-28%), apricot kernel offers a luxurious oil feel to the skin.

Apricot Kernel Oil[10, 11, 12]	
SATURATED FATTY ACIDS	
Palmitic acid (C16:0)	2.93 - 3.42%
Stearic acid (C18:0)	1.06 - 1.69%
MONOUNSATURATED FATTY ACIDS	
Oleic acid (C18:1 n-9)	**62.10 - 71.43%**
POLYUNSATURATED FATTY ACIDS	
Linoleic acid (C18:2 n-6)	**20.5 - 28.86%**
Alpha-linolenic acid (C18:3 n-3)	0.74 - 1.4%
UNSAPONIFIABLE FRACTION	
Sterols 2157 - 9736 mg/kg	Beta-sitosterol (1846 - 4278 mg/kg), campesterol (112 - 487 mg/kg), delta-5-avenasterol (95 - 314 mg/kg), cholesterol (n.d. - 526 mg/kg)
Tocopherols 520 mg/kg	Gamma-tocopherol (330.8 - 520.8 mg/kg), delta-tocopherol (28.5 - 60.2 mg/kg), alpha-tocopherol (14.8 - 40.4 mg/kg)
Squalene	126 - 439 mg/kg; average 230 mg/kg

Formulating with Apricot Kernel Oil

Sensory info: Pale to golden yellow, light texture, almost odorless.
Absorption rate: Wet – absorbs more slowly
Dilution: Can be used 100% or in a blend of other oils.

Therapeutic applications:
All skin types: mature, dry, sensitive, or inflamed skin. Apricot kernel oil protects the skin from free radicals, supports wound healing, and promotes skin barrier homeostasis.[10, 13] A great combination for massage applications is 50% apricot kernel and 50% sunflower oil.

Due to its beta-sitosterol content, apricot kernel is useful for relieving inflammation, itchiness, and dry skin; beta-sitosterol exhibits anti-inflammatory[14] and anti-pyretic activity.[15]

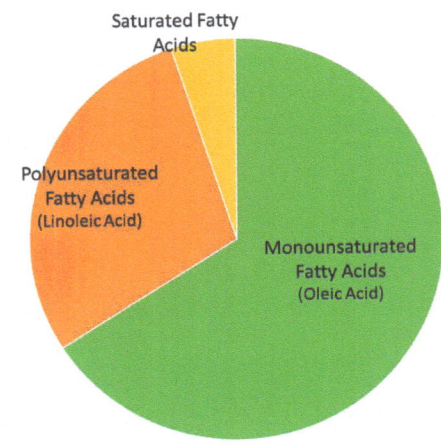

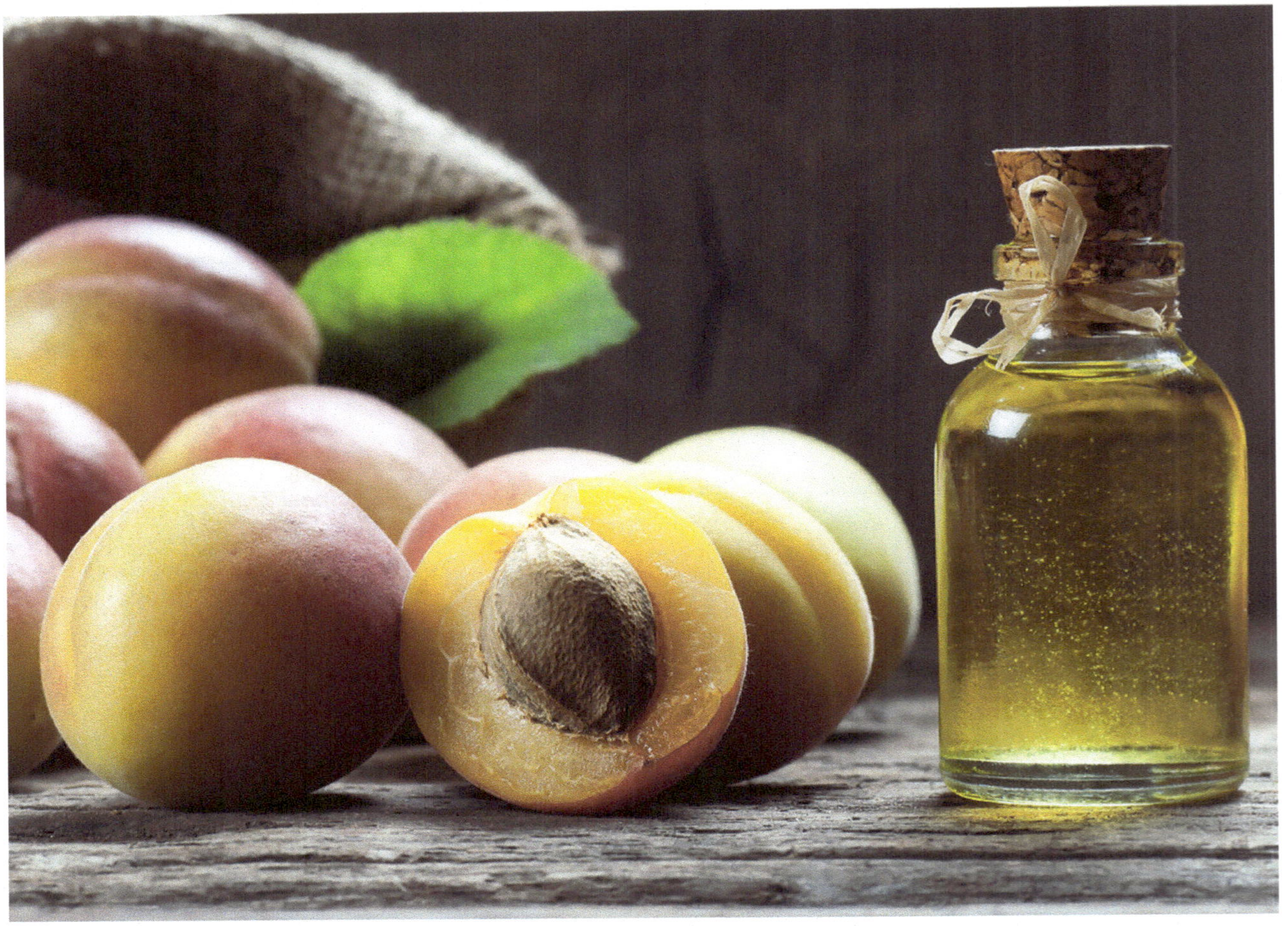

Argan

Argania spinosa

Common name: Argan
Scientific name: *Argania spinosa* (L.) Skeels
Botanical family: Sapotaceae
Conservation status: Not defined

Description: *Argania spinosa* is a large evergreen shrub or small tree in the Sapotaceae family native to Morocco. Its characteristic spiny branches give the tree its species name, "*spinosa*." Argan trees typically grow 15-25 feet tall and spread 25-40 feet wide. Mature trees are characterized by thorny, gnarled trunks; small, green, ovate leaves; rounded crowns; and small, stalkless, yellow-green flowers blooming in axillary clusters. The fruits are plum-sized, with thick, bitter peels and a fragrant pulpy pericarp that envelops a single hard nut, typically containing 2-3 seeds. Fruits require over a year to ripen.

The trees are endemic to a semi-desert, forested region of southwestern Morocco, bordered by the Sahara on the east and the Atlas Mountains to the north. Argan trees serve as a protective ecological buffer against desertification by preventing the incursion of the Sahara Desert west into Morocco.

Argan oil, cold-pressed from the seeds, has a long history of use in food and medicine in Morocco and is used in cooking, much like olive oil. Argan oil was virtually unheard of in the West until the end of the 20th century, when it skyrocketed in popularity as a cosmetics ingredient.

The genus name *Argania* is the Latinized version of the Moroccan name for the tree; the specific epithet *spinosa* is from the Latin, meaning "spiny."[16]

Ethnobotany: Argan oil has been traditionally applied as a moisturizer and to heal pimples and chickenpox scars. It has also been used to treat skin disorders including psoriasis and eczema, heal burns and wounds, ease joint pain, relieve scabies, forestall wrinkles, remedy brittle fingernails, prevent hair loss,

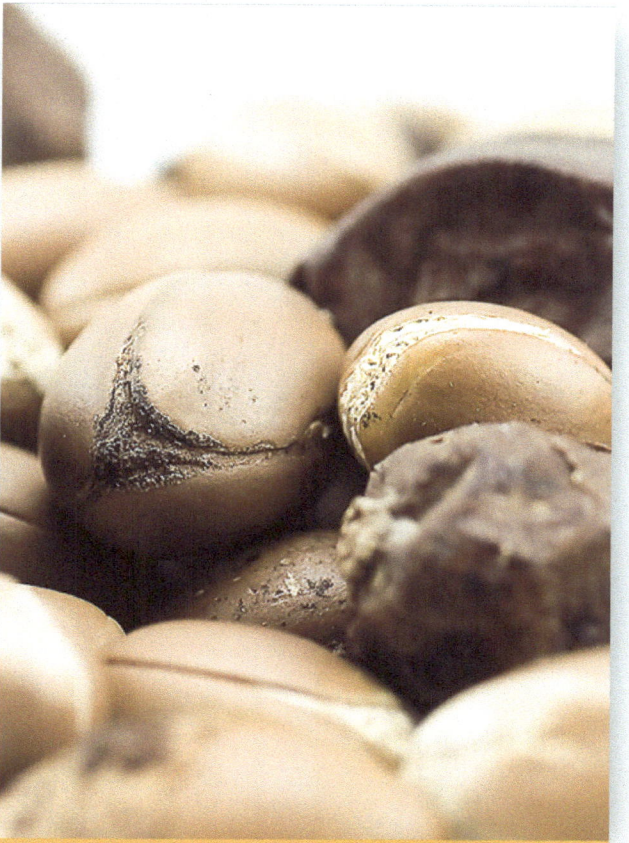

EXTRACTION INFORMATION

Country of origin: Morocco
Part of plant: Nut/fruit, kernel/nut
Oil content: 10-45+% depending on method of extraction and origin of nuts[18]
Extraction method: Expeller pressing

Traditionally, women prepared the argan nuts, manually cracking them open, one by one, between two stones. Further processing would then be done to extract oil.

MANUFACTURING INFORMATION

CAS number: 223747-87-3 / 299184-75-1
EC number: n/a
INCI name: Argania Spinosa (Argan) Kernel Oil
CosIng (functions): Skin conditioning, Skin conditioning - emollient

SHELF LIFE

2 years

and moisturize dry hair.[17]

Sustainability Issue: The argan tree (*Argania spinosa*) is endemic in southwestern Morocco, where it grows over about 320,000 square miles. This slow-growing, spiny tree plays an essential ecological function in this part of Morocco, as it effectively protects the soil against heavy rain or wind-induced erosion and maintains soil fertility.

Unfortunately, people frequently use the wood of *Argania spinosa* for fuel and subsequently accelerate the deforestation problem since populations are generally eager to replace argan groves with plants of higher and more immediate economic benefit. There is currently a program aimed to increase the industrial value of *Argania spinosa* and encourage tree replanting.

NUTRIENT PROFILE

Argan contains approximately 45% monounsaturated fatty acids and 35% polyunsaturated fatty acids.[19] The unsaponifiable fraction, which is comprised of carotenes (37%), tocopherols (8%), triterpene alcohols (20%), sterols (29%), and xanthophylls (5%), constitutes less than 1% of argan oil.[20]

Argan Oil[21, 22, 23, 24, 25, 26]	
Saturated fatty acids	
Palmitic acid (C16:0)	10 - 15.6%
Stearic acid (C18:0)	5.0 - 8.5%
Monounsaturated fatty acids	
Oleic acid (C18:1 n-9)	41.2 - 55%
Palmitoleic acid (C16:1 n-7)	0.3 - 3%
Polyunsaturated fatty acids	
Linoleic acid (C18:2 n-6)	28 - 37.9%
Unsaponifiable fraction - makes up less than 1%	
Sterols 1360 - 2000+ mg/kg	Schottenol (423.5-481.4 mg/kg), spinasterol (361.1-421.1 mg/kg), stigmasta-8.22dien-3b-ol (33.7-58.3 mg/kg)
Tocopherols 633 - 775 mg/kg	Gamma-tocopherol (550 - 640 mg/kg), delta-tocopherol (37.2 - 69 mg/kg), alpha-tocopherol (26.6 - 50+ mg/kg), beta-tocopherol (0.0 - 4.3 mg/kg)
Squalene	3030 - 3210 mg/kg

Formulating with Argan Oil

Sensory info: A nice golden color, light in texture with a slightly nutty aroma. The oil will be a clear, nearly colorless, slightly viscous liquid when refined and deodorized.
Absorption rate: Wet – absorbs slowly
Dilution: Can be used 25-100%

Therapeutic applications:

Argan is a great oil for mature, aging, or damaged skin. Cutaneous application of argan oil can improve skin elasticity and skin hydration in post-menopausal women. Daily dermal application of argan oil may reduce transepidermal water loss and restore a damaged skin barrier.[27,28]

It may be useful in gels or creams to prevent wrinkles or for around the eyes as a nourishing oil or cream. Cultural and historical use indicate argan is appropriate for problematic skin and acne.

Argan oil combined with rosehip seed oil may support healthy scar formation and prevent stretch marks.[29]

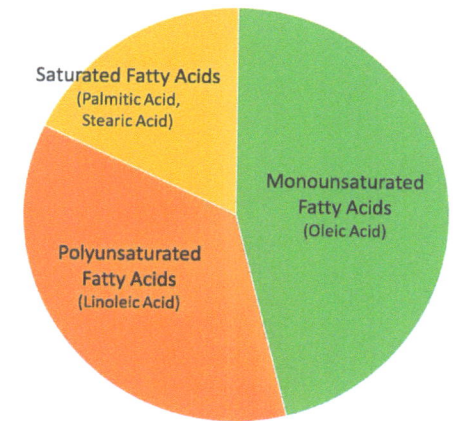

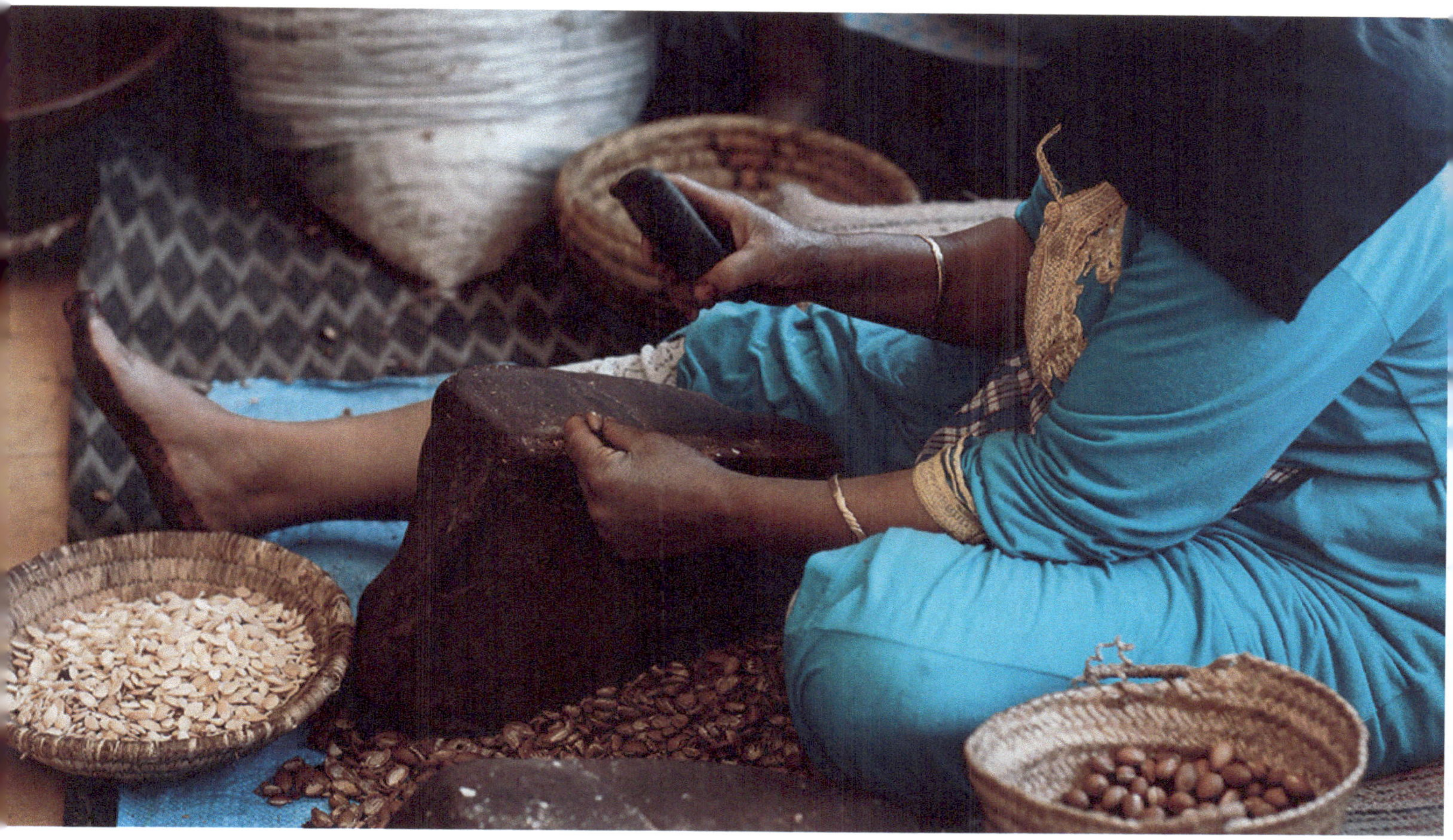

Baobab
Adansonia digitata

Common names: Baobab
Scientific name: *Adansonia digitata* L.
Botanical family: Malvaceae
Conservation status: Not yet assessed

Description: The *Adansonia* genus comprises nine massive, long-lived deciduous tree species in the Malvaceae family. African baobab (*Adansonia digitata*), endemic to mainland Africa and the Arabian Peninsula, is the species most commonly used for its oil. The African baobab is the oldest known angiosperm tree; one baobab in Namibia is over 1,275 years old. The trunk stores water and can reach 18 meters in height and 9 meters in diameter. The trunks of older trees are often hollow, formed by the union of many stems over time. The flowers are pendulous and pollinated by bats and bush babies. The fruit is large, woody, gourd-like, and contains a mucilaginous edible fruit.

Baobab trees are known for their peculiar barrel-like trunks, scraggly root-like branches, and remarkable longevity. According to Arabian legend, "the devil plucked up the baobab, thrust its branches into the earth, and left its roots in the air." As of 2005, nine of the 13 oldest African baobab specimens and five of the six largest trees had died, or their largest/oldest stems had collapsed. This abnormal loss is likely due to climate change.[30]

African baobab bark is smooth, reddish-brown to grey, soft, and characterized by longitudinal fibers. The species is highly branched and features an extensive lateral root system that spreads up to 50 meters from the trunk; root tips are typically tubers. The primary roots of old trees are relatively shallow, and the trees are thus vulnerable to being uprooted in strong winds.

Adult trees produce simple leaves at the beginning of the season, followed by leaves with 2-3 leaflets, which are, in turn, succeeded by mature leaves 20 cm in diameter with 5-9 leaflets.

The inflorescence is composed of one or two flowers

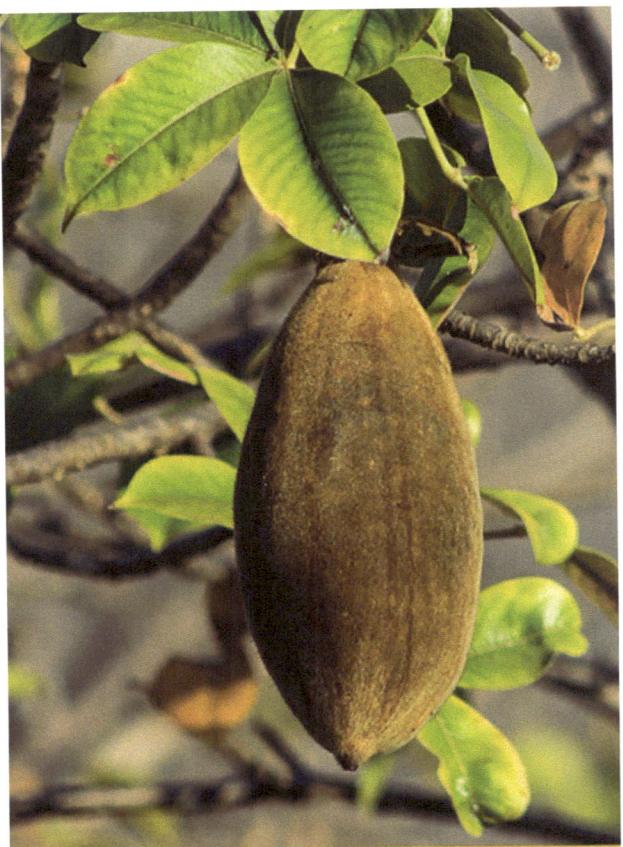

EXTRACTION INFORMATION

Country of origin: Eastern and Southern Africa
Part of plant: Seed
Oil content: 12%
Extraction method: Cold pressing

MANUFACTURING INFORMATION

CAS number: 91745-12-9
EC number: 294-680-8
INCI name: Adansonia Digitata (Baobab) Seed Oil
CosIng (functions): Hair conditioning, Skin conditioning, Skin conditioning - emollient

SHELF LIFE

2-4 years
Extremely stable oil.

positioned in the axils of leaves near the tips of reproductive branches. Flowers are large and showy, white, and pendulous. They bloom at the end of the dry season or just before the first rains, often the same time as the first leaves appear. Flowers open in the late afternoon and fall the following dawn. Their aroma is redolent of sulfur, an aroma that attracts their bat pollinators.

A. digitata grows in the thorn woodlands of African savannahs, which are often at low altitudes with 4-10 dry months per year. The African baobab is typically solitary, but the species sometimes grows in small groups depending on soil factors. The tree is sensitive to waterlogging and frost and does not grow in deep sand. It is found in arid and semi-arid regions.

Ethnobotany: In Africa, baobab has a significant history as food and medicine. The seeds, leaves, roots, flowers, fruit pulp, and bark are all edible. The fruit consists of large seeds embedded in a dry, acidic pulp. The seeds thicken soups, are roasted and eaten as snacks, or can be fermented and used as a flavoring agent. Every part of the tree has been used to treat various ailments, including diarrhea, malaria, and microbial infections.

Baobab has many colorful common names, including "dead-rat tree" (a reference to the fruit's appearance), "monkey-bread tree" (monkeys eat the dry fruit), "upside-down tree" (the bare branches resemble roots), and "cream of tartar tree" (an allusion to the fruit's acidic flavor).[31]

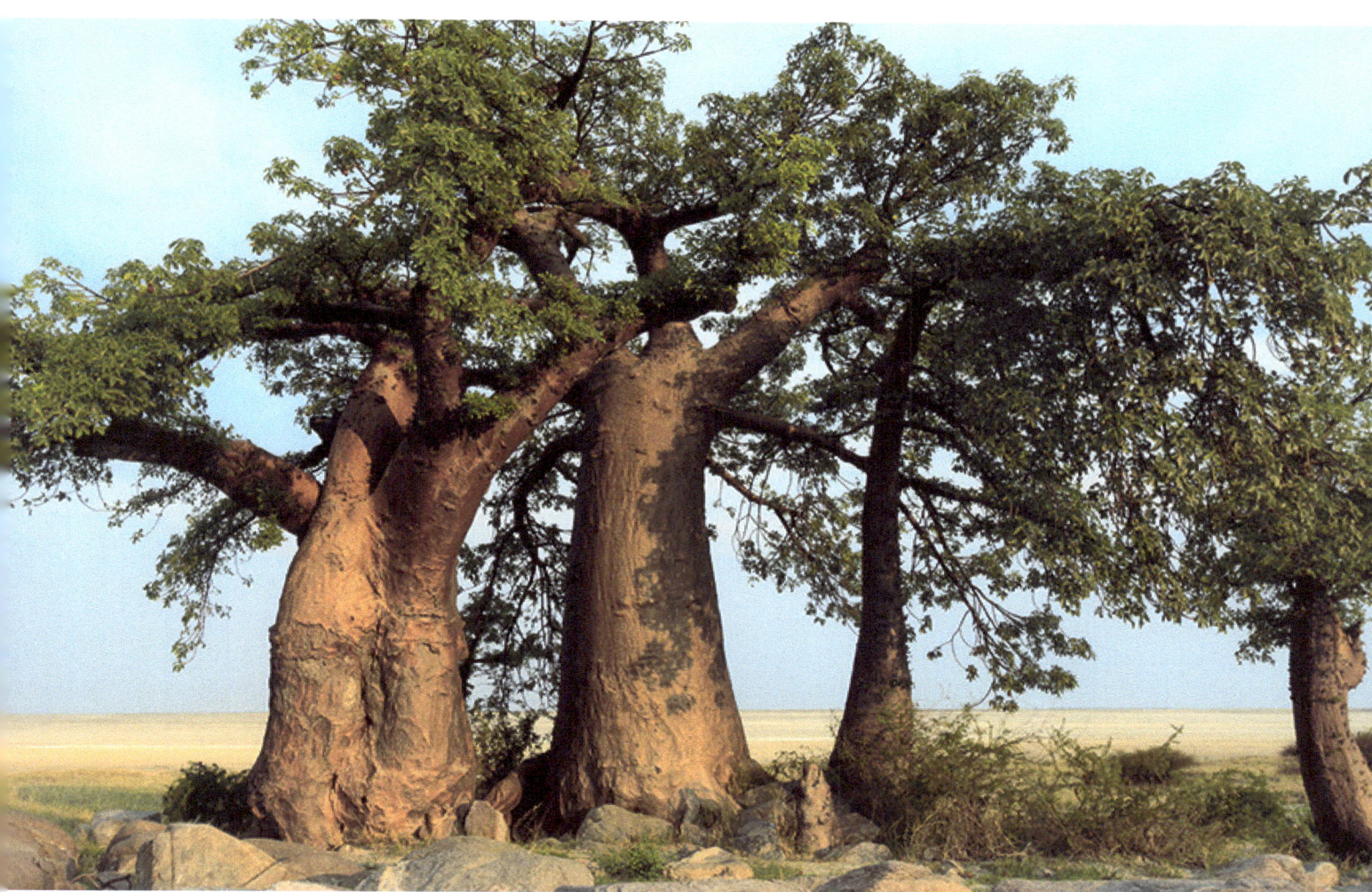

NUTRIENT PROFILE

Baobab oil is especially rich in oleic acid (30-44%), linoleic acid (27-37%), with palmitic acid (18-30%), having reasonably balanced proportions of saturated and unsaturated fatty acids.

Baobab Oil[32, 33, 34]	
SATURATED FATTY ACIDS	
Myristic acid (C14:0)	0.3 - 1.5%
Palmitic acid (C16:0)	**18 - 30%**
Stearic acid (C18:0)	5.1 - 9 %
Arachidic acid (C20:0)	0.5 - 2.0%
MONOUNSATURATED FATTY ACIDS	
Palmitoleic acid (C16:1 n-7)	0.3 - 1.7%
Oleic acid (C18:1 n-9)	**30.0 - 44.0 %**
Gondoic acid (C20:1 n-9)	0 - 3.6%
POLYUNSATURATED FATTY ACIDS	
Linoleic acid (C18:2 n-6)	**27.6 - 37.0%**
Alpha-linolenic acid (C18:3 n-3)	0.3 - 8.0%
UNSAPONIFIABLE FRACTION approx. 2.8-3.8%	
Sterols 2157 - 9736 mg/kg	Beta-sitosterol (≈ 75-80% of the total sterols) is one of the major sterol constituents present in baobab seed oil. Other sterols include campesterol (8.3%) and stigmasterol (2.9%)
Tocopherols 256 mg/kg	Gamma-tocopherol (204 mg/kg), alpha-tocopherol (27 mg/kg), delta-tocopherol (20 mg/kg), beta-tocopherol (4 mg/kg)

Formulating with Baobab Oil

Sensory info: Golden yellow, with a slightly nutty, floral aroma
Absorption rate: Wet - slow to absorb
Dilution: Can be used 100% or in a blend of other oils.

Therapeutic applications:
Baobab oil can improve the skin's elasticity, relieve inflamed skin conditions such as dry eczema and psoriasis, and can be an excellent cell-regenerative oil, as the fatty acids in its profile support epithelial tissue regeneration. Baobab may alleviate pain from burns. It softens and soothes the skin and may improve the appearance of stretch marks and scars. Baobab is also used to improve texture and add shine to hair.

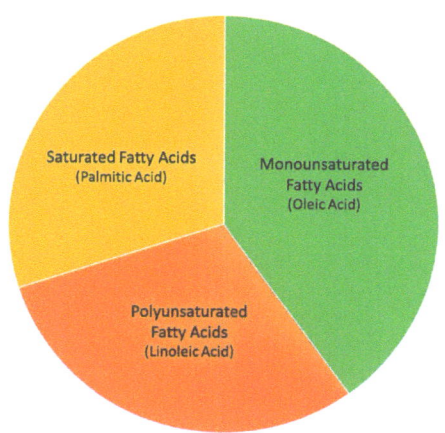

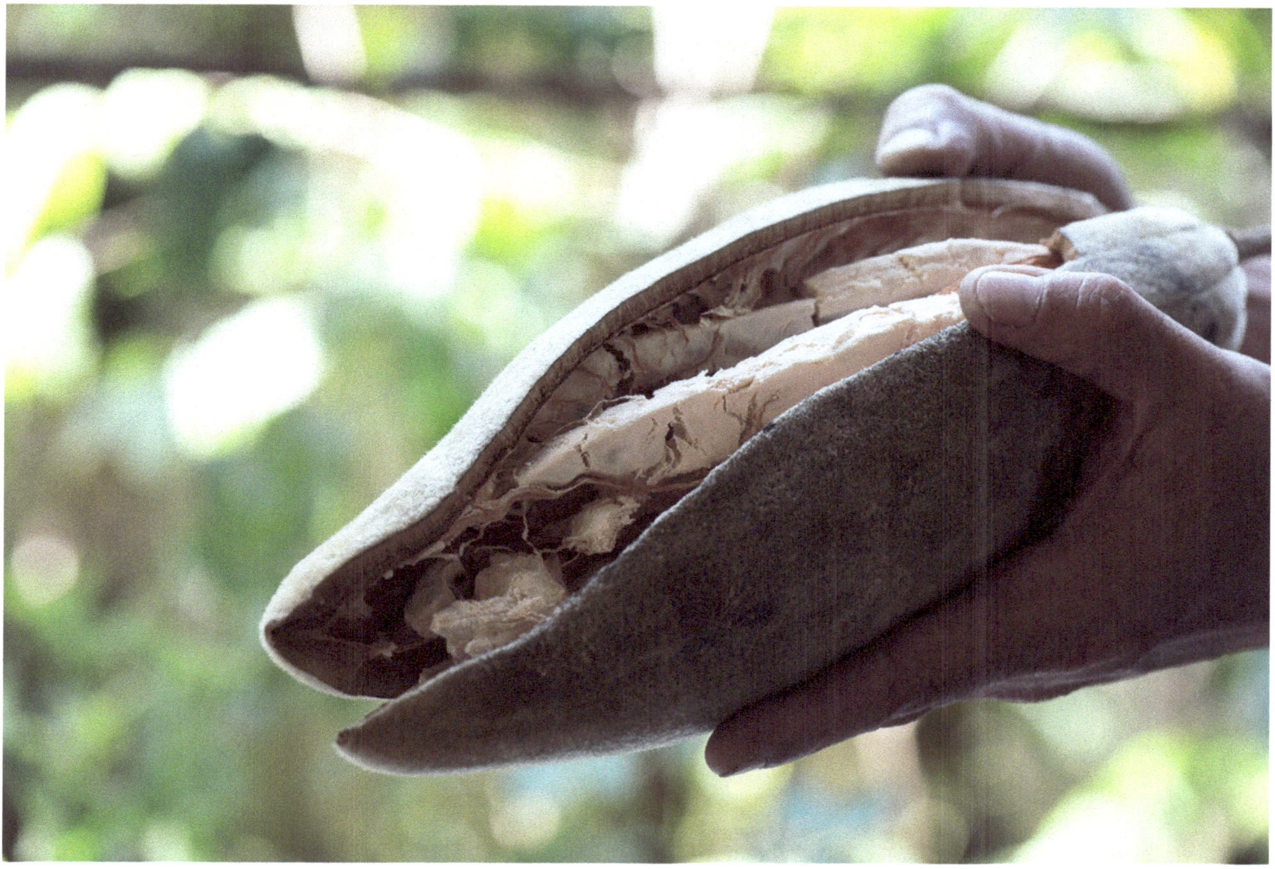

Camelina
Camelina sativa

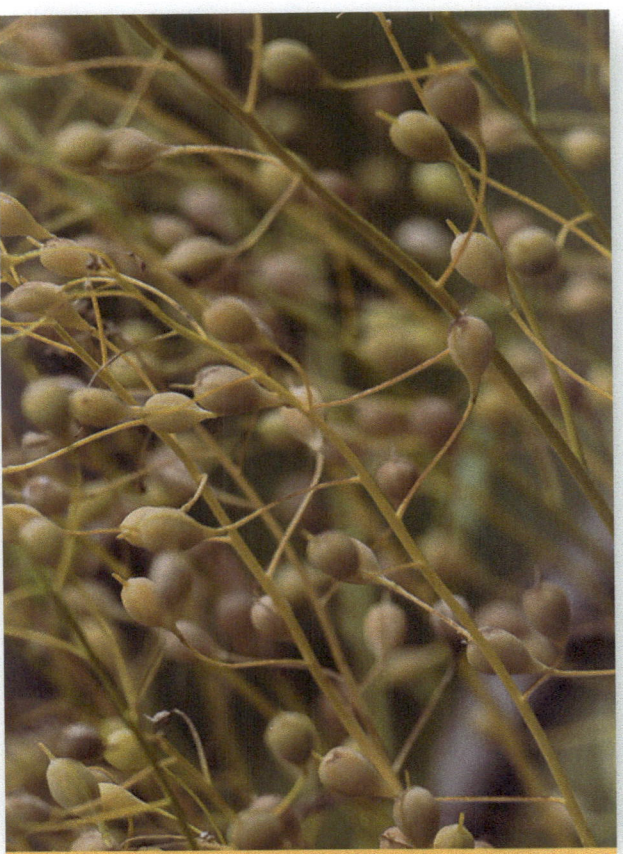

Common names: Camelina, false flax, gold-of-pleasure, Dutch flax, wild flax, German sesame
Scientific name: *Camelina sativa* (L.) Crantz
Synonyms: *Camelina parodii* Ibara & LaPorte, syn. *Myagrum sativum* L.
Botanical family: Brassicaceae
Conservation status: Not yet assessed

Description: Molecular analysis of *Camelina sativa* suggests that it may have originated in southeastern Europe, particularly around Ukraine. Europeans cultivated camelina continuously from the Stone Age until the Middle Ages, when its cultivation declined. It probably moved to the New World as a contaminant of other seeds and crops, particularly flaxseed crops. Canada intentionally introduced camelina in 1863, but it did not become a significant commercial crop until the late 1990s. Today, it grows in most European countries, several Eastern Asian countries, several South American countries, in the northwestern United States, and Tunisia, both as a native and introduced plant. Its range is extensive, as it is fairly drought- and cold-temperature-tolerant. One challenge in its commercial viability is that it is sensitive to most herbicides.

Camelina sativa is a flowering, herbaceous annual plant, growing to 1-3 feet tall (30-90 cm) with branched stems, either smooth or slightly hairy, which become woodier as they mature. The plant's narrow (2-10 mm), lance-shaped leaves (1-3 inches long) lack a petiole and tend to be smooth. Small, yellow flowers exhibit 4 minute petals in racemes with flowers in terminal clusters. These flowers bloom within 4-6 weeks of germination for only 2-3 days, during which time they will often self-pollinate.[35, 36]

The resulting fruits are smooth, 7-9 mm long, pear-shaped siliques, which resemble bolls of flax, giving camelina many of its common names. Small 2-3 mm long seeds are deeply ridged and pale yellow-brown, and each tiny seed weighs less than 1 mg.[37] Several species in the *Camelina* genus look very similar, with only slight distinctions to differentiate *Camelina sativa*

EXTRACTION INFORMATION

Country of origin: United States, Europe, Canada, United Kingdom
Part of plant: Seed
Oil content: 38-43%[41]
Extraction method: Cold pressing

MANUFACTURING INFORMATION

CAS Number: 68956-68-3
EC number: 273-313-5
INCI name: Camelina Sativa (Camelina) Seed Oil
CosIng (function): Skin conditioning

SHELF LIFE

18-24 months

from the other plants.

Ethnobotany: Historically, camelina was grown as food for people and animals. There were many industrial uses of camelina oil; arguably, the most important was using it for lamp oil. Stems were used for their fibers. In Eastern Europe, camelina played a crucial medical role as a folk remedy for stomach ulcers, as a tonic, and as localized treatment of burns, wounds, and eye inflammations.[38]

Camelina sativa has become a valuable source for biofuel production, especially for the commercial airline industry and the military. Camelina oil meal, a by-product of the oil extraction process, is becoming a key component of livestock feed in various sectors. It effectively increases the omega-3 content of the resulting meat, eggs, and dairy products.

Camelina oil is also experiencing renewed popularity as a cooking oil. It has a healthy omega-3: omega-6 fatty acid ratio of 2:1, is high in polyunsaturated fats, relatively high in vitamin E, relatively high in phytosterols, and its smoke-point is 475 degrees F (246 deg. C). These desirable qualities make it easy to use both as a cooking oil and an oil base for non-heated sauces, such as salad dressing.[39,40]

NUTRIENT PROFILE

Camelina oil is high (about 50%) in polyunsaturated fatty acids, which makes camelina oil a rich source of essential fatty acids and an excellent source of omega-3 fatty acids. Overall, there is significant variability in the nutrient profiles of various camelina seed oils, probably based on their varied growing conditions.

Camelina Oil[42]	
SATURATED FATTY ACIDS	
Palmitic acid (C16:0)	5.6 - 7.8%
Stearic acid (C18:0)	2.4 - 3.3%
Arachidic acid (C20:0)	1.0 - 1.6%
MONOUNSATURATED FATTY ACIDS	
Oleic acid (C18:1 n-9)	12.8 - 20.3%
Gondoic acid (C20:1 n-9)	1.10 - 11.9%
POLYUNSATURATED FATTY ACIDS	
Linoleic acid (C18:2 n-6)	16.10 - 23.08%
Alpha-linolenic acid (C18:3 n-3)	31.2 - 53.6%
UNSAPONIFIABLE FRACTION	
Sterols 2533.1 mg/kg	Beta-sitosterol (1440.2 mg/kg), delta-5-campesterol (595.6 mg/kg), a high content of cholesterol (165.6 mg/kg), delta-5-avenasterol (141.7 mg/kg), brassicasterol (123.9 mg/kg), delta-5-stigmastenol (19.4 mg/kg)
Tocopherols 692.5 - 1026.7 mg/kg	Gamma-tocopherol (658.5-888.0 mg/kg), delta-tocopherol (37.8-222.6 mg/kg)
Squalene	15.2-68.9 mg/kg

Formulating with Camelina Seed Oil

Sensory info: Dark gold to light yellow color with a light, green, nutty aroma
Absorption rate: Medium
Dilution: Can be used 100 percent or in a blend of other oils.

Note: Some camelina oil may have a higher erucic acid content. Use blended with other carriers on sensitive skin.

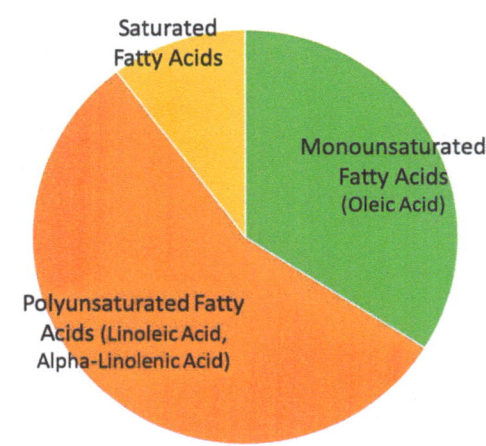

Therapeutic applications:
Camelina seed oil's emollient ability to soothe dry skin and improve skin elasticity and suppleness makes it particularly beneficial for mature skin. It is indicated for Vata.

Camelina oil's high proportion of polyunsaturated fatty acids, particularly the essential fatty acids (EFA) linoleic and alpha-linolenic acid, as well as higher levels of antioxidant tocopherols, make it an excellent choice to address inflammatory conditions, such as eczema or acne, moisturize dry skin that may be an indication of EFA deficiency, enhance the skin's barrier function, and help protect the skin from UV-induced skin damage.[43]

Using camelina on the hair and scalp nourishes and supports healthy hair when used at 0.2-2% dilutions for shampoo and conditioners and 10% for hair masks.[44] It is especially appropriate to address dry, itchy scalp and dandruff.

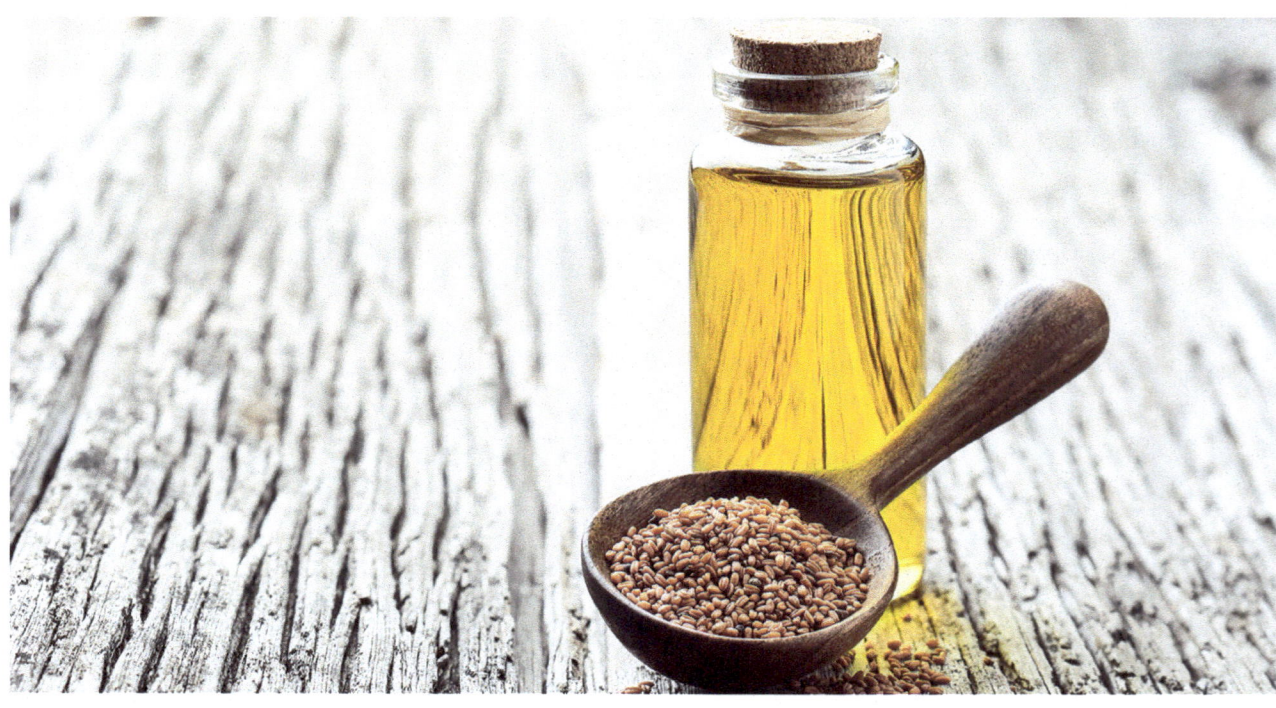

Jojoba
Simmondsia chinensis

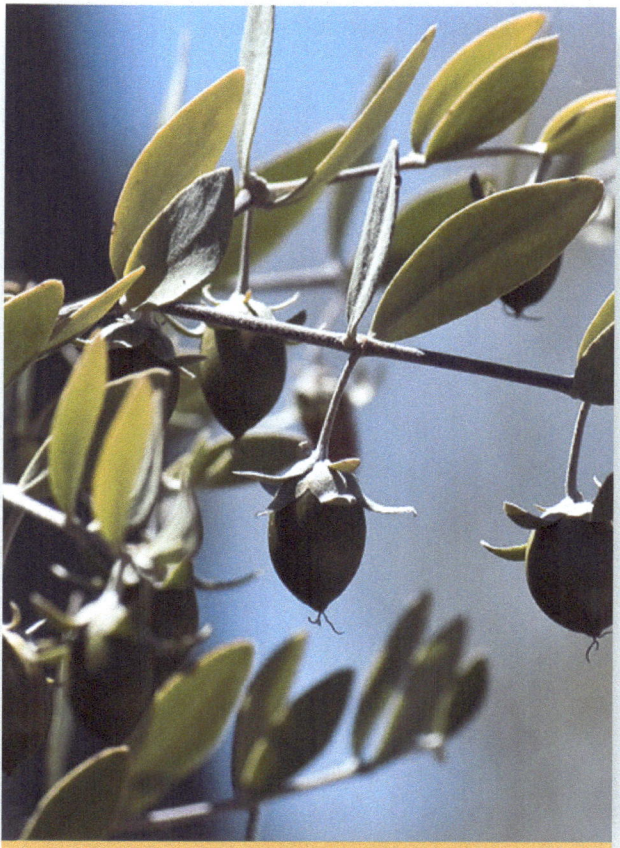

Common names: Jojoba, pig nut, goat nut, deer nut, jojowi, bucknut, coffee nut, coffee bush, coffee berry, lemon leaf, quinine plant, quinine nut, wild hazel, gray box bush
Scientific name: *Simmondsia chinensis* (Link) C.K. Schneid.
Synonyms: *Buxus chinensis* Link, *Simmondsia californica* Nutt.
Botanical family: Simmondsiaceae
Conservation status: Not yet assessed

Description: *Simmondsia chinensis* is a dioecious evergreen desert shrub in the Simmondsiaceae family native to the Sonoran Desert and Baja California regions of North America. Jojoba shrubs are stiff-branched, wide-spreading, with a low mound shape and typically grow 4.5-6 feet tall. Blue-green leaves are simple, opposite, ovate or lanceolate, leathery, and persistent. Flowers are inconspicuous, borne on short axillary stems; acorn-like fruits succeed the pistillate flowers. Jojoba thrives in coarse, well-drained desert soil with limited summer water in full sun to light shade.[45]

The seeds contain a commercially valuable wax, often referred to as an oil, historically used to substitute for sperm whale oil. The common name jojoba (pronounced ho-HO-bah) is derived from the Papago Indian name, a term appropriated by colonial Spaniards.[46]

Jojoba wax is a pale-yellow liquid at room temperature; it is impervious to rancidity and damage caused by prolonged exposure to high temperatures. This wax, and its derivatives, have a wide range of applications from industrial to cosmetic. Skincare lotions, moisturizers, massage oils, hair care products, lipsticks, and nail products often incorporate jojoba oil into their formulations.

Ethnobotany: Indigenous North Americans traditionally ate jojoba seeds raw or roasted. They used various plant parts to treat cancer, kidney disorders,

EXTRACTION INFORMATION

Country of origin: USA
Part of plant: Seed
Oil content: 50%
Extraction method: Cold pressing

MANUFACTURING INFORMATION

CAS number: 90045-98-0 / 61789-91-1
EC number: 289-964-3
INCI name: Simmondsia Chinensis (Jojoba) seed oil
CosIng (functions): Hair conditioning, Skin conditioning, Skin conditioning - emollient

SHELF LIFE

4-5 years
Adding jojoba oil to other carrier oils can enhance their oxidative stability.

colds, dysuria, ocular maladies, obesity, poison ivy, sore throat, warts, wounds, and to facilitate parturition. Modern cosmetic uses of jojoba oil include topically promoting hair growth and relieving dandruff and psoriasis.[47] Additionally, jojoba has many applications in diverse industries, such as pharmaceutical isolation, fire suppression, candle and lamp oil, surfactants, polishes, extraction of radioactive isotopes, and unique lubricants.[48]

NUTRIENT PROFILE[48, 49, 50, 51, 52, 53]

Natural jojoba seed oil is not a triglyceride fat or oil. It is a liquid at room temperature and functions more like a fatty oil than a wax, but its chemistry is more closely related to beeswax. It is primarily a mixture of long-chained, unbranched wax esters that result from the esterification of an omega-9 monounsaturated linear fatty acid and an omega-9 monounsaturated linear fatty alcohol. Jojoba oil from the Arizona deserts is composed almost entirely (97-98%) of wax esters, with the last 2-3% being monounsaturated straight-chain fatty acids, alcohols with high molecular weights, and the unsaponifiable fraction.

Jojoba Oil Fatty Acid and Unsaponifiable Fractions	
SATURATED FATTY ACIDS	
Myristic acid (C14:0)	0.3 - 3.5%
Palmitic acid (C16:0)	1.2 - 9.0%
Arachidic acid (C20:0)	0.3 - 3.8%
Heneicosanoic acid (C21:0)	8.2 - 15.4%
Tricosanoic acid (C23:0)	0.8 - 4.3%
MONOUNSATURATED FATTY ACIDS	
Palmitoleic acid (C16:1 n-7)	0.7 - 2.2%
Oleic acid (C18:1 n-9)	6 - 14.5%
Gondoic acid (C20:1 n-9)	**20.8 - 73.4%**
Erucic acid (C22:1 n-9)	11.8 - 19.3%
Nervonic acid (C24:1 n-9)	1.3 - 4.4%
POLYUNSATURATED FATTY ACIDS	
Linoleic acid (C18:2 n-6)	0.2 - 8.7%
UNSAPONIFIABLE FRACTION	
Sterols 3977 mg/kg	Beta-sitosterol (2732 - 2780 mg/kg), campesterol (672 - 731 mg/kg), stigmasterol (266 - 274 mg/kg), isofucosterol (163 - 238 mg/kg), cholesterol (32 mg/kg)
Tocopherols 412 - 432 mg/kg	Gamma-tocopherol (326 - 330.3 mg/kg), alpha-tocopherol (83 - 84.7 mg/kg), beta-tocopherol (1 - 2 mg/kg)

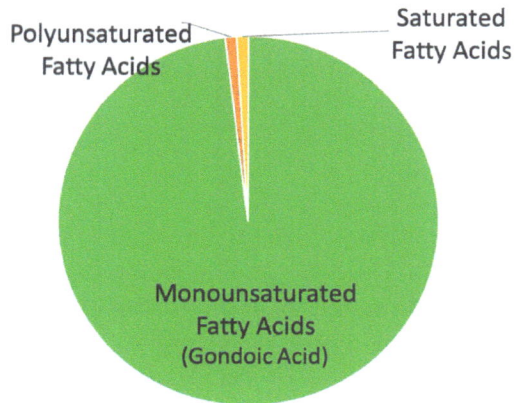

Wax esters can differ in their fatty acid + fatty alcohol combinations yet have the same molecular weight. Categories of wax esters are identified by the total number of carbons in the molecule with no common names. For example, C42:2 is a wax ester with 42 carbon atoms and two double bonds. Wax esters can also be identified as individual, unique molecules, where the fatty acid and fatty alcohol are each identified individually, and these molecules also have common names. For example, C22:1-C20:1 results from the esterification of a C22:1 fatty acid (erucic acid) and a C20:1 fatty alcohol (arachidyl alcohol, syn. 1-eicosanol), producing a molecule called docosenyl eicosenoate. C20:1-C22:1, on the other hand, is the result of a C20:1 fatty acid (gondoic acid) combined with a C22:1 fatty alcohol (erucyl alcohol syn. cis-13-docosen-1-ol), and it is called eicosenyl decosenoate.

Jojoba Oil Wax Esters	
Wax Ester Group (% of oil)	**Wax Esters (% of oil)**
C34:2 — 0.1-0.2%	
C36:2 — 1.4-3%	
C38:2 — 4-10%	Eicosenyl octadecenoate (C20:1-C18:1) 5.5-7.2%
C40:2 — 21-34%	Eicosenyl eicosenoate (C20:1-C20:1) 21.4-30%
C42:2 — 44-51.1%	Docosenyl eicosenoate (C22:1-C20:1) 37.8%, Eicosenyl decosenoate (C20:1-C22:1) 10.7%
C44:2 — 8-15%	Tetracosenyl eicosenoate (C24:1-C20:1) 6.7%
C46:2 — 1-3%	
C48:2 — 0.1-0.4%	

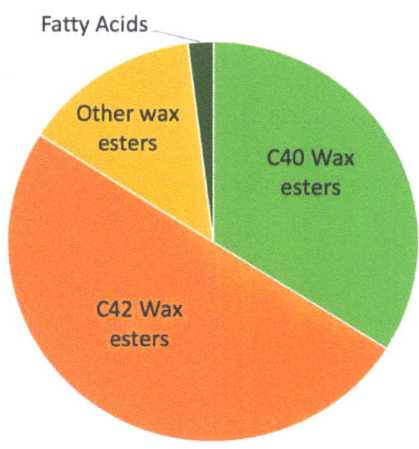

Formulating with Jojoba Oil

Sensory info: Bright yellow liquid with a light, fine texture; very penetrating. Odorless.
Absorption: Dry – readily absorbs into skin
Dilution: Can be used 100 percent or in a blend of other oils

Therapeutic applications:

Jojoba is appropriate for acne-prone skin[54] to dissolve and remove substances clogging pores. It has demonstrated *in vitro*, concentration-dependent, antibacterial[55,56] action against several common pathogenic bacteria and has natural anti-inflammatory[57] properties, making it helpful for eczema, psoriasis, and inflamed skin.

Research also supports jojoba oil's use in wound healing.[58] It is highly recommended for regenerative skincare and preventative aging care. It makes for a great oil in a belly balm or body oil for stretch marks. Wax esters are used primarily for moisture control, protection, and emollience. It is a popular choice for tattoo aftercare.

Jojoba is an excellent oil for the hair, relieving dry scalp and dandruff, and nails and cuticles. A 50/50 combination of jojoba and sesame oil makes a pleasing hair conditioning blend.

Jojoba is a top choice for oily, combination, or acne skin types, although all skin types will benefit. Vata, Pitta, and Kapha Doshas all benefit from jojoba.

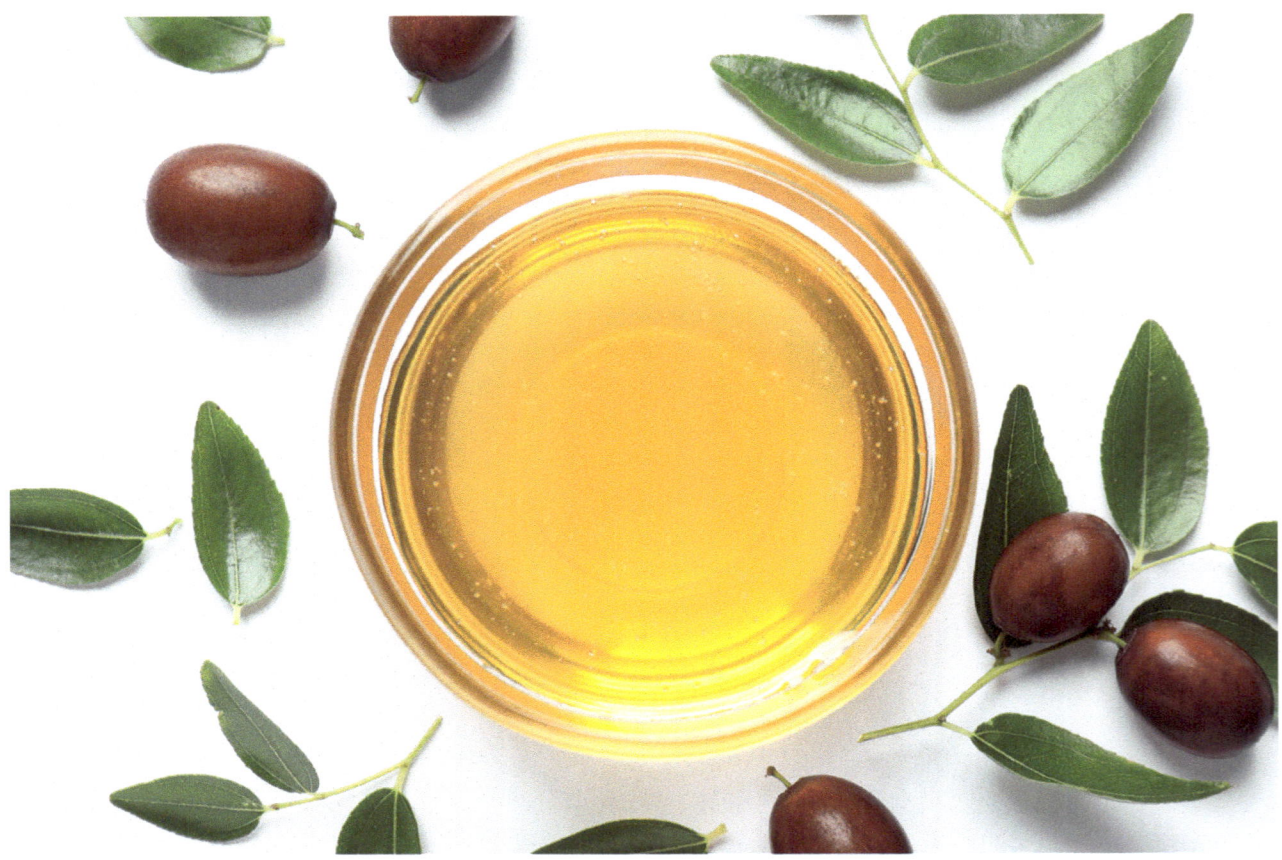

Marula

Sclerocarya birrea

Common names: Marula, cider tree
Scientific name: *Sclerocarya birrea* (A.Rich.) Hochst
Botanical family: Anacardiaceae
Conservation status: Not yet assessed

Description: Commonly known as marula and native to South Africa, *S. birrea* is a medium-sized deciduous tree with an erect trunk. The edible, tough-skinned fruit is yellow and plum-shaped, surrounding a brown, hard seed that contains 2-3 small kernels (nuts), rich in oil. These kernels/nuts are referred to as the "king's nuts" in honor of the nourishment they offer as food to the local people.

Ethnobotany: The fruits have been eaten fresh or used in a range of edible goods, from jelly and jam to juice. The indigenous population also uses marula for a wide range of medicinal uses. Women in the Limpopo region of South Africa have used marula oil to treat various skin conditions, massage babies, and as a lotion for their faces, feet, and hands.[59] In other areas of southern Africa, marula oil protects against dry skin and hair. The oil is also generally used to heal cracked, dry skin.[59]

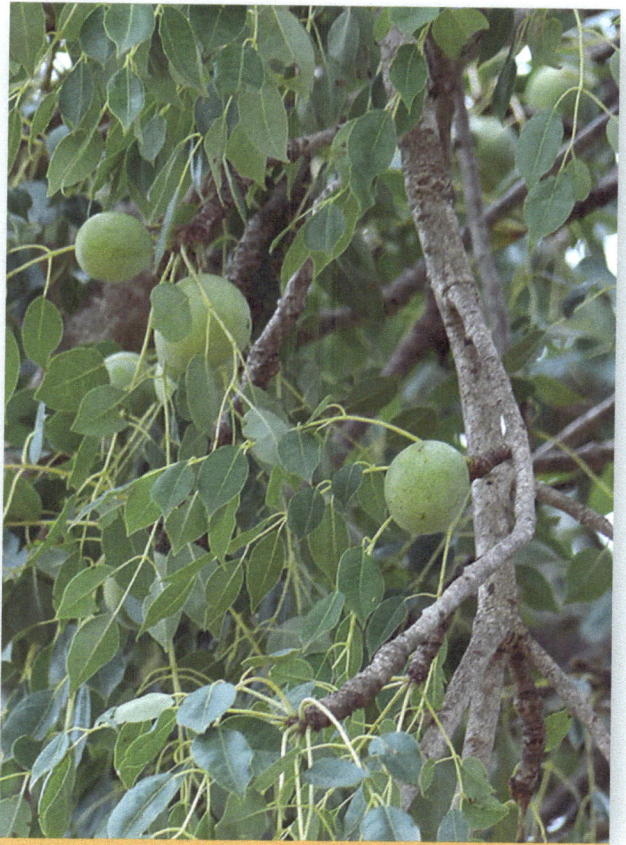

EXTRACTION INFORMATION

Country of origin: South Africa
Part of plant: Seed kernel
Oil content: 53-63%
Extraction method: Cold pressing

MANUFACTURING INFORMATION

CAS number: 68956-68-3
EC number: 273-313-5
INCI name: Sclerocarya Birrea (Marula) Seed Oil
CosIng (functions): Hair conditioning, Humectant

SHELF LIFE

12-24 months

NUTRIENT PROFILE

Marula Oil[59, 60, 61]	
Saturated fatty acids	
Palmitic acid (C16:0)	9 - 12%
Stearic acid (C18:0)	5.0 - 8.0%
Monounsaturated fatty acids	
Oleic acid (C18:1 n-9)	**70 - 78%**
Polyunsaturated fatty acids	
Linoleic acid (C18:2 n-6)	4.0 - 7.0%
Alpha-linolenic acid (C18:3 n-3)	0.1 - 5.0%
Unsaponifiable fraction	
Sterols 2870 mg/kg	Beta-sitosterol (1720 mg/kg), delta-5-avenasterol (48 mg/kg)
Tocopherols 110-990 mg/kg	Alpha-tocopherol (4-710 mg/kg), gamma-tocopherol (112-184 mg/kg), delta-tocopherol (0-40 mg/kg)

Formulating with Marula Oil

Sensory info: Clear, pale, yellowish-brown color oil with a subtle and pleasant nutty aroma, silky texture when applied to the skin

Absorption rate: Wet – medium to slow

Dilution: Can be used 100 percent or in a blend of other oils.

Therapeutic applications:

Marula nourishes and protects the skin, helps heal sunburns, and soothes chapped/irritated skin. It is beneficial for inflamed skin conditions such as dry eczema, dermatitis, and psoriasis and has been used traditionally to prevent stretch marks. It is suitable for all Doshas, particularly Vata. Marula is indicated for dry and cracking skin and dry, damaged, and fragile hair.

Marula oil is commonly used to infuse fragrant flowers. Jasmine-infused marula oil, neroli-infused marula oil, rose-infused marula oil, and vanilla-infused marula oil are available through various aromatherapy companies.

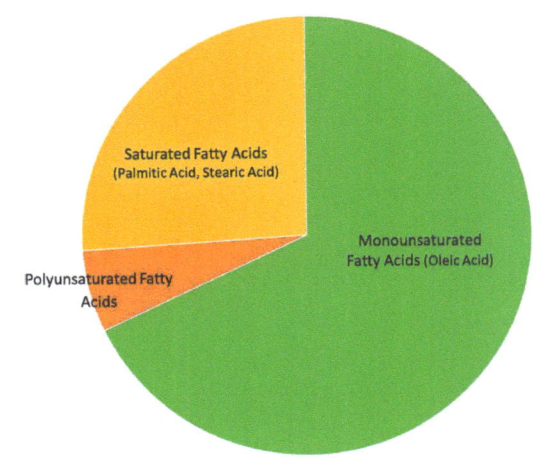

Olive

Olea europaea

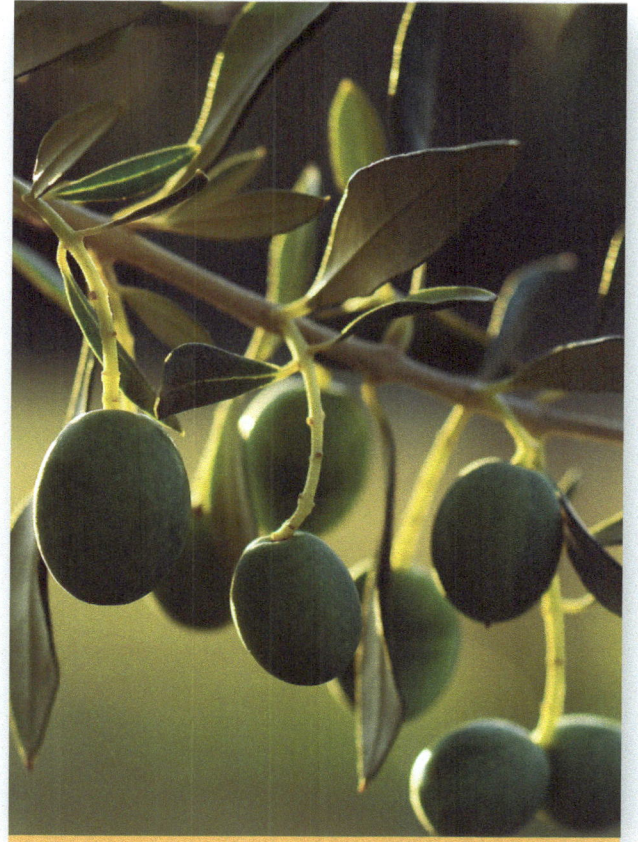

Common name: Olive
Scientific name: *Olea europaea* L.
Botanical family: Oleaceae
Conservation status: Data deficient[62]

Description: *Olea europaea* is a small evergreen tree in the Oleaceae family native to the Mediterranean. Mature olive trees usually reach 20-30 feet tall with rounded crowns. The young trees feature smooth grey bark, although trunks and branches gnarl with age. Leaves are opposite, elliptic to lanceolate, grey-green above and silver-green underneath, 3 inches in length. In the summer, stems from the leaf axils produce small, white, fragrant flowers in 2-inch-long panicles. Flowers are succeeded by green, oval-shaped drupes -- olives -- up to 1.5 inches in length and containing a single pit. These fruits turn black when ripe.

Olive trees grow best in fertile soil that retains moisture but drains well. The plants thrive in Mediterranean climates with a hot-dry summer and mild-wet winter, benefiting from the full sun.[63]

Olives are drupes, botanically similar to other stone fruits. The fruit comprises three layers: a hairless exocarp, or skin, which contains pores called stomata; an endocarp, or pit, which contains the seed; and a middle portion, the mesocarp, the edible flesh of which is eaten and pressed for oil. The size, shape, pit size, and surface morphology of olives are highly variable across cultivars.[64]

O. europaea is one of the oldest cultivated trees on Earth; evidence of cultivation dates back 7,000 years. The Minoans grew olive trees for commercial purposes on Crete in 3,000 BC. The earliest known production of olive oil dates back to 6,500 years ago, off the coast of Haifa, Israel. In 1560 CE, Spanish conquistadors brought cuttings and seeds of olive trees to Peru, where the trees subsequently spread to Mexico and into California by way of Franciscan missionaries.

Olives are not eaten raw due to their extreme

EXTRACTION INFORMATION

Countries of origin: Spain, Greece, Italy, Tunisia
Part of plant: Seed
Oil content: 15-21%
Extraction method: Cold pressing, Decanter centrifugation

MANUFACTURING INFORMATION

CAS number: 8001-25-0
EC number: 232-277-0
INCI name: Olea Europaea (Olive) Fruit Oil
CosIng (functions): Fragrance, Perfuming, Skin Conditioning

SHELF LIFE

12-24 months

bitterness but are typically treated to remove the bitter constituent, oleuropein. They are brined and eaten as table olives or pressed for their oil.[65]

Ethnobotany: All parts of the olive tree, including the bark, fruits, leaves, wood, seeds, and oil, have been used in traditional medicine. The seed oil has been taken internally as a laxative and applied topically to relieve inflammation. Decoctions of dried leaves and fruit treated diarrhea, respiratory and urinary tract infections, stomach and intestinal diseases, and oral hygiene.

Olive leaves taken internally were used to treat stomach and intestinal diseases, asthma, hypertension, and as a febrifuge. In the Mediterranean, olive leaf preparations are a common treatment for gout. In Tunisian folk medicine, the leaves treated gingivitis, infections of the ears and eyes, jaundice, cough, sore throat, hemorrhoids, and rheumatism. Moroccans used a decoction of the leaves to treat hypertension and diabetes. Olive oil mixed with lemon juice may clear gallstones.

In the United States, people took olive oil internally to treat various maladies from hypertension and agitation to use as a laxative and vermicide. The oil was valued as a skin cleanser and was applied topically to fractured limbs. Topical applications of olive oil were used to prevent hair loss.[66]

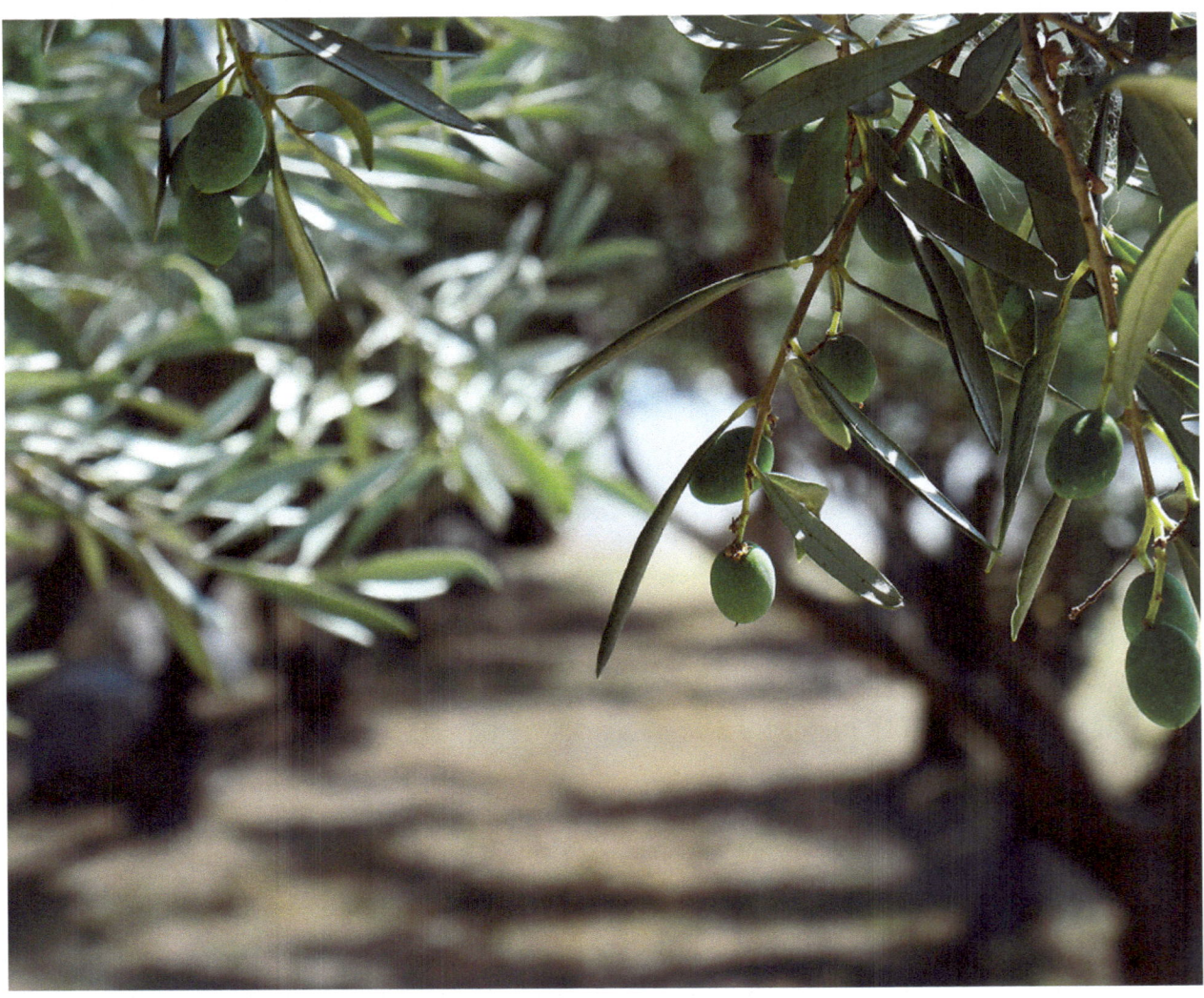

NUTRIENT PROFILE

Rich in the monounsaturated fatty acid oleic acid (55 - 83%), olive oil contains vitamin E (alpha-tocopherol), squalene, and carotenoids. Although alpha-tocopherol concentrations in olive oil are relatively low, the oil is highly resistant to oxidative degradation. This resistance is due, in part, to the relatively low content of polyunsaturated fatty acids and the high concentration of polyphenolic antioxidants (oleuropein and its by-product hydroxytyrosol), particularly in extra virgin olive oil.[67]

Olive Oil[68,69,70]	
SATURATED FATTY ACIDS	
Palmitic acid (C16:0)	7 - 20%
Stearic acid (C18:0)	1.8 - 3.1%
MONOUNSATURATED FATTY ACIDS	
Palmitoleic acid (C16:1 n-7)	0.3 - 3.5%
Oleic acid (C18:1 n-9)	**55.0 - 83.0%**
POLYUNSATURATED FATTY ACIDS	
Linoleic acid (C18:2 n-6)	3.5 - 21.0%
UNSAPONIFIABLE FRACTION	
Sterols Virgin or Refined: 1000 mg/kg	Cholesterol (5 mg/kg), campesterol (<40m g/kg), delta-5-avenasterol, beta-sitosterol, delta-5-avenasterol, delta-5-23-stigmastadienol, clerosterol, sitostanol and delta-5-24-stigmastadienol (combined make up 930 mg/kg)
Tocopherols 97 - 520 mg/kg	Alpha-tocopherol (92 - 250 mg/kg)
Squalene	800-12000 mg/kg[71]

Polyphenols (PP) are potent antioxidants and are essential for the stability as well as the flavor characteristics of bitterness and pungency in olive oil. The amount of PP in the oil can vary from 0 to 1000 mg/kg or more. Usually, the range is from 60 to 400. Oils can be categorized into "Low," around 50–200; "Mild," 200–400; and "High," at > 400 mg/kg.

Polyphenols comprise a very diverse group (several thousands of compounds) of plant secondary metabolites, including flavonoids, isoflavonoids, phenolic acids, proanthocyanidins and other tannins, and lignans with different biological activities. The major polyphenols in olive oil are phenolic acids (e.g., hydroxytyrosol and tyrosol), secoiridoids (e.g., oleuropein) and lignans (e.g., pinoresinol).

Formulating with Olive Oil

Sensory info: Pale yellow to greenish-yellow liquid
Absorption rate: Wet – absorbs more slowly
Dilution: Can be used at 100% percent or in a blend of other oils.

Therapeutic applications:
Olive oil is appropriate for wound healing, dry skin, eczema, antioxidant, aging skin, hair care, and can be used as a skin cleanser. It has been used to maintain skin and muscle suppleness, heal abrasions, and soothe sun and water's burning and drying effects. Olive oil has excellent antioxidant activity.

Olive oil serves as a penetration enhancer,[72] making it a helpful carrier for essential oils.

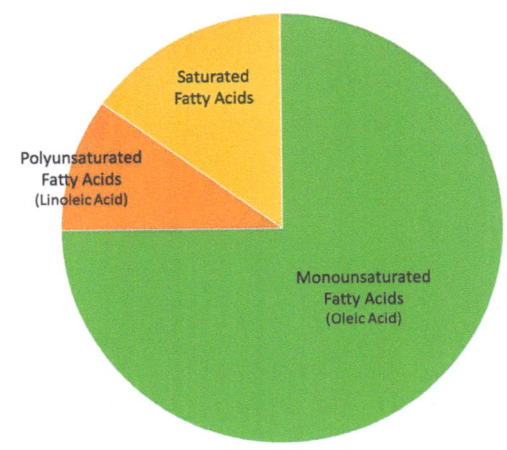

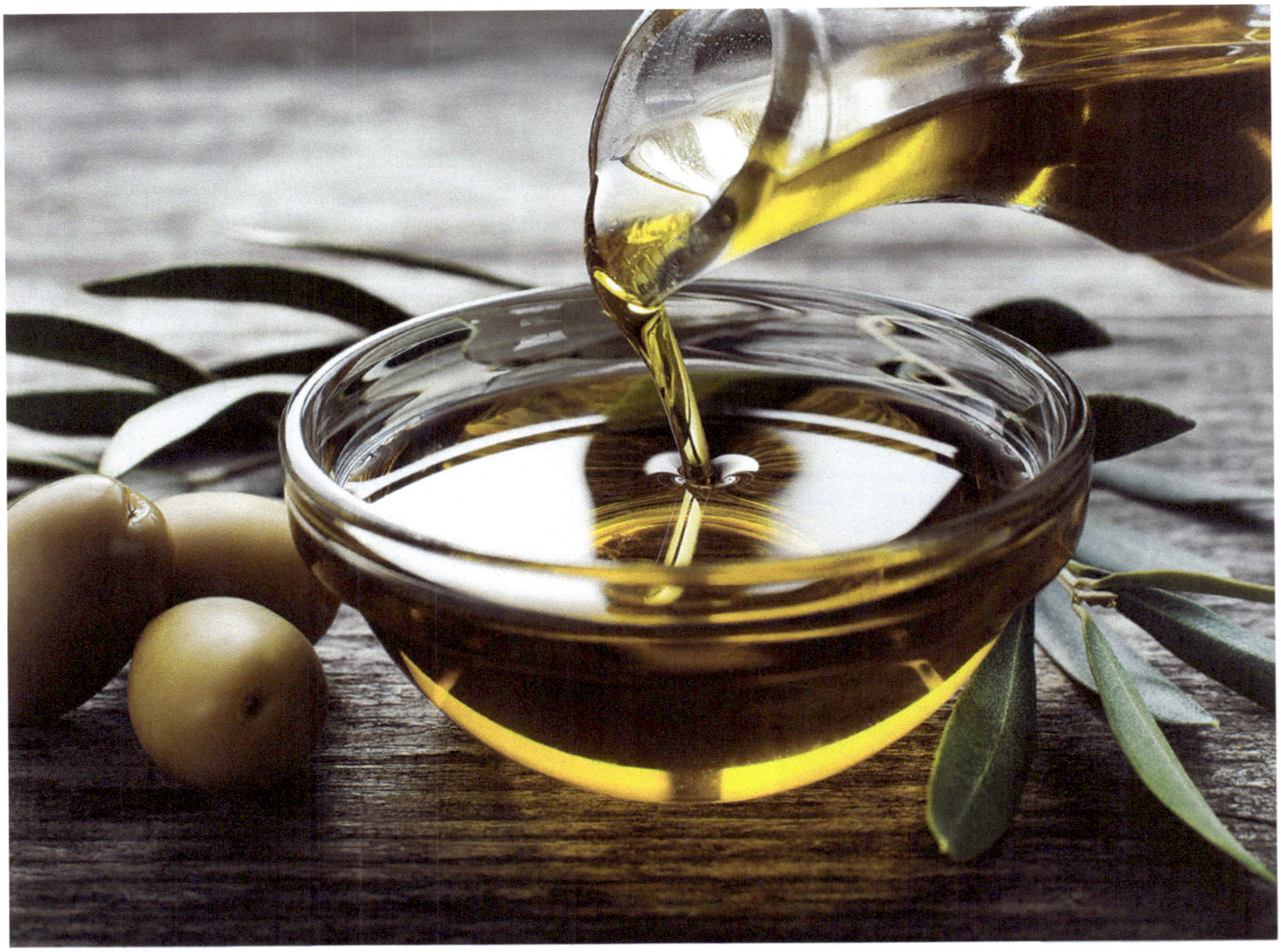

Safflower
Carthamus tinctorius

Common name: Safflower, false saffron
Scientific name: *Carthamus tinctorius* L.
Botanical family: Asteraceae syn. Compositae
Conservation status: Not yet assessed

Description: Safflower is a thistle-like, flowering annual in the Asteraceae family native to Western Asia and widely cultivated in China, India, Iran, and Egypt. *Carthamus tinctorius* is erect, bushy, and herbaceous with a sturdy stem and many branches, which are often spiny. The plant typically grows 180 cm tall and features a deep taproot that can reach 2.5 meters down into the soil. Sunny yellow to orange flowers bloom at the terminus of each branch.

Safflower thrives in semi-arid subtropics, though many developed cultivars of the species are hardy in more temperate zones and at higher elevations in the tropics. *C. tinctorius* requires well-drained soil and full sun. The plant prefers heavy clays with water-retaining capacity but will also grow in deep sandy or clay loams with good drainage.

Safflower is one of the oldest cultivated plants, valued for the dye obtained from the flowers and its oil-rich seeds.[73]

Ethnobotany: Safflower has a long history of use as food, dye, and medicine. Iranians consume raw safflower. The specific epithet *tinctorius* likely refers to its dye application, as safflower has been invaluable in Eastern European carpet weaving industries and as a flavoring and dye ingredient in Italian, French, and British cuisines. Archaeologists have found Ancient Egyptian mummies buried with safflower seeds and floral garlands.

Traditional and folkloric Indian, Chinese, and Iranian medicine have used safflower to treat conditions from scabies, arthritis, breast pain, amenorrhea, gastric tumors, diabetes, and wounds to baldness, phlegm, melancholy, and colic. Persian traditional medicine uses safflower seed infusions topically to ease menstrual

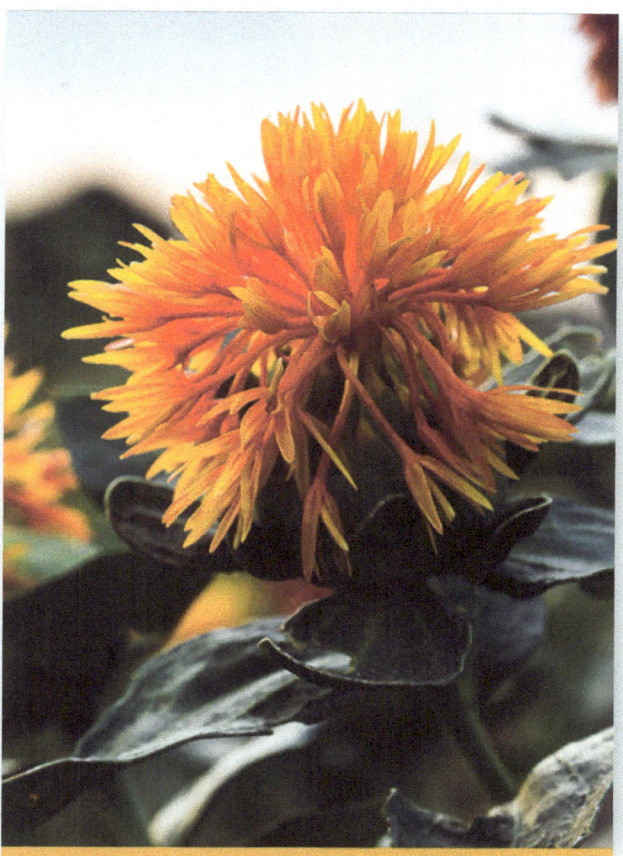

EXTRACTION INFORMATION

Country of origin: USA, Mexico, Australia, Ethiopia
Part of plant: Seed
Oil content: 20–45%[75]
Extraction method: Cold pressing

MANUFACTURING INFORMATION

CAS number: 8001-23-8
EC number: 232-276-5
INCI name: Carthamus Tinctorius (Safflower) Seed Oil
CosIng (functions): Fragrance, Skin conditioning

SHELF LIFE

- **Oleic acid-rich:** 12-24 months
- **Linoleic acid-rich:** 6-9 months

pain and constipation while recommending internal infusions of the dried floret to treat coronary heart disease, angina pectoris, stroke, and hypertension.

In some regions of Asia and Africa, safflower was used as an antidote to poison and as a medicinal oil to enhance sweating and cure fevers. All parts of the plant have been used in Pakistan and India and were considered aphrodisiacal. However, there is also evidence that safflower can negatively affect the reproductive system, particularly in women.[74]

NUTRIENT PROFILE

Safflower oil has two versions readily available in the market. One is rich in linoleic acid, and the other is rich in oleic acid. The linoleic acid-rich safflower oil readily absorbs into the skin, while the oleic acid-rich oil absorbs more slowly. Both oils have a rich content of sterols and tocopherols.

Safflower Oil		
	Linoleic acid-rich[5,76,77]	**Oleic acid-rich**[5]
SATURATED FATTY ACIDS		
Palmitic acid (C16:0)	5.3 - 8.0%	3.6 - 6.0%
Stearic acid (C18:0)	1.9 - 3.0%	1.5 - 2.4%
MONOUNSATURATED FATTY ACIDS		
Oleic acid (C18:1 n-9)	8.4 - 21.3%	**70.0 - 83.7%**
POLYUNSATURATED FATTY ACIDS		
Linoleic acid (C18:2 n-6)	**67.8 - 83.2%**	9.0 - 19.9%
UNSAPONIFIABLE FRACTION		
Sterols	Total: 2100 - 4600 mg/kg Beta-sitosterol (40.2 - 50.6 mg/kg), delta-7-stigmastenol (13.7 - 24.6 mg/kg), campesterol (9.2 - 13.3 mg/kg), stigmasterol (4.5 - 9.6 mg/kg), delta-7-avenasterol (2.2 - 6.3 mg/kg), delta-5-avenasterol (0.8 - 4.8 mg/kg)	Total: 2000 - 4100 mg/kg Beta-sitosterol (40.2 - 50.6 mg/kg), delta-7-stigmastenol (13.7 - 24.6 mg/kg), campesterol (9.2 - 13.3 mg/kg), stigmasterol (4.5 - 9.6 mg/kg), delta-7-avenasterol (2.2 - 6.3 mg/kg), delta-5-avenasterol (0.8 - 4.8 mg/kg)
Tocopherols	Total: 240 - 670mg/kg Alpha-tocopherol (234 - 660 mg/kg), beta-tocopherol (n.d. - 17 mg/kg), gamma-tocopherol (n.d. - 12 mg/kg)	Total: 250 - 700 mg/kg Alpha-tocopherol (234 - 660 mg/kg), gamma-tocopherol (n.d. - 44 mg/kg), beta-tocopherol (n.d.-13 mg/kg)

Formulating with Safflower Oil

Sensory info: Pale yellow. Light texture, good penetrating power.
Absorption rate:
    Linoleic acid-rich: Dry - readily absorbs
    Oleic acid-rich: Medium-slow, with a slightly oily finish
Dilution: Can be used 100% percent or in a blend of other oils.

Therapeutic applications:

Linoleic acid-rich safflower oil

It is especially good for remediating EFA deficiency, thereby improving skin barrier function.[78]

It is appropriate for all skin types, including oily or acne-prone skin. It has a great, lighter texture for massage, skincare, and bath preparations.

Linoleic acid-rich safflower oil is recommended for inflamed, irritated skin, atopic dermatitis, and eczema due to its anti-inflammatory and skin-soothing properties.

Oleic acid-rich safflower oil

A useful carrier when applying an essential oil or other product that does not cross the skin barrier easily as oleic acid behaves as a skin penetration enhancer.[79]

Use as a hair oil for thicker, shinier, stronger hair. Use on the scalp to eliminate dandruff.

It is appropriate for dry, aging skin, decreasing the appearance of premature wrinkles and lines.

Best used in a blend with lower-oleic acid oils to mitigate skin barrier disruption and TEWL.

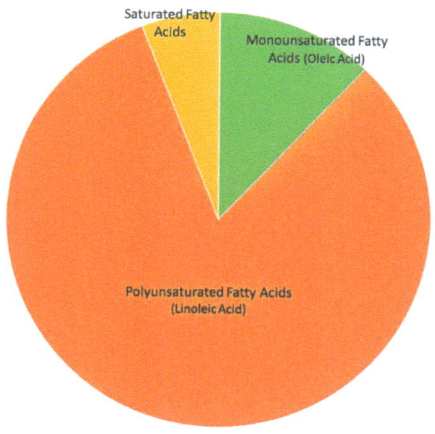
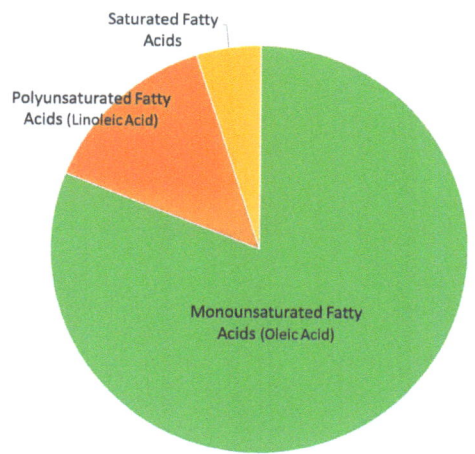

Sesame
Sesamum indicum

Common name: Sesame
Scientific name: *Sesamum indicum* L.
Botanical family: Pedaliaceae
Conservation status: Not yet assessed

Description: Sesame is an erect annual in the Pedaliaceae family, endemic to East Africa and Asia, which grows 0.5-2.5 meters tall. Some *S. indicum* plants feature branches, while others do not. Leaf axils bear one to three flowers each. Seed capsules open when dry, allowing the seeds to scatter. When hulled, sesame seeds are pearly white, 3 mm long, with a flattened pear shape.

Sesame seeds have a long and widespread history of use in food and medicine. Ancient Egyptians ground the seeds for flour, while the Romans ground sesame seeds together with cumin to make a spread for bread. Sesame was thought to possess magical powers, as evidenced by its use as a password in the Arabian Nights tale of "*Ali Baba and the Forty Thieves*." The Chinese have used sesame since 3,000 BE, and for centuries they burned the oil to make soot for fine ink blocks.[80]

Ethnobotany: *S. indicum* is widely cultivated in most tropical, subtropical, and southern temperate regions of the world. Sesame oil is used for culinary purposes and in manufacturing soaps, pharmaceuticals, lubricants, and cosmetics ingredients. Its historical use in Chinese medicine dates back to the 16th century. The oil, valued for its wound healing properties, has been used in India, Africa, and North America as a substitute for olive oil in making liniments, ointments, plasters, and other topical preparations. Sesame seed has been taken internally as a mild laxative for dry constipation, particularly in the elderly. It has also been used to promote menstruation.

In Ayurvedic medicine, sesame oil is valued as a healing tonic. It is applied to the head to relieve headache and dizziness, to the face to treat acne, and to the skin to keep the skin supple and heal minor abrasions. In

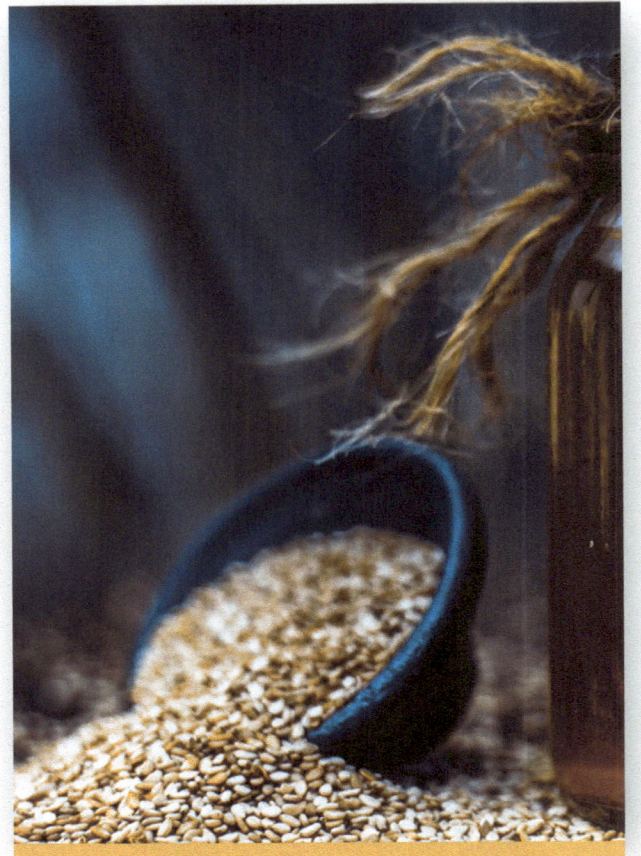

EXTRACTION INFORMATION

Country of origin: India, China, Mexico, Egypt
Part of plant: Seed
Oil content: 18-25%
Extraction method: Cold pressing

MANUFACTURING INFORMATION

CAS number: 8008-74-0
EC number: 232-370-6
INCI name: Sesamum Indicum (Sesame) Seed Oil
CosIng (functions): Fragrance, Hair conditioning, Skin conditioning, Skin conditioning - Emollient

SHELF LIFE

24 months
A relatively stable oil, sesame is one of the oils most resistant to oxidation because it contains the powerful natural antioxidants sesamolin and sesamin.

traditional Middle Eastern medicine, sesame oil is used to eradicate lice infestations, treat skin infections, and in applications used to relieve diaper rash. When swabbed inside the nose, it is thought to prevent colds; additionally, sesame oil nose drops have been used to treat chronic sinusitis.[81]

NUTRIENT PROFILE

The sesame seeds are 50 - 60% oil. Sesame seed oil contains two antioxidant lignans, sesamolin (0.3 - 0.6%) and sesamin (0.5 - 1.1%), which give sesame oil a relatively long shelf life by preventing oxidation and rancidity. Adding sesame oil to other oils can enhance their oxidative stability.

Sesame Seed Oil[82, 83]	
SATURATED FATTY ACIDS	
Palmitic acid (C16:0)	7.9 - 12.0%
Stearic acid (C18:0)	4.8 - 6.1%
MONOUNSATURATED FATTY ACIDS	
Oleic acid (C18:1 n-9)	35.9 - 42.3%
POLYUNSATURATED FATTY ACIDS	
Linoleic acid (C18:2 n-6)	41.5 - 47.9%
UNSAPONIFIABLE FRACTION	
Sterols 5400 mg/kg	Beta-sitosterol (577 - 620 mg/kg), campesterol (101-200 mg/kg), delta-5-avenasterol (62 - 78 mg/kg), delta-7-avenasterol (12 - 56 mg/kg), stigmasterol (34 - 64 mg/kg), delta-7-stigmastenol (5 - 76 mg/kg), cholesterol (1 - 5 mg/kg)
Tocopherols 446 mg/kg	Gamma-tocopherol (403.6 mg/kg), delta-tocopherol (32.6 mg/kg), alpha-tocopherol (9.8 mg/kg)

Formulating with Sesame Oil

Sensory info: Light to medium-dark yellow with a very light nutty aroma
Absorption rate: Average absorption rate; slightly oily feeling
Dilution: Can be used 100% percent or in a blend of other oils.

Therapeutic applications:
Sesame seed oil demonstrates skin restructuring and emollient properties while also reinforcing the integrity of the skin. Sesame is a free-radical scavenging oil, making it appropriate to use where an antioxidant is needed. Ayurvedic medicine uses sesame oil specifically to pacify Vata due to the oil's warming properties. Sesame is particularly effective in dry and/or cold climates because it is heavy and penetrates the skin, going deep into the tissue, where it is very nourishing and prevents the skin from getting excessively dry. Sesame oil massaged into the scalp once a week is an excellent way to nourish the scalp and restore hair's natural balance and luster.

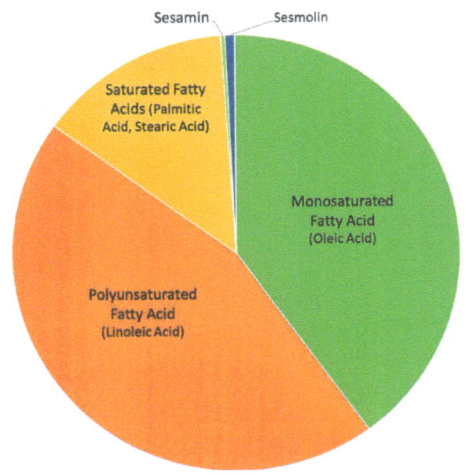

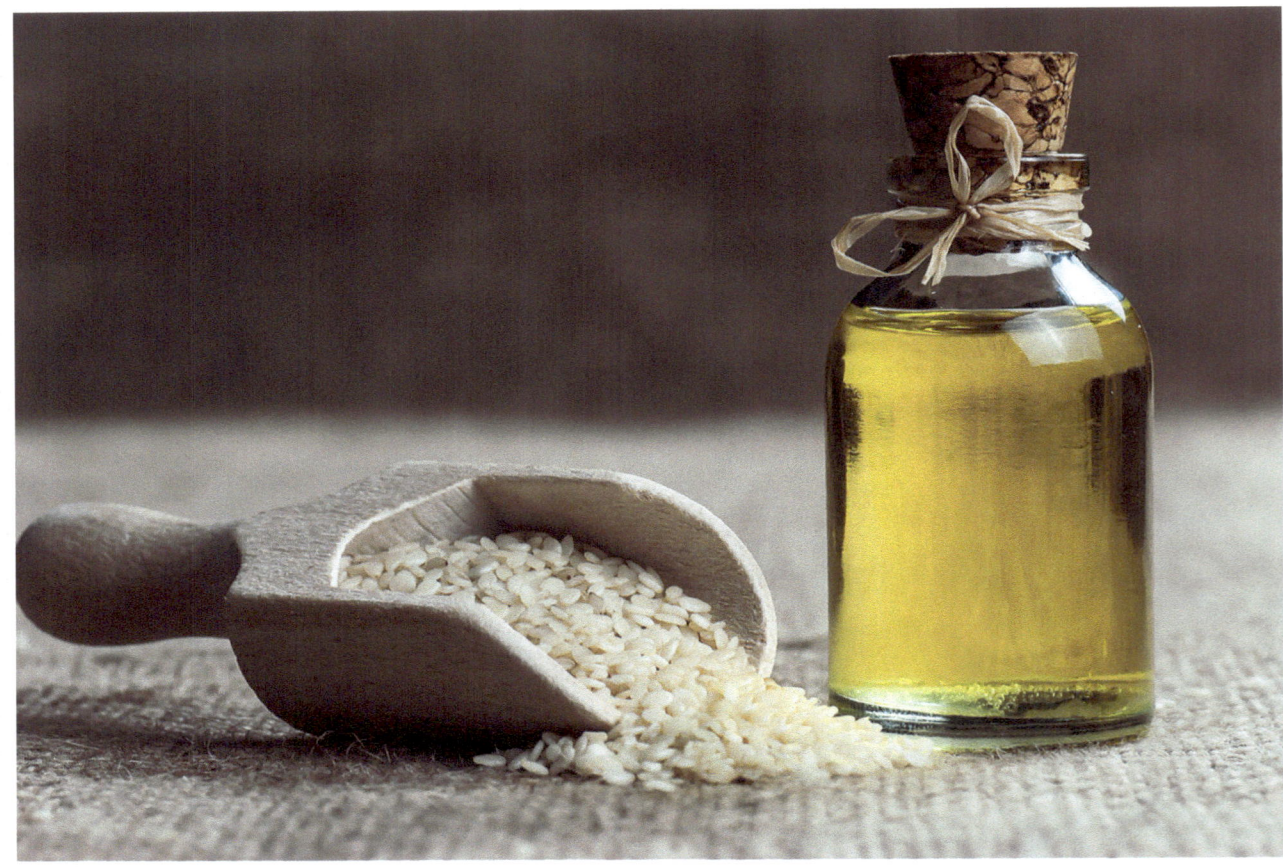

Sunflower
Helianthus annuus

Common name: Sunflower
Scientific name: *Helianthus annuus* L.
Botanical family: Asteraceae
Conservation status: Not yet assessed

Description: Sunflowers are herbaceous annuals in the Asteraceae family native to the Americas. *H. annuus* features a rough, hairy stem and spirally-arranged, coarsely-toothed, rough leaves 3-12 inches (7.5 – 30 cm) in length. Sunflowers grow 3 - 15 feet (1 - 4.5 m) tall and 1.5 - 3 feet (0.4 - 1 m) wide. The flower heads are showy and grow 3 – 6 inches (7.5 -15 cm) in diameter in wild species and as large as 12+ inches (30+ cm) across in certain cultivars. The disk-shaped flowers at the center are brown, yellow, or purple, while the surrounding ray flowers are yellow. The sunflower bears a single-seeded achene as its fruit.[84]

Helianthus annuus is among the top five oilseed crops in the world today.[85] The plant requires fertile soil and moderate rainfall to thrive; the adaptation of various cultivars to different climatic and soil conditions has allowed for its commercial cultivation throughout the world.

Ethnobotany: Sunflowers are one of the most significant agronomic crops to originate in the Americas, where the Native Americans bred and domesticated the plant, possibly even before they domesticated corn. Europeans took sunflower seeds back to Europe with them, and in the 1800s, the Russians developed them into a commercial crop. The flower returned to North America as a cultivated crop in the early 1900s.[86] There is evidence that Native Americans used sunflowers extensively as a food crop, using the seeds whole, cracked, ground, or pounded and the oil to make bread. They used the plant in various ceremonies and the flowers to produce dyes, which they used to decorate textiles and paint their bodies.[86]

The modern common sunflower has many applications. There are two primary seed types: oilseed, processed

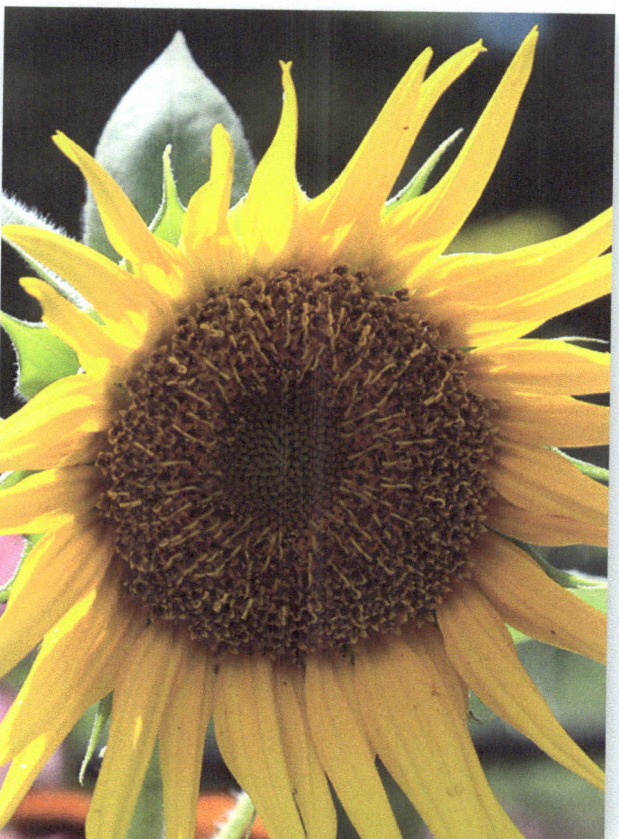

EXTRACTION INFORMATION

Country of origin: Russia, USA, India, China, Mexico
Part of plant: Seed
Oil content: 35-42%
Extraction method: Cold pressing, Warm pressing, Solvent extraction

MANUFACTURING INFORMATION

CAS number: 8001-21-6
EC number: 232-273-9
INCI name: Helianthus Annuus Seed Oil
CosIng (functions): Fragrance, Skin Conditioning, Skin Conditioning - Emollient

SHELF LIFE

- **Oleic acid-rich:** 12-24 months
- **Linoleic acid-rich:** 6-9 months

into sunflower oil and meal and included in birdseed mixes, and non-oilseed type, the white-striped seeds people most commonly associate with sunflower seed snacks. The seeds used as food are dried, roasted, and ground into nut butter for human consumption and included in birdseed mixes. Oil-producing seeds are pressed to extract a sweet yellow oil used for culinary and cosmetic purposes. The oil is also used for industrial applications and as an ingredient in soap and paint. Sunflower oil cake and sunflower leaves are fed to poultry and livestock. The flower itself is considered a beautiful ornamental.[84]

There are three types of sunflower oil on the market: a high oleic acid (80%+) version, a mid-oleic acid version, and a high linoleic acid version (low oleic), which is the original, traditional sunflower oil. The other versions result from conventional agricultural selective breeding and hybridization methods; currently, there are no Genetically-Modified-Organism (GMO) or transgenic sunflower plants. All versions of the oil have good alpha-tocopherol content and medium sterol content.[87]

Sunflower has been used in traditional medicine to treat dysentery, diarrhea, coughs and colds, heart disease, bronchial, laryngeal, and pulmonary infections, including whooping cough, skin rashes, diarrhea, sores, and snakebite.[85]

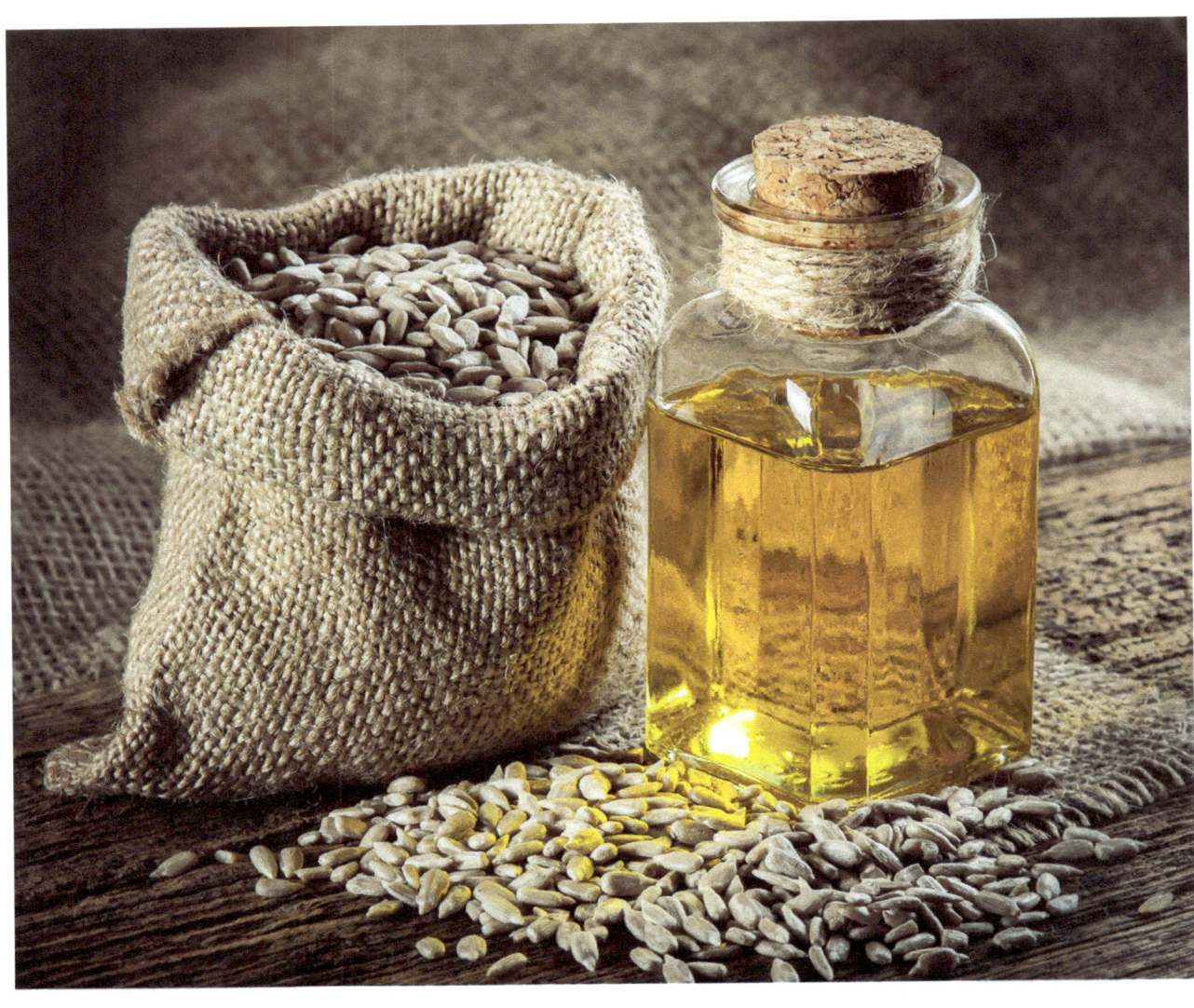

NUTRIENT PROFILE

Sunflower oil has two versions readily available in the market. One is rich in linoleic acid, and the other is rich in oleic acid. The linoleic acid-rich sunflower oil readily absorbs into the skin, while the oleic acid-rich form absorbs more slowly. Both oils have a rich content of sterols and tocopherols.

Sunflower Oil[95, 96]		
Saturated fatty acids	**Linoleic acid rich**	**Oleic acid rich**
Palmitic acid (C16:0)	5.0 - 7.6%	2.6 - 5.0%
Stearic acid (C18:0)	2.7 - 6.5%	2.9 - 6.2%
Behenic acid (C22:0)	0.3 - 1.5%	0.5 - 1.6%
Monounsaturated fatty acids		
Oleic acid (C18:1 n-9)	14.0 - 39.4%	**80 - 90.7%**
Polyunsaturated fatty acids		
Linoleic acid (C18:2 n-6)	**48.3-74.0%**	2.1-17%
Unsaponifiable fraction		
Sterols	**Total:** 2400 - 5000 mg/kg Beta-sitosterol (1200 - 3500 mg/kg), delta-7-stigmastenol (156 - 1200 mg/kg), campesterol (156 - 306.5 mg/kg), stigmasterol (144-306.5 mg/kg), delta-7-avenasterol (72 - 375 mg/kg), delta-5-avenasterol (n.d. - 345 mg/kg)	**Total:** 1700 - 5200 mg/kg Beta-sitosterol (714 - 3640 mg/kg), delta-7-stigmastenol (110.5 - 1248 mg/kg), campesterol (85 - 676 mg/kg), stigmasterol (76.5 - 676 mg/kg), delta-7-avenasterol (n.d. - 468 mg/kg), delta-5-avenasterol (255 - 358.8 mg/kg)
Tocopherols	**Total:** 440 - 1520 mg/kg Alpha-tocopherol (403 - 935 mg/kg), beta-tocopherol (n.d.- 45 mg/kg), gamma-tocopherol (n.d. - 34 mg/kg), delta-tocopherol (n.d. - 7.0 mg/kg)	**Total:** 450 - 1120 mg/kg Alpha-tocopherol (400 - 1090 mg/kg), beta-tocopherol (10 - 35 mg/kg), gamma-tocopherol (3 - 30 mg/kg)

Formulating with Sunflower Oil

Sensory info: Light yellow color, clear, odorless
Absorption rate:
   Linoleic acid-rich: Dry - readily absorbs
   Oleic acid-rich: Medium-slow, with a slightly oily finish
Dilution: Can be used 100% percent or in a blend of other oils.

Therapeutic applications:

Linoleic acid-rich sunflower oil

It is especially good for remediating EFA deficiency, thereby improving skin barrier function.[97]

In an *in vivo* study, high linoleic acid sunflower improved wound healing speed.[98]

It is appropriate for all skin types, including oily or acne-prone skin. Sunflower oil blends well with apricot kernel oil, and it has a great, lighter texture for massage, skincare, and bath preparations.

Sunflower oil has anti-inflammatory properties, making it especially appropriate for inflamed skin conditions such as acne, atopic dermatitis, and dry, aging skin. Sunflower oil also helps address bacterial and fungal skin infections.

Oleic acid-rich sunflower oil

A useful carrier when applying an essential oil or other product that does not cross the skin barrier easily as oleic acid behaves as a skin penetration enhancer.[99]

Use as a hair oil for thicker, shinier, stronger hair. Use on the scalp to eliminate dandruff.

It is appropriate for dry, aging skin, decreasing the appearance of premature wrinkles and lines.

Best used in a blend with lower-oleic acid oils to mitigate skin barrier disruption and TEWL.

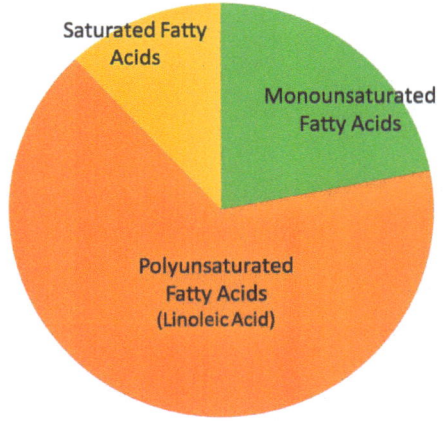
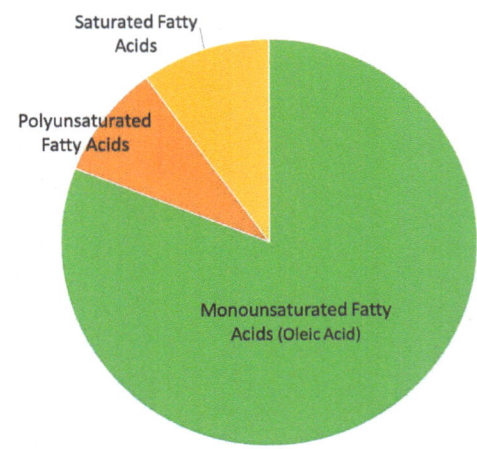

Part Four:
The Enhancer Carrier Oils

The Enhancer Carrier Oils

We commonly use enhancer carrier oils at a lower percentage (1% to 25%) than the core carrier oils. The enhancer carrier oils tend to be rich in polyunsaturated fatty acids. Due to the relatively short shelf life of the polyunsaturated fatty acid-rich carrier oils, it is valuable to add an antioxidant into formulations that contain these oils. You can also add an antioxidant to individual polyunsaturated fatty acid-rich carrier oils to stabilize them and extend their shelf lives.

About Antioxidants

An antioxidant extends the shelf life of polyunsaturated fatty acid-rich carrier oils by preventing oxidation. Oxidation is a naturally occurring chemical process when molecules lose electrons (to another substance), lose hydrogen atoms, or replace hydrogen atoms with oxygen atoms. Heat, oxygen, and light can all cause oxidation reactions to occur, which is why we caution you to keep carrier oil containers cool, sealed, and away from direct light. When carrier oils oxidize, they often smell sour or off, and we say the carrier oil is "rancid." Adding antioxidant ingredients can help lengthen the shelf life of the polyunsaturated fatty acid-rich carrier oils.

Choice of Antioxidants

Mixed Tocopherols: T50 Vitamin E is the most commonly available mixed tocopherol product (CAS # 1406-18-4, INCI: Tocopherol). This product usually comprises 50% vitamin E (d-alpha-tocopherol, d-beta-tocopherol, d-gamma-tocopherol, d-delta-tocopherol) and 50% (GMO-Free) refined soybean oil. T-50 Vitamin E is viscous, a golden yellow to reddish color, and has a very slight nutty aroma. ECOCERT GREENLIFE approves it, and it conforms to the COSMOS Standards.

To prolong the shelf life of an individual polyunsaturated fatty acid-rich carrier oil, add 0.04 - 0.5% T50.

For oil-based formulations, add T50 at 0.5 - 1.5% to improve shelf life.

Rosemary CO_2 Extract Antioxidant: This is a standardized, oil-soluble CO_2 extract from rosemary (*Salvia rosmarinus*) leaves in 60-65% sunflower oil (organic or non-organic depending on supplier). It is considered a more potent antioxidant than mixed tocopherols and is also ECOCERT and COSMOS Standards approved. Rosemary CO_2 extract antioxidant has a very slight aroma and a dark green color; due to the low dilution in formulations, it is unlikely to alter the aroma or the color of the product significantly. Rosemary CO_2 extract antioxidant has a shelf-life of up to five years. (CAS #8001-21-6 / 84604-14-8, INCI: Helianthus Annuus Seed Oil and Rosmarinus Officinalis Leaf Extract).

Use rosemary CO_2 extract antioxidant at 0.2 – 0.5% of the total oil-based formulation.

Cold-Pressed Oils vs. CO2 Extracts

Two methods are used to extract most of the enhancer carrier oils – cold- or expeller pressing and SFE CO2 extraction. It is important to understand the strengths and weaknesses of each extraction method to select the best carrier oil for your product.

Cold pressing is a physical process, which often yields only a relatively small part of the fat contained in the seed or fruit. Constituents in minute quantities in the plant may not show up in the extract, and producers cannot manipulate the process to tailor the product to a particular chemical profile. However, the resulting oil contains multiple unadulterated, beneficial constituents from both the saponifiable and unsaponifiable fractions, including fatty acids, carotenoids, tocopherols, vitamins, phenols, hydrocarbons, and pigments. It tends to be safe for most people.

SFE CO2 extraction could be considered a form of solvent extraction since the oil dissolves in the carbon dioxide. However, unlike with most solvent extraction processes, CO2 extracts do not contain toxic solvent residues; the inert carbon dioxide completely evaporates away when the process is complete. SFE is considered to be green technology for extracting a wide variety of material from plants. SFE also uses a low temperature and short extraction time, so the extraction process minimizes degradation and oxidation of the oil constituents. Thus, SFE CO2 extracts are another safe choice for carrier oils. The SFE CO2 extraction process can also be manipulated to optimize the balance of constituents by manipulating the temperature, time (solvent flow rate), and pressure parameters for each specific oil.[1]

The two processes may yield somewhat different amounts for any given constituent, but the final proportions are often within the same range.[2] However, one notable difference is the amount of carotenoids and pigments that each process can extract. Carotenoids come through in cold-pressed oils, resulting in brightly colored oils, but carotenoids, and other molecules over 500 g/mol, are only slightly soluble in supercritical carbon dioxide due to their large molecular masses (beta-carotene and lycopene are 536.9 g/mol). By comparison, alpha-tocopherol has a mass of 430.7 g/mol, and arachidic acid (C20:0) is 312.5 g/mol. For a reasonable proportion of carotenoids to be in a CO2 extract, the extraction process must include an additional solvent (a modifier or co-solvent), often ethanol.[3]

Both cold pressing and SFE CO2 produce high-quality carrier oils containing many desirable compounds. These carrier oils all provide the fatty acids we seek when selecting a particular carrier oil. When selecting an enhancer oil for a specific non-fatty acid, bioactive constituent, you will want to be sure the extract you choose contains the constituent you seek.

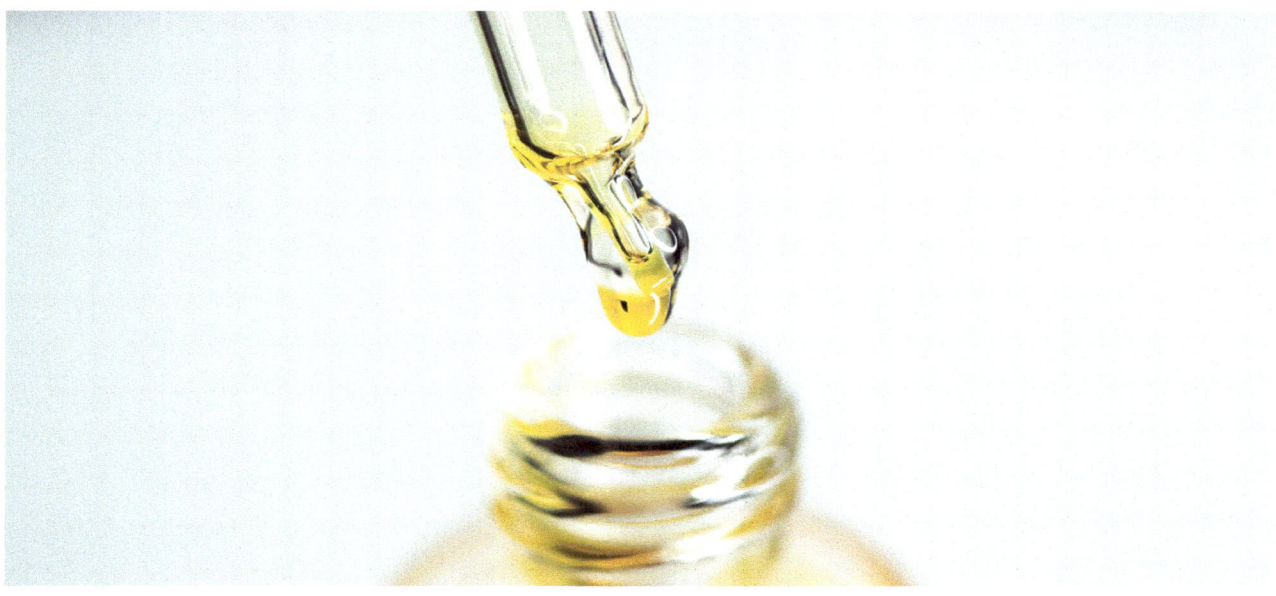

Avocado
Persea americana

Common names: Avocado
Scientific name: *Persea americana* Mill.
Synonym: *Persea gratissima* Gaertn.
Botanical family: Lauraceae
Conservation status: Least concern[4]

Description: Avocado is a broadleaf evergreen tree in the Lauraceae family native to Mexico, Central America, and South America. *Persea americana* typically grows 30-60 feet tall. Leaves are 4-8 inches long, elliptic-to-ovate, glossy, and dark green. Small greenish-yellow flowers grow on panicles; green-skinned pear-shaped fruits succeed these flowers. Each fruit contains a large central seed or pit enveloped by an edible pulp. Mature fruits ripen off the tree, and the flesh turns buttery and yellow.

P. americana grows best in rich, loose, evenly moist, well-drained soils and full sun. The trees thrive in warm and sunny climates and are somewhat tolerant of light shade but not of frost.

Avocados are vitamin-rich and commonly eaten as a vegetable in salads and guacamole. The genus name comes to us from the Greek name *persea* for an Egyptian tree (*Cordia myxa*), and the specific epithet *americana* means "of the Americas." The word "avocado" reportedly arises from the Aztec word for "testicles," an apparent riff on the fruit's shape.[5]

Ethnobotany: Avocados are a dietary staple across Mexico and Central America. According to archaeological records, avocados are one of Mexico's most ancient food plants, dating back to 8000 BCE.

Likewise, avocado leaves, seed oil, seeds, and fruit pulp, have a long history of traditional medicine use. A 16th-century codex describes avocado's medicinal applications based on observations and interviews with indigenous Aztecs. Tea made from the leaves treated coughs and colds, relieved diarrhea, promoted menstrual flow, and treated hypertension. Topically, leaves were applied to heal bruises. The seed oil was used as an astringent treatment to heal sores, skin

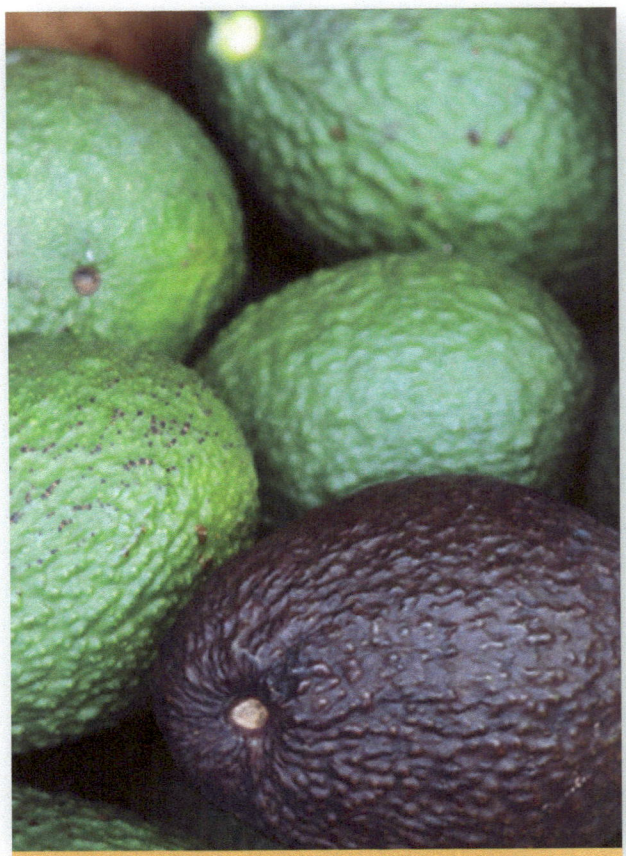

EXTRACTION INFORMATION

Country of origin: Mexico, South America, United States, South Africa, and Austria
Part of plant: Fleshy fruit/pericarp of the fruit
Oil content: 25 - 50%
Extraction method: Solvent extraction, Cold pressing

While most producers have used solvent extraction and high temperatures to extract avocado oil, recent, twenty-first-century producers have developed a cold-pressing process like that used in olive oil production. Much of the cosmetic industry avocado oil is also refined.[7]

MANUFACTURING INFORMATION

CAS number: 8024-32-6
EC number: 232-428-0
INCI name: Persea Gratissima (Avocado) Oil
CosIng (functions): Skin conditioning

eruptions, and scars. The powdered seed was a topical remedy for infected teeth, dandruff, and arthritic pain. Both the Aztecs and the Maya thought the avocado affected reproductive health, either to promote fertility or as an aphrodisiac. The avocado fruit was also eaten for spiritual protection.

In Nigeria, people eat avocado fruit pulp to ease hypertension, body aches, inflammation, and infection. They also eat the ground seed to treat dysentery and whitlows.[6]

SHELF LIFE

- **Unrefined avocado oil:** 6-9 months
- **Refined avocado oil:** 12 months
  * Solidifies when refrigerated.

NUTRIENT PROFILE

Avocado oil is a monounsaturated oil rich in oleic acid. It also contains appreciable quantities of the saturated fatty acid palmitic acid and the polyunsaturated fatty acid linoleic acid. The green color of the unrefined oil is due to the presence of chlorophyll, which degrades when exposed to sunlight, turning the oil a brown color. The fatty acid composition can vary tremendously depending on the variety and age of the avocado used to produce the oil.[8]

Avocado Oil[7, 9, 10, 11]	
Saturated fatty acids	
Palmitic acid (C16:0)	12.16 – 28.21%
Stearic acid (C18:0)	0.24 - 0.98%
Monounsaturated fatty acids	
Oleic acid (C18:1 n-9)	**47.20 - 67.69 %**
Palmitoleic acid (C16:1 n-7)	1.60 - 12%
Gondoic acid (C20:1 n-9)	0.16 - 1.29%
Polyunsaturated fatty acids	
Linoleic acid (C18:2 n-6)	10.6 - 18.7%
Alpha-linolenic acid (C18:3 n-3)	0.72 - 2.14%
Unsaponifiable fraction 2-11%	
Sterols 2906 - 5955 mg/kg	Beta-sitosterol (73.9 - 3280 mg/kg), campesterol (200 - 770 mg/kg), delta-5-avenasterol (67 - 339 mg/kg), stigmasterol (n.d. - 496 mg/kg)
Tocopherols 49 - 130 mg/kg	Alpha-tocopherol (40.05 - 130 mg/kg), gamma-tocopherol (3.84 - 20.35 mg/kg), beta-tocopherol (0.82 - 1.57 mg/kg), delta-tocopherol (0.04 - 5 mg/kg)
Pigments	Chlorophyll (13.3 - 73.8 mg/kg), carotenoids (1.9 - 48.7 mg/kg)
Squalene	190 – 1327.33 mg/kg[12]

Formulating with Avocado Oil

Sensory info: Dark green to light green to almost colorless, depending on the processing and refining process. Thick, heavy oil, but very penetrating, easily absorbed.

Absorption rate: Dry – readily absorbs into skin
Dilution: Can be used 5 - 25% in a blend of other carrier oils.

Research
- Dermal application of avocado oil increased collagen synthesis and reduced inflammation during wound healing (*in vivo*).[11,13]
- Skin readily absorbs refined avocado oil.[14]
- Dermal application of avocado oil can reduce itchiness in the skin.[15]

Therapeutic actions: moisturizing, antibacterial, antiwrinkle, antioxidant, cell regenerating

Therapeutic applications:
Avocado is moisturizing, emollient, and penetrates the skin easily. Repeated massage applications with avocado and sesame oils reveal an increase in hydration of the upper layers of the skin and an improvement in the skin's elasticity properties.[8]

The cosmetic industry values avocado for its skin-penetrating, antibacterial, antiwrinkle, revitalizing, antioxidant, and cell-regenerating properties. It is suitable for all skin types, especially post-menopausal, dry, dehydrated, fragile, mature skin, or skin experiencing premature aging. Avocado oil is also helpful for dry eczema or psoriasis.

The unsaponifiable fraction of avocado oil contributes significantly to its therapeutic properties through its sterol content and other lesser-known molecules. The high chlorophyll and carotenoid content in cold-pressed avocado oil produce its bright or emerald green color, which turns yellow or brown when it oxidizes. Avocado oil can oxidize quickly, so it is vital to protect it from light and oxygen by storing it in dark glass or stainless-steel bottles.[16]

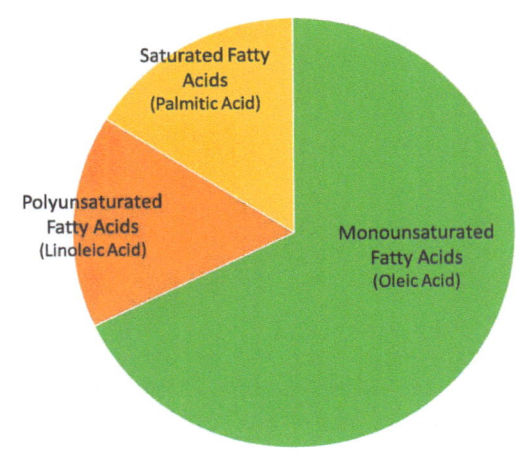

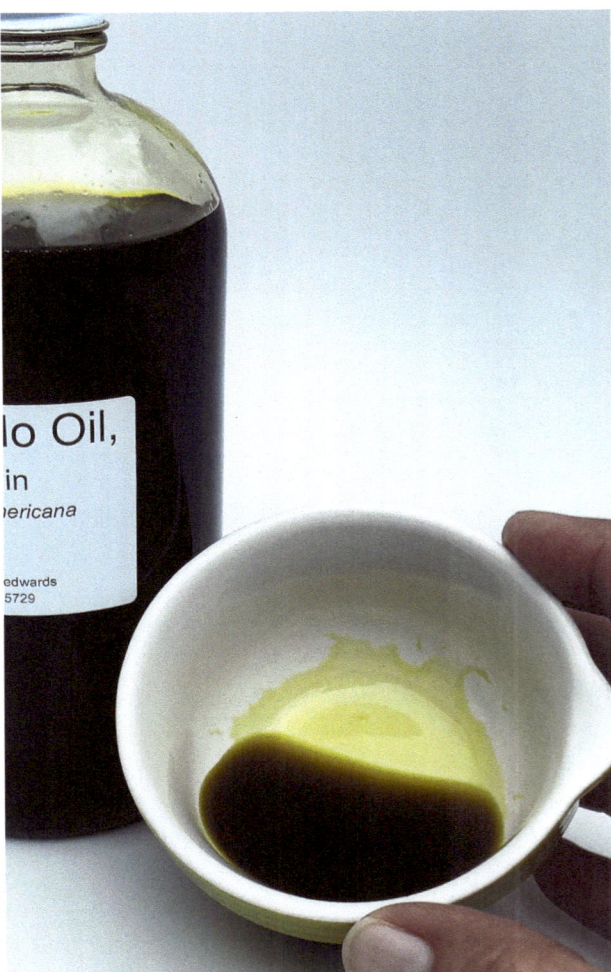

Black Cumin
Nigella sativa

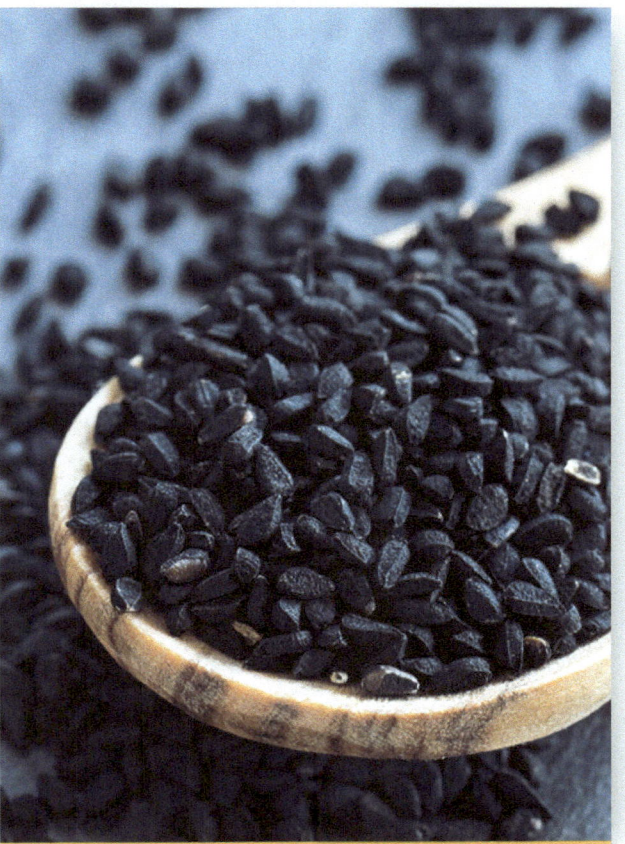

Common name: Black cumin, kalonji/kalanji, black seed, black caraway, charnushka, black onion seed
Scientific name: *Nigella sativa* L.
Synonym: *Nigella cretica* Mill.
Botanical family: Ranunculaceae
Conservation status: Not yet assessed

Description: *Nigella sativa* is a hardy, flowering annual in the Ranunculaceae family, native to Southern Europe, North Africa, and Southwest Asia. It is presently cultivated in the Mediterranean, southern Europe, India, Pakistan, Syria, Turkey, and Saudi Arabia. *N. sativa* and its seeds are commonly called black cumin seed, black caraway seed, black seed, and kalonji (Hindi).

The plant grows 8-24 inches tall and features a developed taproot. Leaves are finely divided with feathery, thread-like leaflets. Flowers are white, yellow, pink, light blue, or lavender, with 5-10 petals. The fruit is a large, inflated capsule with 3-7 follicles containing many bitter, aromatic seeds. The seeds are tiny (2-3.5 mm long and 1-2 mm wide), black on the outside and white inside.[17]

Ethnobotany: Black cumin seeds and their oil have a long history as food and traditional medicine, especially throughout Southeast Asia, North Africa, and the Middle East. Some scholars have speculated that when the Old Testament prophet Isaiah speaks of cumin (Isaiah 28: 25,27), he refers to what we now know as *Nigella sativa*. The pharmacopeias of Ayurveda, Siddha, and Unami Tibb medicine all contain references to *Nigella*. Muslims consider *Nigella* to be "Habbatul barakah," or "seed of blessing";[18] according to the Prophet Muhammad, "The black seed can heal every disease, except death."[19]

Both formal and folk medicine have used *N. sativa* to treat headaches, migraines, toothaches, intestinal worms, asthma, bronchitis, rheumatism, indigestion, backache, hypertension, loss of appetite, diarrhea, dropsy, amenorrhea, dysmenorrhea, skin eruptions,

EXTRACTION INFORMATION

Country of origin: Egypt, India, Pakistan, Middle East
Part of plant: Kernel or seed
Oil content: 28 - 39%
Extraction method: Cold pressing, SFE CO_2

MANUFACTURING INFORMATION

CAS number: 90064-32-7
EC number: 290-094-1
INCI name: Nigella Sativa (Black Cumin) Seed Oil
CosIng (functions): Perfuming, Skin conditioning, Skin conditioning - Emollient

SHELF LIFE

24 months

vomiting, and intestinal worms.[20] When the oil is applied topically, it has served as an antiseptic and local anesthetic. In "The Canon of Medicine" (completed 1025 AD), Persian Muslim physician-philosopher Avicenna recommended black cumin seed to promote energy and aid in recovery from fatigue and "dispiritedness."[17]

Black cumin seeds are redolent of fennel, with an intense flavor akin to nutmeg. The seeds are used widely for culinary purposes in India, the Middle East, and North Africa; they are typically roasted then ground into a powder used to season curries, rice, bread, and confections. *N. sativa* is sometimes cultivated as an ornamental due to its attractive flowers.[21]

NUTRIENT PROFILE

Black cumin oil is a polyunsaturated oil rich in linoleic acid with a rich sterol and tocopherol content.

Black Cumin Oil[22, 23, 24]	
Saturated fatty acids	
Palmitic acid (C16:0)	11.94 - 13.1%
Stearic acid (C18:0)	2.29 - 3.34%
Arachidic acid (C20:0)	0.2 - 1.1%
Monounsaturated fatty acids	
Oleic acid (C18:1 n-9)	20.51 - 24.64%
Polyunsaturated fatty acids	
Linoleic acid (C18:2 n-6)	56.17 - 63.97%
Unsaponifiable fraction	
Sterols 1660 - 2915 mg/kg	Beta-sitosterol (592.8 - 1428.4 mg/kg), stigmasterol (243.0 - 536.4 mg/kg), campesterol (169.2 - 381.9 mg/kg), delta-5-avenasterol (n.d. - 361.5 mg/kg), delta-7-avenasterol (n.d. - 61.5 mg/kg)
Tocopherols 1718 - 1745 mg/kg	Gamma-tocopherol (935.9 - 941.1 mg/kg), alpha-tocopherol (110.8 - 113.4 mg/kg), beta-tocopherol (3.5 - 4.1 mg/kg), delta-tocopherol (3.5 - 5.5 mg/kg)

Formulating with Black Cumin Oil

Sensory info: Pale yellow to dark amber, slightly bitter aroma

Absorption rate: Slow-to-average, leaving a slight oily feeling on the skin

Dilution: Recommended up to 10% for cosmetic/topical use

Caution: Black cumin seed may be skin sensitizing.[25]

Therapeutic actions: antioxidant, emollient, anti-inflammatory, antimicrobial, skin penetration enhancer, reduce hyperpigmentation

Therapeutic applications:

Black cumin seed contains a unique chemical, thymoquinone (1.78 mg/ml[26] - 7.2 mg/ml[27] in cold-pressed oil), a potent antioxidant, antinociceptive, and anti-inflammatory agent. Scientists have studied it extensively, demonstrating how the black cumin seed oil offers even more powerful benefits than other carrier oils with similar fatty acid profiles.

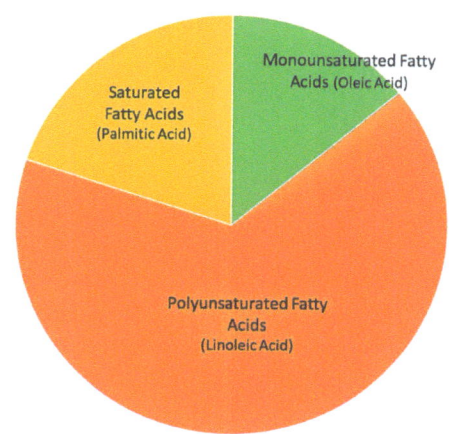

Black cumin seed oil is soothing, emollient, and nourishing to the skin. Its anti-inflammatory and potent antioxidant activity make it especially suited for products to address eczema, psoriasis, acne, injured skin, dry skin, aging skin, and in after-sun care products.

It also contributes to products addressing inflammation and pain in the joints, such as in arthritis. In one study, elderly patients with osteoarthritis massaged their knees with 1 ml of black cumin seed oil every 8 hours for three (3) weeks. The study determined that black cumin seed oil effectively reduced pain compared to no treatment.[28]

Black cumin seed oil is antimicrobial, making it an appropriate ingredient in products for acne[30] and fungal skin infections. *In vitro* research shows it may also work synergistically with some antibiotics.[31,32] Additionally, black cumin seed oil has demonstrated its skin penetration enhancement abilities, which the scientists thought to be due to its linoleic acid content.[32]

Black cumin seed oil also improves the health of both scalp and hair, reducing scalp inflammation and irritation, damage from UV radiation and pollution, and hair loss while moisturizing hair strands. Use it in deep-conditioning oil treatments and conditioners.

Black seed oil may be effective in treating vitiligo. A small group of patients in Iran experienced improved skin appearance after applying a black seed oil medication twice a day for six months.[33]

When purchasing black cumin seed carrier oil, be sure to read the product descriptions carefully. The fatty carrier oil may be either cold-pressed or CO2 extracted, but a steam-distilled black cumin seed essential oil also exists.

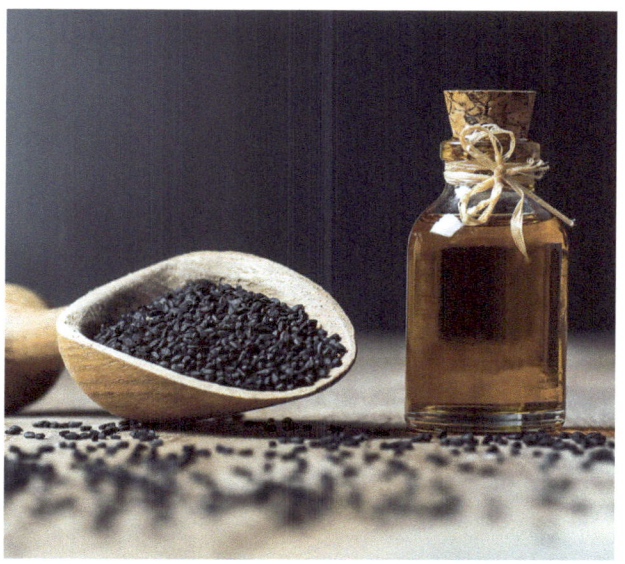

Borage
Borago officinalis

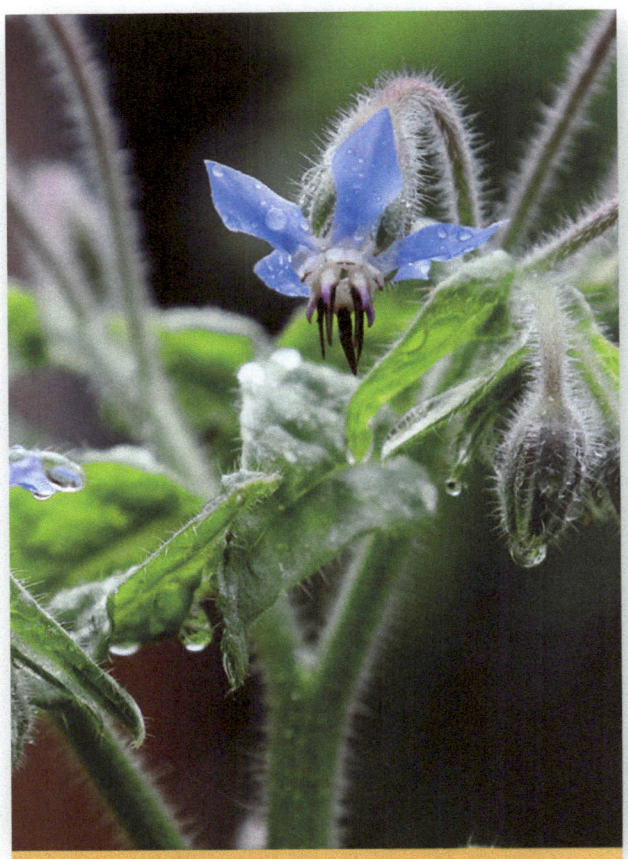

Common names: Borage, common borage, starflower, tailwort
Scientific name: *Borago officinalis* L.
Botanical family: Boraginaceae
Conservation status: Least concern[34]

Description: *Borago officinalis* is a sprawling, herbaceous annual in the Boraginaceae family, native to the Mediterranean. Borage grows 70 - 100 cm tall. Its stems are hairy, straight, hollow, often branched, and covered in tough fibers. Leaves are alternate, simple, and hairy. Flowers are typically blue but sometimes appear white or rose-colored. The fruit is a small, wrinkled, brownish, oval nutlet. Borage grows best in moist, well-drained soils in full sun and is tolerant of cold temperatures.

Ethnobotany: *B. officinalis* has long been cultivated for medicinal and culinary purposes, later developing into a popular commercial crop to produce borage seed oil.[35]

In Germany, borage is an ingredient in sauces, while the Italians use it to prepare a traditional ravioli. In some regions of Spain, borage is boiled and sautéed with garlic and served with potatoes. Borage was thought to bring courage and was used in traditional medicine to treat swellings and inflammation, respiratory ailments, and melancholy. In Iran, borage tea would be made to treat flu, bronchitis, rheumatoid arthritis, and kidney inflammation. Women have used borage as a remedy for premenstrual syndrome and menopause symptoms, including hot flashes.[36]

The genus name *Borago* is thought to arise from the Latin word *burra*, which means "hairy garment," referring to the hairy leaves of some species.[37]

EXTRACTION INFORMATION

Country of origin: Canada, New Zealand, England, Poland, The Netherlands
Part of plant: Seed
Oil content: 22 - 40%
Extraction method: Cold pressing, SFE CO2

MANUFACTURING INFORMATION

CAS number: 225234-12-8 / 84012-16-8
EC number: 281-661-4
INCI name: Cold-pressed oil: Borago Officinalis (Borage) Seed Oil **CO2 extract:** Borago Officinalis (Borage) Seed Extract
CosIng (functions): Skin conditioning, Skin conditioning - emollient

SHELF LIFE

6-9 months
* Store in the refrigerator.

NUTRIENT PROFILE

Highly valued for its rich linoleic acid and gamma-linolenic acid (GLA) contents.

Borage Seed Oil		
	Cold-Pressed[38, 39, 40, 41]	CO2 Extract[42]
SATURATED FATTY ACIDS		
Palmitic acid (C16:0)	7.64 - 10%	11.3 - 12.89%
Stearic acid (C18:0)	3.08 - 6.4%	3.84 - 4.4%
Arachidic acid (C20:0)	0.2-1.4%	
MONOUNSATURATED FATTY ACIDS		
Oleic acid (C18:1 n-9)	14.23 - 18.5%	16.51 - 17.68%
Gondoic acid (C20:1 n-9)	4.2%	3.53 - 4.11%
Erucic acid (C22:1)	2.06 - 2.3%	2.36 - 2.8%
POLYUNSATURATED FATTY ACIDS		
Linoleic acid (C18:2 n-6)	34.23 - 37.9%	37.13 - 38.01%
Gamma-linolenic acid (C18:3 n-6)	21.1 - 24.79%	22.77 - 24.27%
UNSAPONIFIABLE FRACTION (COLD-PRESSED OIL)		
Sterols 1820 - 4990 mg/kg	Campesterol (838.9 mg/kg), delta-5-avenasterol (811.4 mg/kg), beta-sitosterol (309.7 mg/kg)	
Tocopherols[43] 1019 - 1359 mg/kg	Delta-tocopherol (921 - 1320 mg/kg), gamma-tocopherol (98 - 659 mg/kg)	
Squalene	87 mg/kg	

Formulating with Borage Seed Oil

Sensory info: Clear to Pale yellow
Absorption rate: Dry - absorbs quickly into the skin
Dilution: Can be used 10 - 20% percent in a blend of other oils.

Note: It is best to add borage seed oil only to a cool phase or near the end of skincare product preparation. Heat can damage its health benefits.

Antioxidant use: Recommend a 0.5% mixed tocopherols or rosemary CO2 extract antioxidant to support shelf life and stability when using borage seed oil in a formulation.

Therapeutic actions: anti-inflammatory, moisturizing, emollient

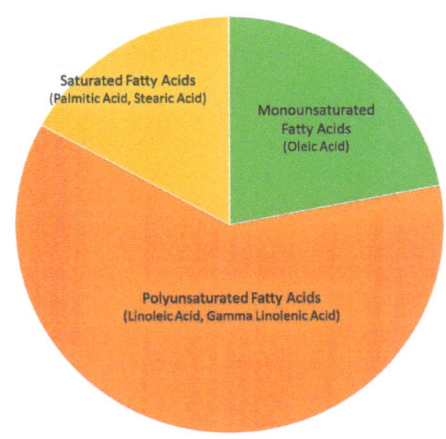

Therapeutic applications:
Borage seed oil is recommended for premature aging, dry and devitalized skin, psoriasis, sensitive skin, and eczema. Due to its rich gamma-linolenic acid content and other essential fatty acids, borage seed oil is a beneficial anti-inflammatory carrier oil.[44] Borage seed oil has been shown to reduce TEWL and treat atopic dermatitis.[45]

Borage seed oil does not contain any pyrrolizidine alkaloids (PA), which are in the borage leaf.[46] The seed oil is a suitable ingredient for infant and children's skincare products.

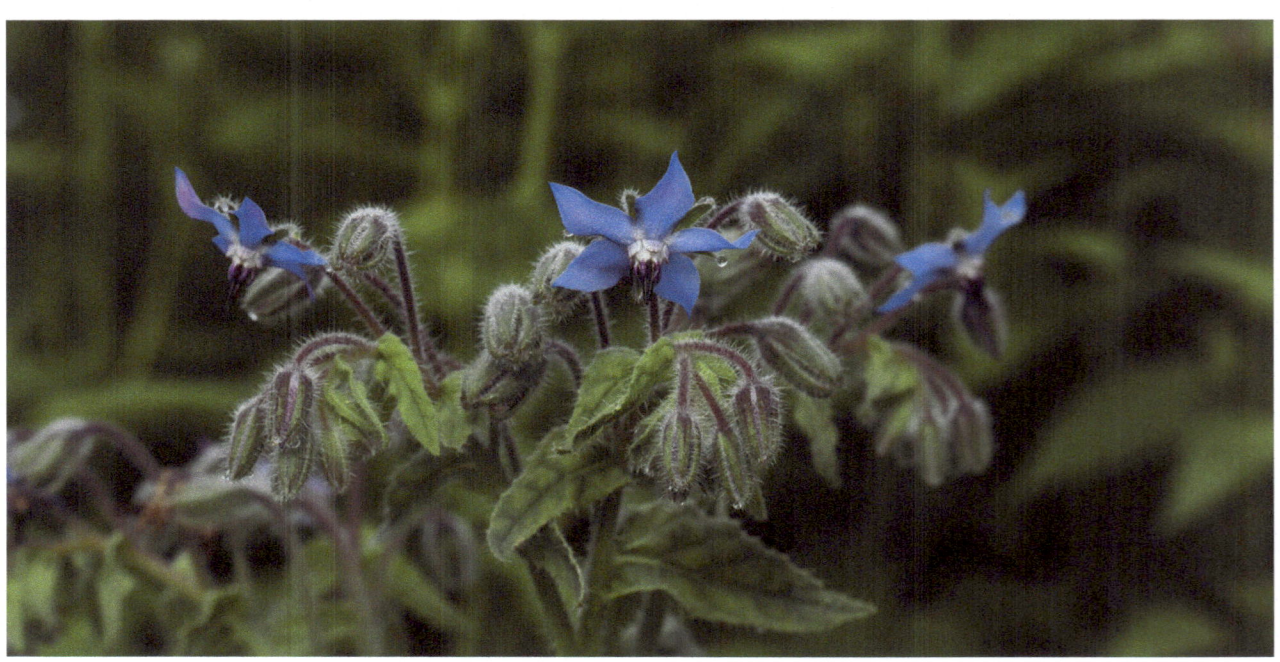

Castor
Ricinus communis

Common name: Castor
Scientific name: *Ricinus communis* L.
Botanical family: Euphorbiaceae
Conservation status: Not yet assessed

Description: *Ricinus communis*, the castor bean or castor oil plant, is a large perennial in the Euphorbiaceae family native to tropical Africa. Castor bean plants grow 10-13 m tall in the tropics and 1.5-2.5 m as annuals in temperate climates. The giant leaves are fan-like, with 12 lobes. Bristly, bronze-to-red clusters of fruit bear mottled, bean-like seeds. Castor beans contain a toxic protein called ricin, making them inedible.

Castor bean plants are predominantly cultivated in India, China, and Brazil as a commercial source of castor oil.[47] Castor oil has myriad commercial applications in manufacturing soaps, lubricants, and coatings. It is one of the oldest cultivated crops, and global demand has skyrocketed in recent years.

Ethnobotany: Archeologists have found castor bean seeds in Egyptian tombs dating back to 4,000 BC. The oil was reportedly used to treat eye irritations, and the Greeks used it in ointments. Castor seed oil has been used as a laxative in India since 2,000 BC, and Chinese folk medicine used castor oil to stimulate childbirth and the expulsion of the placenta. Persians used the oil to treat epilepsy. In Western traditional medicine, castor oil is best known for two primary applications, first as a potent laxative and second as "castor packs." To make a castor pack, one soaks several layers of flannel fabric in castor oil then places the oil-infused fabric on top of the area receiving the treatment.[48] In modern-day Western allopathic medicine, castor oil is used as a vehicle to deliver pharmaceutical drugs.[49]

The genus name *Ricinus* is Latin for "tick," referring to the resemblance of the seed to those parasitic arachnids.[50]

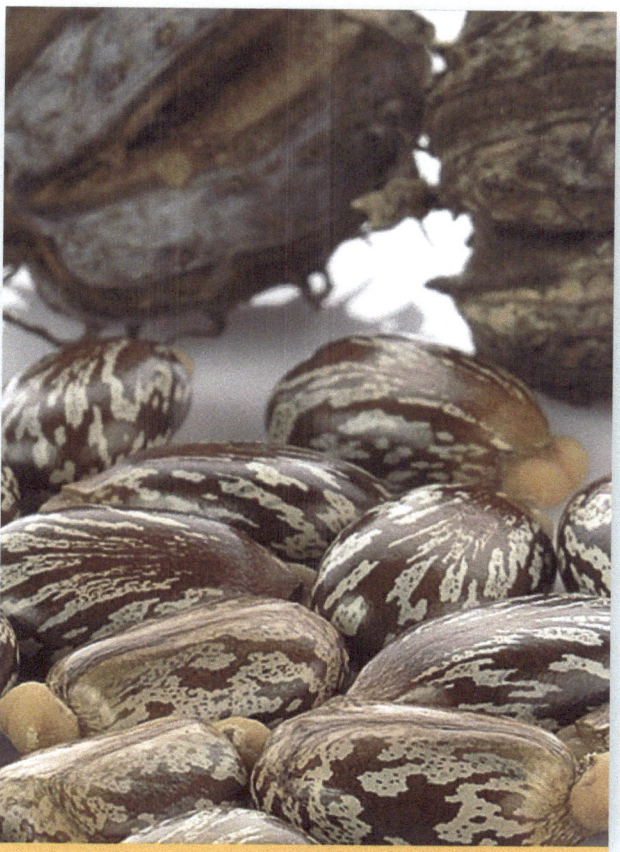

EXTRACTION INFORMATION

Country of origin: India, Brazil, China, Russia
Part of plant: Seed
Oil content: 30 - 51.90%
Extraction method: Cold pressing

MANUFACTURING INFORMATION

CAS number: 8001-79-4
EC number: 232-293-8
INCI name: Ricinus Communis (Castor) Seed Oil
CosIng (functions): Fragrance, Perfuming, Skin conditioning

SHELF LIFE

12 - 24 months

NUTRIENT PROFILE

Chemically, castor oil is a triglyceride characterized by a high ricinoleic acid content, which is responsible for many of castor oil's therapeutic properties. Ricinoleic acid is a hydroxy omega-9 fatty acid.

Castor Oil[51, 52]	
SATURATED FATTY ACIDS	
Palmitic acid (C16:0)	0.56 - 2.77%
Stearic acid (C18:0)	0.9 - 2.7
MONOUNSATURATED FATTY ACIDS	
Oleic acid (C18:1 n-9)	2.05 - 7.7%
Ricinoleic acid (C18:1-OH)	**75.0 - 94.59%**
POLYUNSATURATED FATTY ACIDS	
Linoleic acid (C18:2 n-6)	4.2 - 9.7%
Alpha-linolenic acid (C18:3 n-3)	0.2-1.0%
UNSAPONIFIABLE FRACTION	
Sterols 1520.4 - 2209 mg/kg	Beta-sitosterol (661.4 - 1040.8 mg/kg), stigmasterol (324.1 - 406.6 mg/kg), delta-5-avenasterol (357.9 - 383.1 mg/kg), campesterol (104.9 - 249.7 mg/kg), delta-7-avenasterol (n.d. - 8.83 mg/kg), delta-7-stigmastenol (4 - 4.41 mg/kg), cholesterol (n.d. - 4.41 mg/kg)[51]
Tocopherols 183 - 461.3 mg/kg	Gamma-tocopherol (52.7 - 395.32 mg/kg), delta-tocopherol (43.1 - 47.42 mg/kg),[55] alpha-tocopherol (2.8 mg/kg)

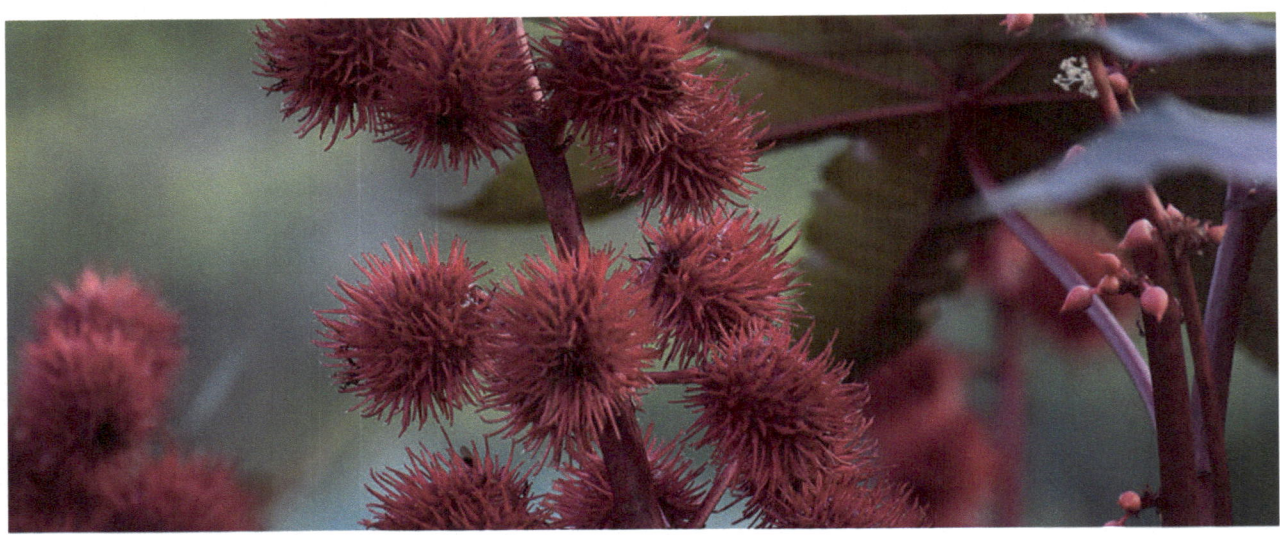

Formulating with Castor Oil

Sensory info: Pale yellow, viscous, clear liquid; may feel slightly tacky
Absorption rate: Wet - slow to absorb
Dilution: Can be used 100 percent or, more commonly, at a 10 - 15% dilution in a blend of other oils.

Therapeutic actions: emollient, antinociceptive, analgesic, anti-inflammatory

Therapeutic applications:
Although castor oil is an excellent emollient, it is seldom used in aromatherapy practices or products besides adding shine to lip balms. It may be useful for brown patches (age spots), liver spots, or blemishes.[8] Castor packs may make bowel movements easier to pass during episodes of constipation.[54]

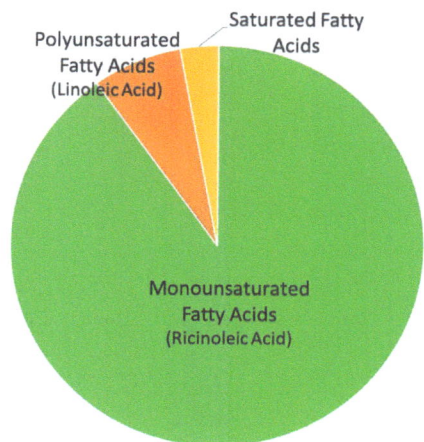

Ricinoleic acid has demonstrated antinociceptive[55], analgesic, and anti-inflammatory activity.[56] Castor oil may be a suitable ingredient in formulations for muscular aches and pains or to address general tension in the body.

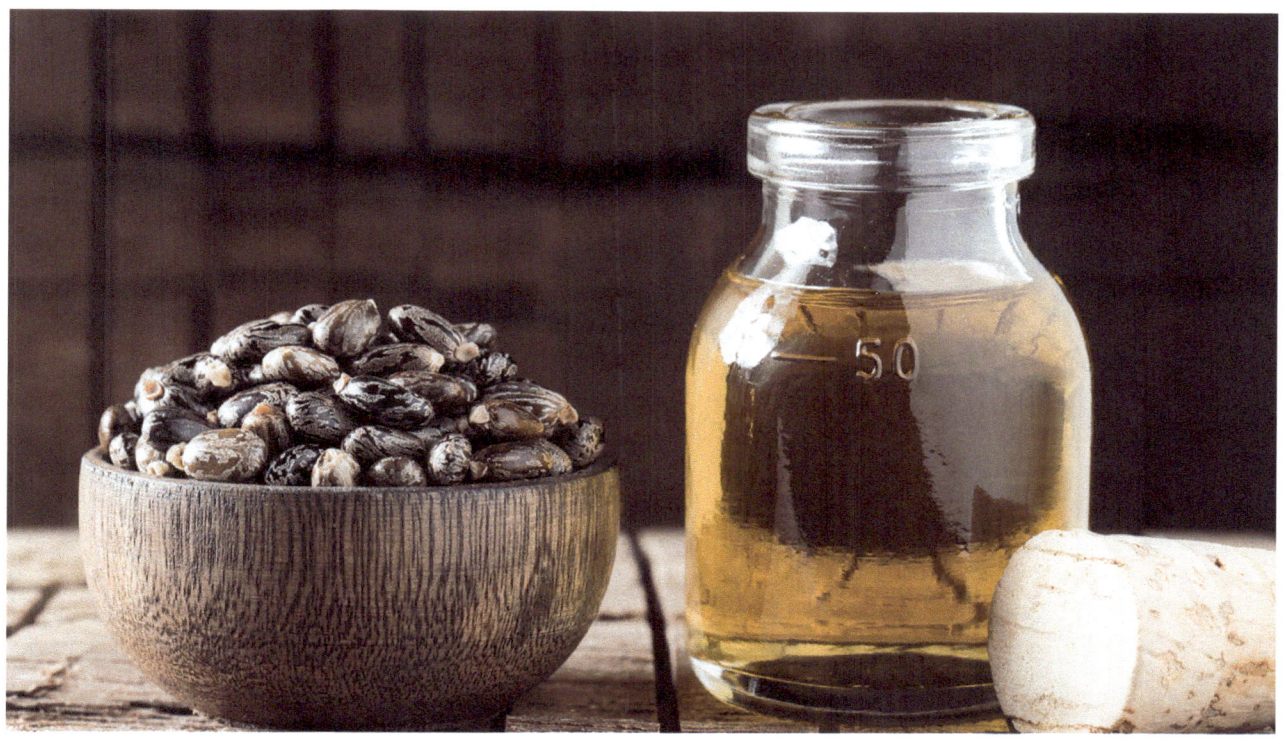

Evening Primrose
Oenothera biennis

Common name: Evening Primrose
Scientific name: *Oenothera biennis* L.
Botanical family: Onagraceae
Conservation status: Not yet assessed

Description: Evening primrose is an upright biennial in the Onagraceae family native to North America. In the 1600s, evening primrose plants were exported to Europe, where they now grow as well. Evening primrose grows naturally in open grassy areas, disturbed areas edging forests, and along roadsides and railroads. The commercial popularity of evening primrose for its valuable seed oil has led to its formal cultivation in many countries.

In its first year, evening primrose stays close to the ground as a rosette of toothed, lanceolate, light green to olive-green leaves, approximately 4-8 inches long and 2 inches wide. In its second year, the blooming and fruiting year, the plant sends up a rigid, hairy, purple-tinged, 3- to 5-foot-tall flower stem. Leaves spiral up the stem from the center of the basal rosette. From June to September, the top of the stem produces bowl-shaped four-petaled bright yellow flowers, which are borne on multi-flower terminal panicles, as well as in panicles at the tips of primary stems. A single flower blooms at the base of each upper leaf-like bract. The fruits are narrow seed pods 1.5 inches long, which, when ripe, rupture to release up to 100 seeds per capsule.

The provenance of the genus name *Oenothera* is uncertain but may be derived from the Greek words *oinos* and *theras*, meaning "wine-seeker," which is likely an allusion to the ancient practice of using the *Oenothera* species' roots to scent wine.[57] The common name "evening primrose" describes how the flowers open at dusk and close at dawn.

Ethnobotany: Europeans also called evening primrose "King's Cure-All" and "Fever-Plant," referring to its medicinal value. Indigenous North Americans ate the roots as food and used evening primrose

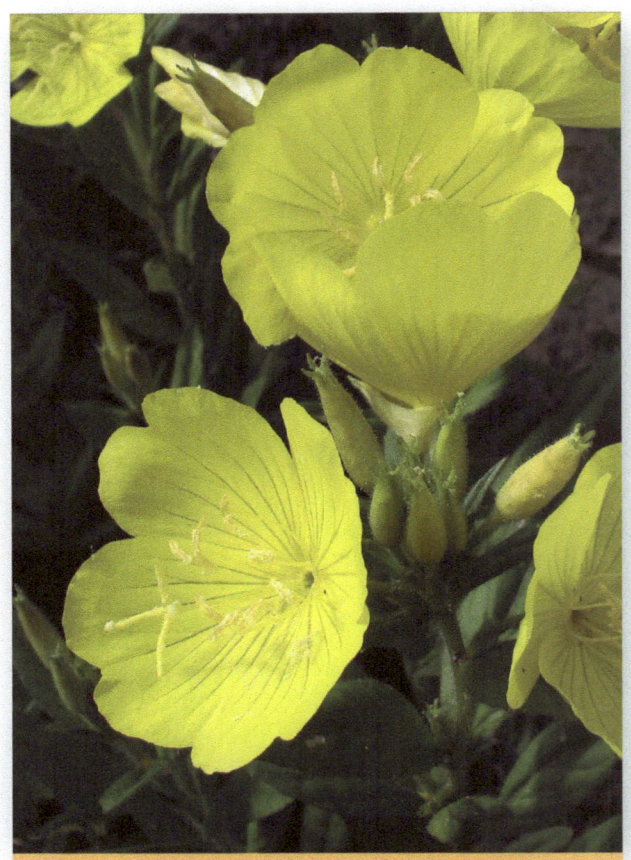

EXTRACTION INFORMATION

Country of origin: North America, Europe, Asia, China
Part of plant: Seed
Oil content: 18 - 25%[60]
Extraction method: Cold pressing

MANUFACTURING INFORMATION

CAS number: 90028-66-3
EC number: 289-859-2
INCI name: Oenothera Biennis (Evening Primrose) Oil
CosIng (functions): Skin conditioning- emollient

SHELF LIFE

6 - 12 months
* Store in the refrigerator.

medicinally. They would make teas from the leaves to combat emotional disorders such as laziness and make hot poultices from various plant parts to apply to skin conditions such as bruises, piles, and boils. They also used the plant to combat internal pains, such as menstrual and bowel pains.[58] Traditional evening primrose seed oil use includes treatments for eczema, asthma, rheumatoid arthritis, premenstrual and menopausal syndrome, and other inflammatory disorders.[59]

NUTRIENT PROFILE

Evening primrose oil (EPO) is valued for its rich content of linoleic acid and gamma-linolenic acid (GLA), which are metabolic precursors of anti-inflammatory mediator molecules. The unsaponifiable fraction also plays a valuable role in the EPO's therapeutic properties.[61]

Evening Primrose Oil[60, 62, 63]	
Saturated fatty acids	
Palmitic acid (C16:0)	5.5 - 10.0%
Stearic acid (C18:0)	1.5 - 3.15%
Monounsaturated fatty acids	
Oleic acid (C18:1 n-9)	6.6 - 18%
Polyunsaturated fatty acids	
Linoleic acid (C18:2 n-6)	65 - 80%
Gamma-linolenic acid (C18:3 n-6)	9.24 - 27%
Unsaponifiable fraction	
Sterols 6024 - 10390 mg/kg	Beta-sitosterol (5450.2 - 7952 mg/kg), campesterol (531.4 - 883.3 mg/kg), delta-5-avenasterol (354.4 - 504.8 mg/kg), sitostanol (127.23 - 206.8 mg/kg), clerosterol (120 mg/kg), delta-5-24-stigmastadienol (88.9 - 101 mg/kg), delta-7-stigmasterol (38.17 – 43.2 mg/kg), delta-7-avenasterol (11.8-43.80 mg/kg)[64, 65]
Tocopherols 280 - 415 mg/kg	Gamma-tocopherol (187 - 335 mg/kg), alpha-tocopherol (16 - 76 mg/kg), delta-tocopherol (n.d. - 15 mg/kg)

Formulating with Evening Primrose Oil

Sensory info: Yellow/yellow-green, clear, oily liquid
Absorption rate: Dry - absorbs quickly into the skin
Dilution: Can be used 5 - 15% in a blend of other carrier oils.

Note: It is best to add evening primrose seed oil only to a cool phase or near the end of skincare product preparation. Heat can damage its health benefits.

Antioxidant use: Recommend a 0.5% mixed tocopherols or rosemary CO2 extract antioxidant to support shelf life and stability when using evening primrose seed oil in a formulation.

Therapeutic actions: skin regeneration, anti-inflammatory, moisturizing, emollient

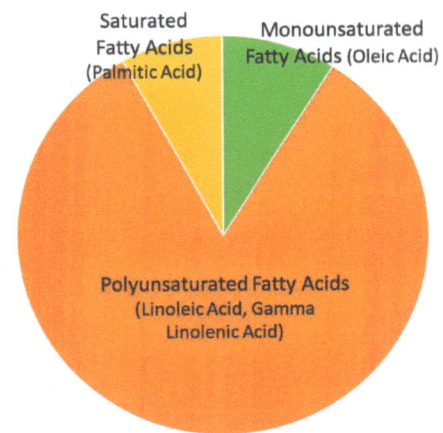

Therapeutic applications:
Evening primrose oil strengthens the epidermal barrier, normalizes excessive water loss through the epidermis, regenerates skin, and improves smoothness after topical and oral applications.[66]

Suitable for premature skin aging, dry and devitalized skin, psoriasis, eczema, regenerative skin care, and where there is a loss of skin elasticity.[8] It is an excellent oil for facial serums or specialty oil blends. Evening primrose's cooling and anti-inflammatory activities make it an appropriate choice to combat atopic dermatitis.[15] Suitable for Vata and Pitta skin types.

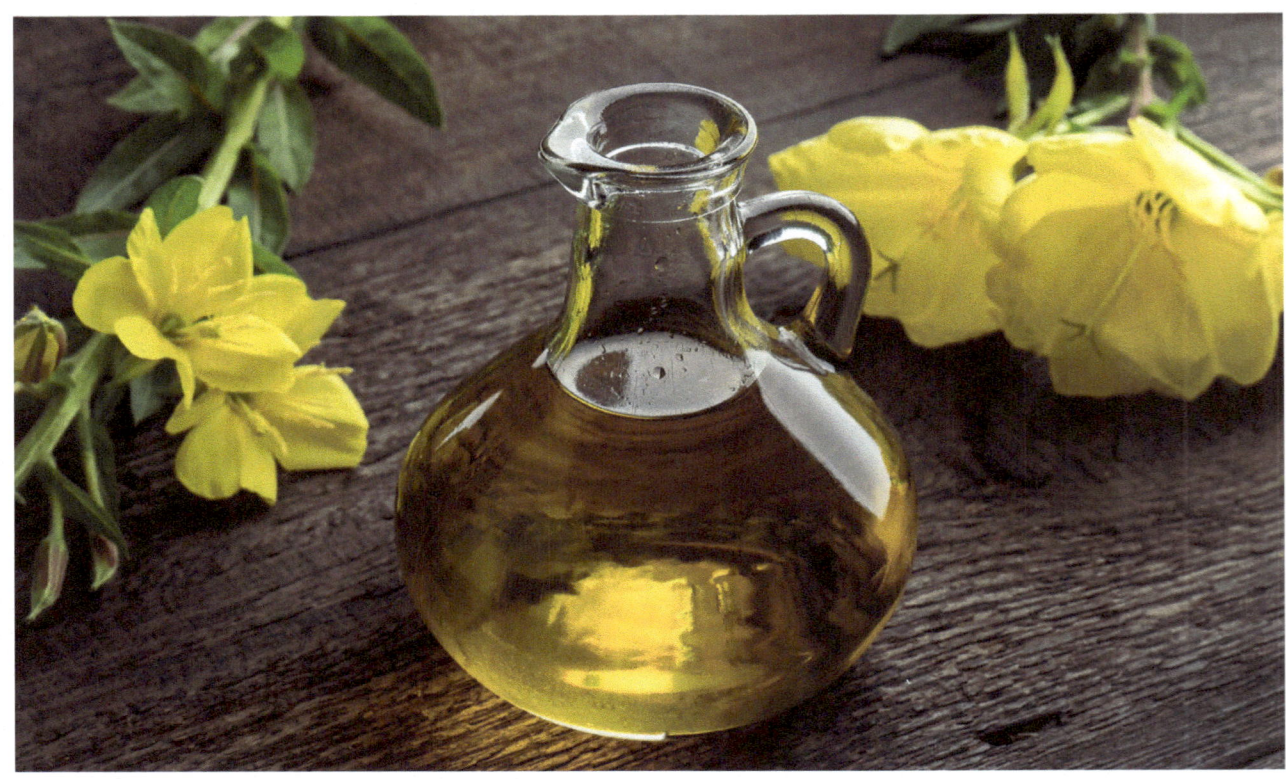

Hemp
Cannabis sativa

Common name: Hemp
Scientific name: *Cannabis sativa* L.,
Synonyms: *Cannabis indica* Lam., *Cannabis ruderalis* Janisch.[67]
Botanical family: Cannabaceae
Conservation status: Not assessed

Description:[68] Cannabis is an annual herb, growing 1-5 m tall, originating in central Asia. It has a yearly 2-10-month growth period, flowering in the fall. As the plant matures, its hollow stem elongates without developing branches, and the leaves become more complex. The plant has one large taproot with smaller lateral roots.

The first true leaves are single leaflets, and the second pair has three leaflets per leaf. Each new generation of leaves is increasingly palmately compound, up to a maximum of eleven leaflets per leaf, each averaging 92-136 mm long. These leaflets are what give hemp plants their feathery appearance.

The hemp plant is dioecious, with female plants outliving the male plants by 3-5 weeks. Male flowers appear first, at the base of the petioles. The male flowers consist of five fused tepals, which open to release five hanging anthers. The axillary and terminal female flowers are smaller and more compact, each containing a pair of white styles associated with a single ovary.

Hemp fruits are round, dark red-brown hemp achenes, 2-5 mm in diameter, covered by two pericarp layers. The seed endosperm contains approximately 25-30% oil, 25-30% protein, and 30-40% fiber.

Cannabis produces a unique class of chemicals, the cannabinoids, synthesized and stored in stalked, secretory epidermal glands called trichomes. Trichomes are located primarily on the female plant's flowers, with fewer being present on leaves and stems. However, there are no trichomes on the fruit or seeds, so any cannabinoids appearing in seed products result from contamination from contact with other parts of the

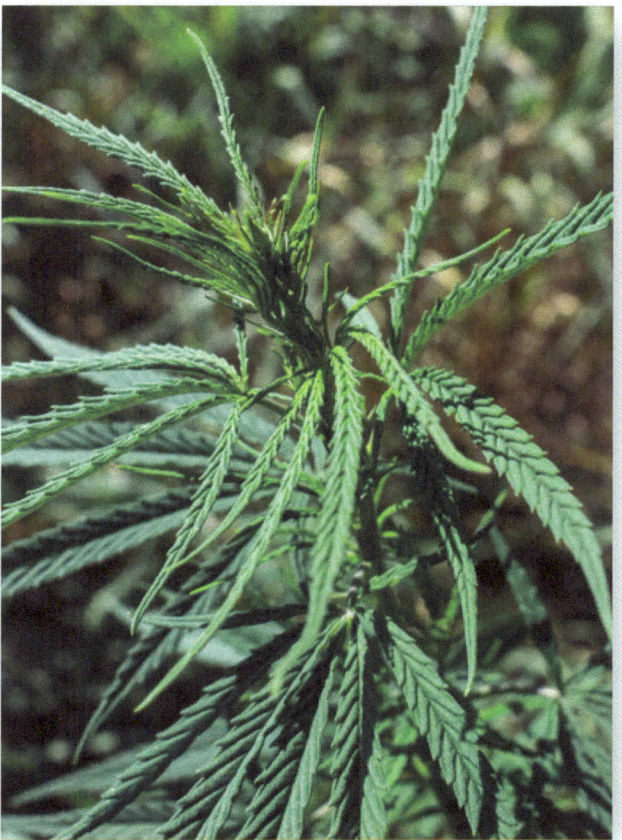

EXTRACTION INFORMATION

Country of origin: Canada
Part of plant: Seed
Oil content: 25 - 35%
Extraction: Cold pressing

MANUFACTURING INFORMATION

CAS number: 8016-24-8 (oil) / 89958-21-4 (hemp extracts, including seed oil)
EC number: 289-644-3 (hemp extracts, including seed oil)
INCI name: Hempseed (Cannabis Sativa) Oil, Cannabis Sativa (Hemp) Seed Oil
CosIng (functions): Emollient, Skin conditioning

SHELF LIFE

8-12 months
* Store in the refrigerator.

plant.

Ethnobotany:[69, 70, 71] Humans have utilized hemp plant products in multiple industries for millennia, including fiber production, cosmetics, food, medicine, and drugs. Archeological evidence shows that the Chinese cultivated hemp as an economic crop as early as 4500 BC. Hemp fibers appear in paper, and the oldest known written record of medicinal hemp use is in an ancient Chinese herbal.

Cannabinoids in *C. sativa* interact with specific receptors on the surface of human cells, particularly in the central nervous system. *C. sativa* plants containing high amounts of the psychoactive cannabinoid THC (tetrahydrocannabinol), also known as marijuana or hashish, have played important recreational, spiritual, and medicinal roles and developed an infamous reputation in the last century. There is archaeological evidence of cannabis drug use from Ancient Egypt and Ancient Persia. The name "hashish" comes from the Arabic *hashish al kief*, or "herb of pleasure."

However, the hemp plant varieties containing very little or no THC have also been vitally important in the history of humankind. During the Age of Exploration, tall ships sailed worldwide using hemp canvas sails. Hemp also provided the fibers for paper, fine clothing, and household linens. Hemp continues to be important in the paper industry, providing fiber for specialty paper, such as tea bags, cigarettes, and paper currency. The oil from hemp seeds was also crucial in the paint industry.

The hemp industry in the United States has struggled since implementing The Marijuana Tax Act of 1937, which criminalized commercial hemp dealings, effectively eliminating industrial hemp production in the United States. The U.S. revived commercial hemp production during World War II but stopped again at the war's end. The result of this prohibition on hemp cultivation has been to exclude the hemp plant and its extracts from significant industrial or nutritional research.

Canada reinstituted licensed hemp cultivation in 1998, and the high demand has required the market to expand since then. Canada currently supplies a significant portion of the world's hemp and hemp seed products and materials, followed by several countries in the European Union.

Hemp seed oil, marijuana, CBD oil, and hemp oil all come from the *C. sativa* plant, but the individual plant's chemistry determines its usefulness. THC is the primary cannabinoid produced in "marijuana" plants, while, in the United States, "hemp" must have a female flower dry weight THC level below 0.3%. There may also be some physiological differences between the hemp and marijuana plants. These differences may be adequate to claim they are from different subspecies, but the morphological or phylogenetic differences are insufficient to distinguish the plants as separate species.

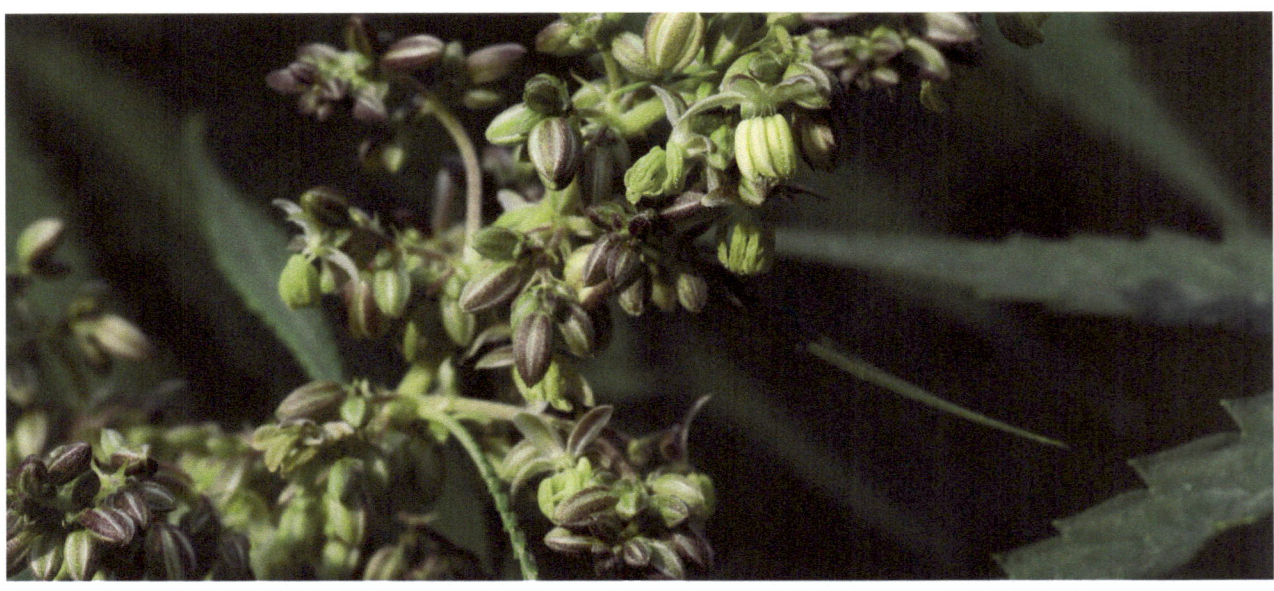

NUTRIENT PROFILE

Hemp seed oil is an excellent source of essential fatty acids and has an omega-6 to omega-3 fatty acid ratio of approximately 3:1. It is also a significant source of carotenoids.

Hemp Seed [68, 70, 72, 73, 74, 75, 76]	
SATURATED FATTY ACIDS	
Palmitic acid (C16:0)	5 - 9%
Stearic acid (C18:0)	2 - 3%
MONOUNSATURATED FATTY ACIDS	
Oleic acid (C18:1 n-9)	6 - 12%
POLYUNSATURATED FATTY ACIDS	
Linoleic acid (C18:2 n-6)	**50 - 70%**
Alpha-linolenic acid (C18:3 n-3)	**15 - 25%**
Gamma-linolenic acid (C18:3 n-6)	1 - 6%
UNSAPONIFIABLE FRACTION	
Sterols 2571 - 2794 mg/kg	Beta-sitosterol (1846 - 1964 mg/kg), stigmasterol (92.7 - 107.7 mg/kg), campesterol (473 - 537 mg/kg), phytol (165 - 169 mg/kg), delta-5-avenasterol (135.1 – 150.5 mg/kg), cycloartenol (87 - 94 mg/kg)
Tocopherols 600 - 1350 mg/kg	Gamma-tocopherol (216 - 762 mg/kg), alpha-tocopherol (25.6 - 246.2 mg/kg), delta-tocopherol (12.8 - 41.5 mg/kg)
Pigments	Chlorophyll (39.5 - 99.6 mg/kg), Carotenoid (31.46 - 78 mg/kg)
Squalene	80.52 mg/kg
Polyphenols	22.1-160.8 mg GAE/g

Formulating with Hemp Seed Oil

Sensory info: Pale green, transparent liquid.
Absorption rate: Dry - absorbs quickly into skin
Dilution: 3 - 10% of the formulation
Note: It is best to add hemp seed oil only to a cool phase or near the end of skincare product preparation. Heat can damage its health benefits.

Antioxidant use: Recommend a 0.5% mixed tocopherols or rosemary CO2 extract antioxidant to support shelf life and stability when using hemp seed oil in a formulation.

Therapeutic actions: 3:1 omega-6 to omega-3 fatty acid ratio, address EFA deficiency, anti-inflammatory, skin-regeneration, antioxidant, moisturizing, emollient

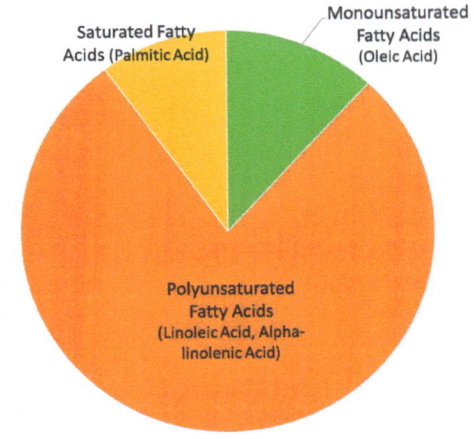

Therapeutic applications:
Hemp seed oil has a healthy balance of an approximately 3:1 ratio of omega-6 to omega-3 fatty acids. This ratio and the high percentage of essential fatty acids in hemp seed oil make it an appropriate choice for nutrient-deficient, dry, flaky skin and to lighten UV-hyperpigmented skin. Linoleic acid, alpha-linolenic acid, and gamma-linolenic acid contents indicate hemp seed oil to be anti-inflammatory and skin regenerative, making it appropriate for dermatitis, eczema, psoriasis, acne, rosacea, arthritis, and wound care. It has very low antibacterial action against Gram-positive bacteria,[77] so formulations to address acne and rosacea would benefit from blending hemp seed oil with a more potent antibacterial carrier oil.

Hemp seed oil is appropriate for anti-aging formulations to reduce fine lines and wrinkles and reduce skin photodamage.[78] It is moisturizing and emollient.

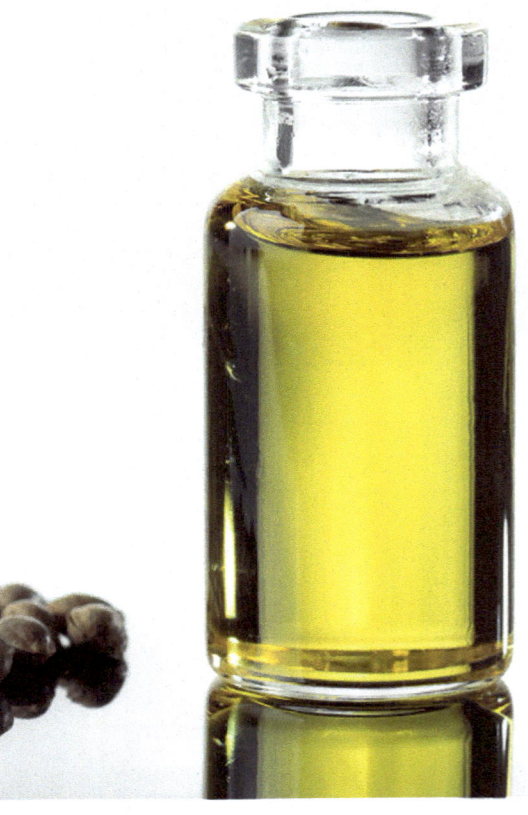

Meadowfoam
Limnanthes alba

Common name: Meadowfoam, white meadowfoam
Scientific name: *Limnanthes alba* Hartw. ex Benth. (syn. *Floerkea alba* Greene)
Botanical family: Limnanthaceae
Conservation status: Commercial, cooperative farms, using ecologically sound farming practices.[79]

Description:[80, 81, 82, 83] Meadowfoam is native to the United States Pacific Northwest, grown in California and Oregon in the United States and British Columbia in Canada. The commercial crop grows on multiple local family farms. One acre of 120 million flowers can support up to 100,000 bees, meadowfoam's insect pollinators, and produces 950 lbs. of seed, which can yield up to 250 lbs. of oil.

Meadowfoam plants grow as a winter annual 10-18 inches (8-40 cm) tall. The plants have 1-4 inch (2-10 cm) long, shallowly to deeply pinnate leaves with 5-9 oblong blades. Bowl-shaped flowers are perfect on axillary peduncles. The flowers are mostly white with a yellow ring around the center of the five petals, 4-8 mm long. When the plants are in full bloom, the white flowers that blanket the area resemble seafoam, especially when the wind blows through them, which is how meadowfoam got its name. Limnanthes means "marsh flower."

In the 1950s, the United States Department of Agriculture (USDA) studied meadowfoam seed oil during its search for new renewable industrial oils, leading to the oil's commercial development in 1980. Meadowfoam is uniquely interesting in that it is over 90% long-chain fatty acids (C20 - C22), including three uncommon fatty acids. Of particular interest are the omega-5 fatty acids (C20:1, C22:2).

Meadowfoam seed oil fatty acid esters can transform the oil into a liquid wax like jojoba oil. This liquid wax is also valuable as a renewable substitute for sperm whale oil, which had been a leading cosmetic ingredient and industrial oil through the late 20th century.

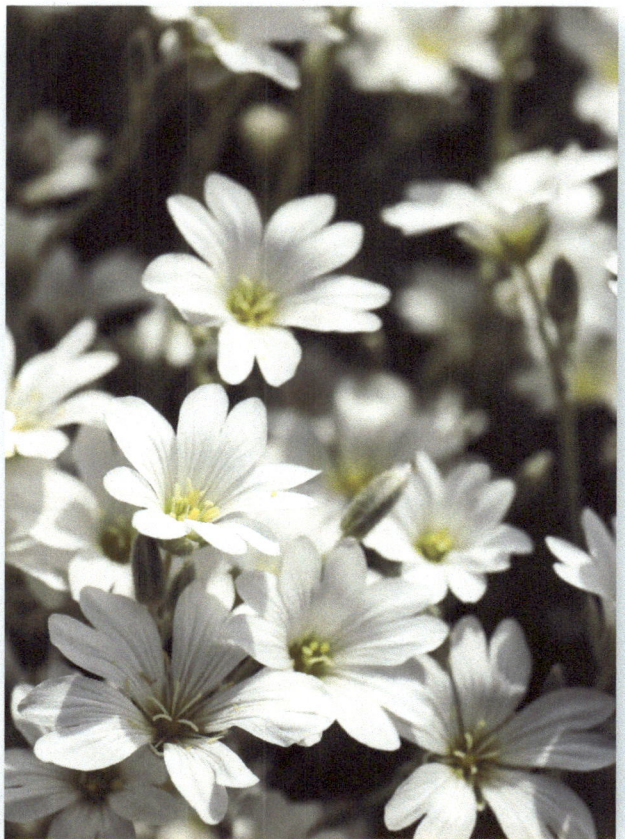

EXTRACTION INFORMATION

Country of origin: Oregon, USA; California, USA
Part of plant: Seed
Oil content: 20 - 30%,[79] with 20 - 25% being common
Extraction method: Cold pressing, Expeller pressing, Solvent extraction

MANUFACTURING INFORMATION

CAS number: 153065-40-8
EC number: 604-884-4
INCI name: Limnanthes Alba (Meadowfoam) Seed Oil; Limnanthes Alba Seed Oil
CosIng (functions): Skin Conditioning, Skin Conditioning - Emollient

SHELF LIFE

Up to 5 years[85]
Adding meadowfoam oil to other carrier oils can enhance their oxidative stability.

Derivatives of meadowfoam oil have great industrial potential, and the USDA is currently researching this precious oil for use in multiple industries. Its non-cosmetic industrial uses include specialty lubricants, inks, detergents, and plasticizers, often placing meadowfoam seed oil in direct competition with rapeseed oil.

Both cold-pressed and refined meadowfoam seed oils (MSO) are available to use in natural care products. Refining removes MSO's natural color and aroma without changing its oxidative stability and emollient properties.[92] There are at least two forms of the refined MSO, and some retailers label their refined MSO as "cold-pressed" without mentioning the refining process. Be sure to select the oil that meets your needs before purchasing.

MSO also contains a high proportion of erucic acid, present in seed oils from the Brassicaceae family, most notably rapeseed and mustard. People who consume high levels of erucic acid can develop health problems, so MSO is for topical use only. Canola oil, which is a low erucic acid version of rapeseed oil, by regulation, cannot contain more than 2% (U.S.) - 5% (EU) (by weight) erucic acid.

NUTRIENT PROFILE

Long-chain fatty acids (C:20 and C:22) predominate in the meadowfoam profile.

Meadowfoam Seed Oil[86, 87, 88, 89]	
Saturated fatty acids	
Arachidic acid (C20:0)	0.8 - 0.92%
Monounsaturated fatty acids	
Oleic acid (C18:1 n-9)	1-1.89%
Gondoic acid (C20:1 n-9)	**58-65%**
Erucic acid (C22:1 n-9)	**10-20%**
Polyunsaturated fatty acids	
5,13 – Docosadienoic acid (C22:2 n-9,17)	10 - 21%
Unsaponifiable fraction	
Tocopherols 515 - 563 mg/kg	Gamma-tocopherol (443 - 534 mg/kg), alpha-tocopherol (29 - 54 mg/kg), delta-tocopherol (15 - 17 mg/kg), beta-tocopherol (3 mg/kg)

Formulating with Meadowfoam Seed Oil

Sensory info:
- **Cold-pressed:** red-orange colored; earthy aroma; non-greasy, silky, slight powdery, dry feeling
- **Refined (cold-pressed oil):** light-colored and odorless

Absorption rate: Dry, fast absorption
Dilution: up to 100%

Therapeutic actions: skin conditioning, emollient, extend carrier oil blend shelf life, antioxidant, all skin types

Therapeutic applications:
The cosmetics industry values meadowfoam seed oil's exceptional qualities for skincare and haircare applications, benefiting all skin types from oily or acne-prone skin to dry, mature skin. Meadowfoam blends well with other products, is very shelf-stable, has a non-greasy feel, and is highly moisturizing.

Combine meadowfoam with other carrier oils, especially costly oils that oxidize quickly, such as borage and evening primrose oil, to increase their overall oxidative stability and shelf-life.[90] MSO's antioxidant capacity may counteract free radicals in the skin, helping repair photodamage and slow the effects of skin aging. MSO is also an appropriate substitute for argan oil, making it is a more-sustainable ingredient choice.[81]

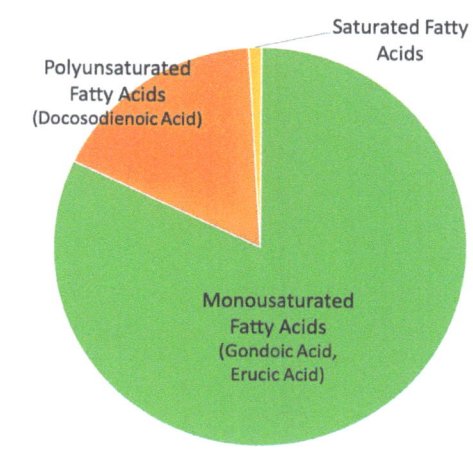

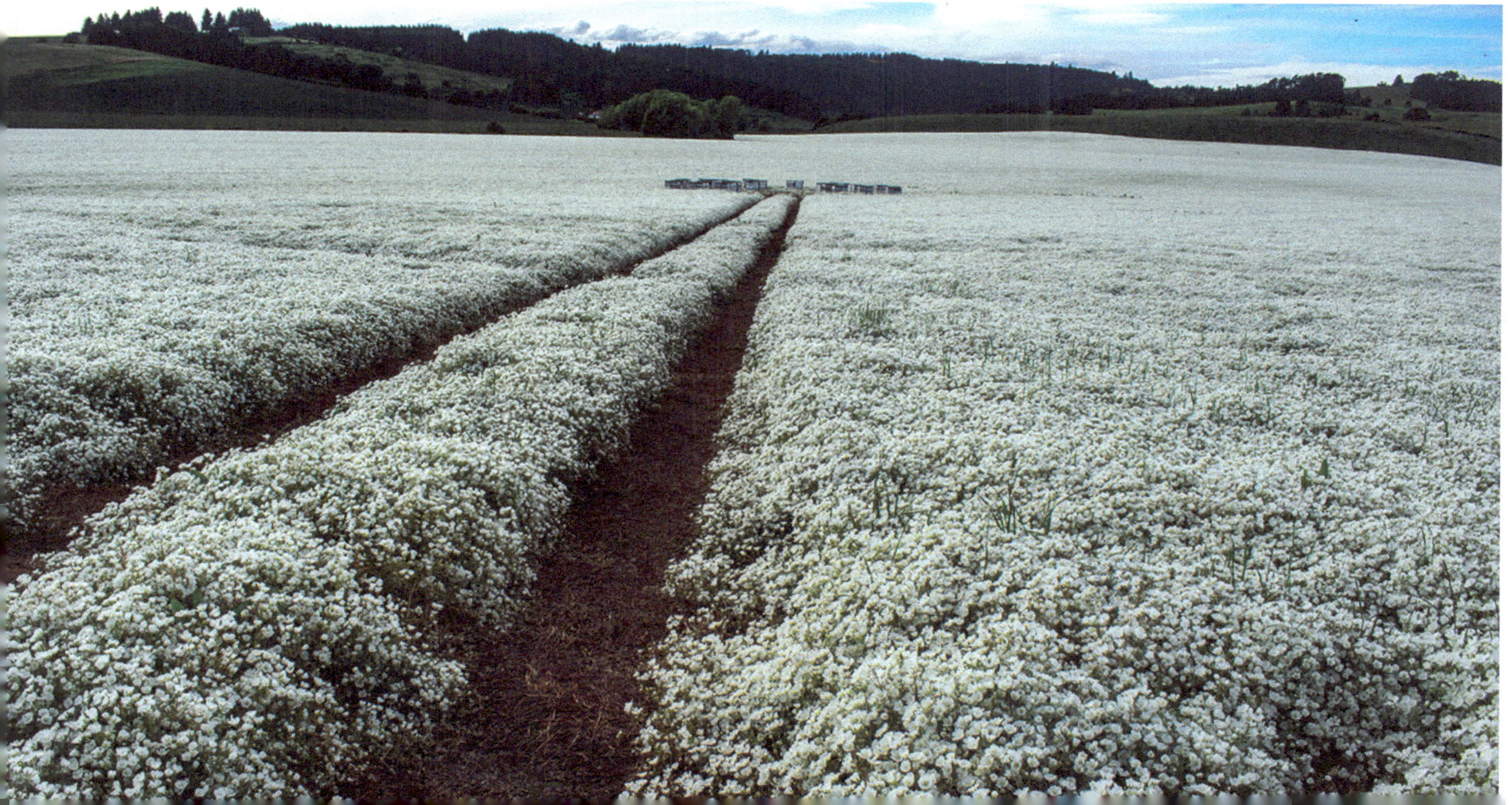

Neem

Azadirachta indica

Common name: Neem, margosa tree, nimtree, Indian lilac
Scientific name: *Azadirachta indica* A. Juss., syn. *Melia azadirachta*
Botanical family: Meliaceae, the mahogany family
Conservation status: Least concern[91]

Description: Neem, an evergreen tree in the mahogany family, flourishes in hot, arid, and semi-arid climates. It grows primarily on the Indian subcontinent, and its cultivation has spread to other Southeast Asian and African countries. The largest single plantation of neem trees grows in Saudi Arabia. The trees grow quickly and may reach 30 m tall, usually 15-20 m, with trunk diameters of 2.5 m. The many pinnately compound leaves containing 9-19 leaflets crowd near the ends of the tree branches. The leaflets themselves are toothed, irregularly and deeply serrated, sharply pointed, and the leaflet's upper surface is shiny. Many of the leaflets have a distinctive curve, giving them an asymmetrical appearance. The small, white, fragrant flowers form clusters at the leaf axils. The fruit is a drupe, which turns from dark purple to yellow when ripe. Each round drupe contains one seed.[92, 93]

Ethnobotany: Neem is a fundamental herb in Ayurveda and virtually every aspect of health and wellness in India, where it is called the "free tree of India,"[105] "healer of all ailments," and the "village pharmacy." Records of neem's use extend back at least to Siddha medicine, over 4,500 years ago.[93]

While one could write whole book chapters about the myriad medicinal and therapeutic uses of various parts of the neem plant, the list of therapeutic remedies attributed only to the neem oil is still significant and diverse. Neem oil is an ingredient in folk remedies to combat leprosy, intestinal worms, respiratory disorders, constipation, rheumatism, sores from chronic syphilis, ulcers, and skin infections. It is also considered a valuable general tonic.[95] Modern uses include neem oil in shampoos, toothpaste, soaps, cosmetics, mosquito repellents, creams and lotions, and pet products such

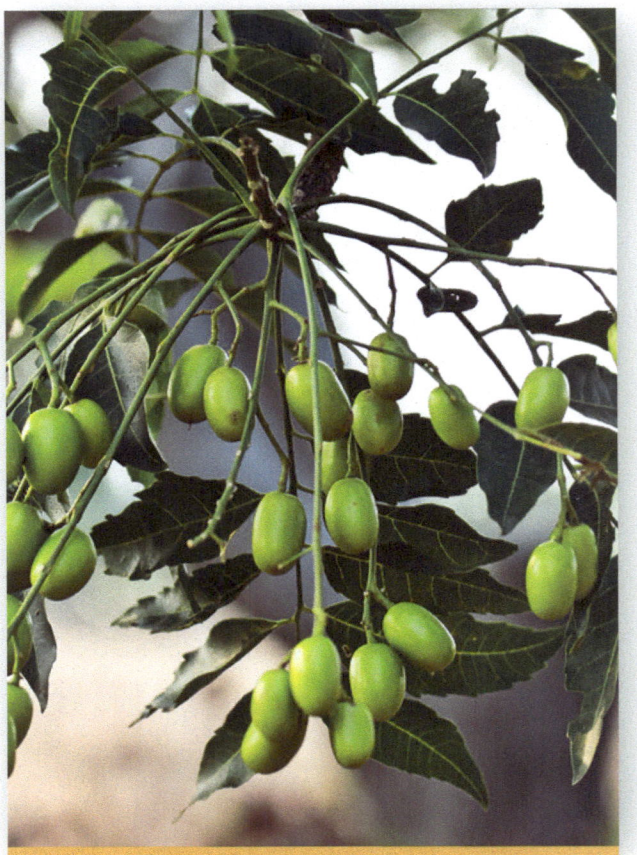

EXTRACTION INFORMATION

Country of origin: India
Part of plant: Seed
Extraction: Expeller pressing, Solvent extraction

MANUFACTURING INFORMATION

CAS number: 8002-65-1 / 84696-25-3 (Other neem extracts, including neem seed oil)
EC number: 290-052-2
INCI name: Melia Azadirachta (Neem) Seed Oil, Azadiracta Indica Seed Oil
CosIng (functions): Skin conditioning – emollient
Additional commercial oil name: Margosa oil, Margose oil

SHELF LIFE

24 months

as pet shampoo.

In addition to neem oil's many medicinal and therapeutic uses, it is also a registered pesticide,[96] categorized as a repellent, growth regulator, and insecticide. Neem oil contains several bioactive compounds, the critical constituent in its use as a pesticide being a limonoid (C26) known as azadirachtin. Azadirachtin acts in various ways to negatively impact the reproductive cycles of mature adults and the development of immature arthropods, effectively reducing current and future populations.[97] Scientists have investigated this chemical's various effects on parasitic and destructive arthropods from multiple families. As a result, neem oil pesticides are a relatively non-toxic alternative to the many home and garden pesticides that carry a significant risk to humans (or their mammalian pets) in addition to the pests they target.

The scientific studies that have directly addressed azadirachtin and neem oil effects on ticks, lice, and mosquitoes, especially from the *Anopheles* genus, the vector for malaria, are promising. One study in an Ethiopian village compared the effectiveness of a neem oil blend to DEET in repelling the *Anopheles arabiensis* mosquito. Neem oil was as effective as DEET as a repellent; only the protection time was much shorter, lasting only 3 hours compared to DEET's 8-hour protection time.[98] Another study against *A. gambiae* found that the 40% (v/v) concentration was most effective for repellent effects.[99]

Other bioactive limonoids in neem oil include nimbidin and several of its chemical relatives and metabolites. These compounds have demonstrated human spermicidal, anti-inflammatory, antibacterial, and antipyretic activity.[100]

NUTRIENT PROFILE

Neem's most unique constituents are its limonoids, especially azadirachtin (0.1 - 0.3% of neem seeds).[101] Its fatty acid profile is balanced between oleic and linoleic acids.

Neem Oil[102, 103]	
SATURATED FATTY ACIDS	
Palmitic acid (C16:0)	6.7 - 18.2%
Stearic acid (C18:0)	3.3 - 17.2%
Arachidic acid (C20:0)	0.27 - 1.3%
MONOUNSATURATED FATTY ACIDS	
Oleic acid (C18:1 n-9)	18.9 - 52.0%
POLYUNSATURATED FATTY ACIDS	
Linoleic acid (C18:2 n-6)	13.6 - 69.2%
UNSAPONIFIABLE FRACTION	
Sterols 2856.2 mg/kg	Beta-sitosterol (1905.1 mg/kg), campesterol (445.6 mg/kg), delta-5-avenasterol (188.5 mg/kg), stigmasterol (148.5 mg/kg), delta-7-stigmasterol (33.1 mg/kg), delta-7-avenasterol (28.8 mg/kg)
Tocopherols 276 mg/kg	Gamma-tocopherol (163.4 mg/kg), alpha-tocopherol (98.3 mg/kg), delta-tocopherol (14.1 mg/kg)

Formulating with Neem Oil

Sensory info: Yellow, brown, or red color with a potent, bitter, sulfuric aroma. May be very thick at room temperature but will thin out with gentle warming. Retailers may blend neem with another carrier oil to help with ease of use.
Absorption rate: Slow to absorb
Dilution: Can be used 100% but recommended at 10 - 25% due to powerful aroma.

Therapeutic actions: antibacterial, antifungal, anti-inflammatory, insect repellent, pesticide, emollient

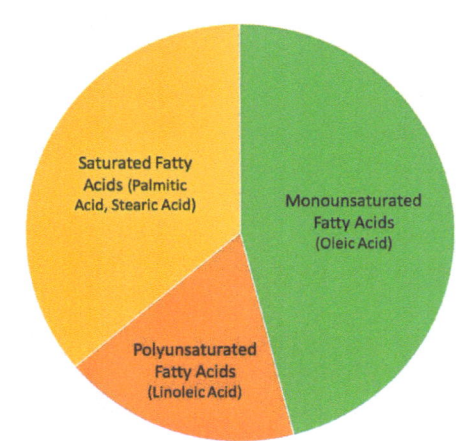

Therapeutic applications:
Neem is used for many skin conditions and is an ingredient in many skincare preparations. It has antibacterial, antifungal, and anti-inflammatory activity and is indicated for acne, eczema, yeast infections, foot fungus, scabies, and seborrheic dermatitis. It is also appropriate for treating dandruff or dry, itchy scalps and restoring dry, damaged hair.[104]

Neem oil is an effective treatment for lice[105, 106] and as a mosquito repellent.[98] It may effectively address various parasitic infestations, such as chiggers, ticks, fleas, scabies, and swimmer's itch. One study found that a blend of 20% neem oil in coconut oil was as effective as the conventional potassium permanganate (KMnO4) treatment against sand flea tungiasis in Kenyan children. The children receiving the neem/coconut oil mixture reported less pain, and the fleas in the test group aged faster than in the control group.[107]

When using pure neem for dandruff and lice, massage about one (1) teaspoon on the scalp, then wash it off after 30-60 minutes. When applying pure neem to the face, apply a few drops, then wash it off after 10 minutes.[94]

In Ayurveda, neem oil balances Kapha and Pitta Doshas. It is safe to use for children and mammalian pets.

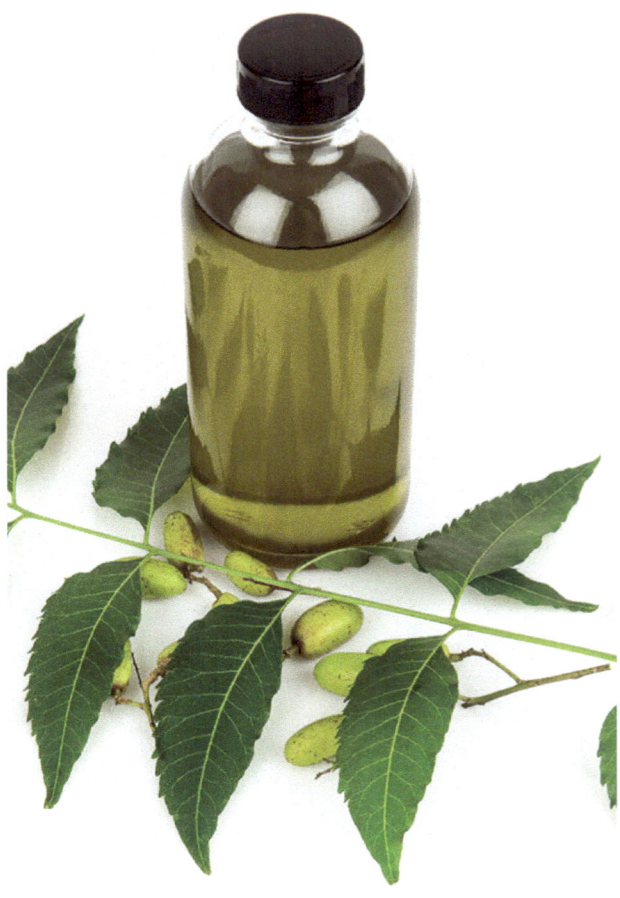

Pomegranate
Punica granatum

Common name: Pomegranate
Scientific name: *Punica granatum* L.
Botanical family: Lythraceae (formerly known as the Punicaceae family)
Conservation status: Least concern[108]

Description: *Punica granatum* is a small tree or large shrub in the Lythraceae family native to Iran and neighboring countries. The tree has long been cultivated throughout the Mediterranean, the Arabian Peninsula, Afghanistan, and India. Cultivation has since spread to the Americas, stretching from the United States' warmer to Chile. *P. granatum* grows best in deep, heavy loams in full sun, with high temperatures and a dry climate during the ripening period.

Pomegranate typically grows 5-7 meters tall, with bright green, elliptic-to-lanceolate leaves 7.5 cm long. Flowers are orange-red in color, axillary, and develop near the ends of branchlets. The fruit is a rounded hexagonal berry, about the size of a hand, with reddish leathery skin. It is subdivided into several chambers, which contain thin, transparent arils of dark red, edible pulp. Each pomegranate fruit holds approximately 600 arils, each containing one angular seed.[109]

The genus name *Punica* is a contraction of the Latin *punicum malum*, meaning the "Carthaginian apple." The specific epithet *granatum* means "many-seeded."[110]

Ethnobotany: Pomegranate has a long history of use as food and medicine. Traditional medicine uses the fruit extensively to treat dysentery, diarrhea, hemorrhage, respiratory ailments, and eradicate intestinal worms. The fruit's dried pericarp and the juice have been used to relieve colic, colitis, menorrhagia, pinworm infestations, headache, acne, hemorrhoids, allergic dermatitis, and oral maladies.[111]

Ayurvedic medicine considers the pomegranate a pharmacy unto itself. The bark and roots are valued for their anthelmintic and vermifuge properties, while the peels are used as a potent astringent and cure for

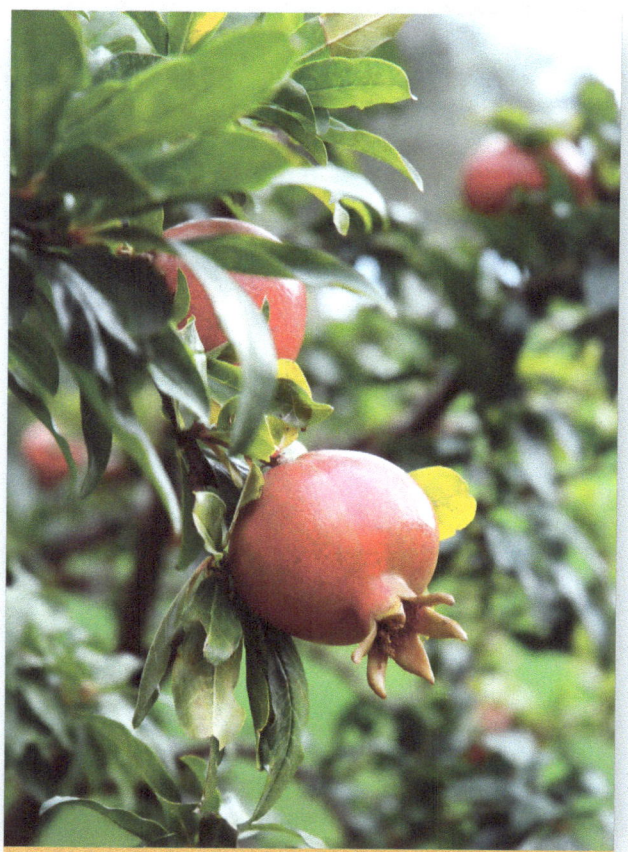

EXTRACTION INFORMATION

Country of origin: China, India, Iran, Turkey
Part of plant: Seed
Oil yield: 7.9% - 16%
Extraction method: Cold pressing
Extraction method: SFE CO_2
CO_2 yield: 14%[113]

MANUFACTURING INFORMATION

CAS Number: 84961-57-9
EC number: 284-646-0
INCI name: Cold-pressed oil: Punica Granatum (Pomegranate) Seed Oil **CO_2 extract:** Punica Granatum (Pomegranate) Seed Extract
CosIng (functions): Skin Conditioning - emollient

SHELF LIFE

12-24 months
*Refrigeration is recommended.

diarrhea and oral ulcers. The juice is thought to be a tonic for the blood. In Unani medicine, pomegranate flowers are a remedy for diabetes mellitus.

Pomegranate is powerfully symbolic. The fruit is referenced in a Kabbalistic text dating back to 1287 CE, *Sefer ha Rimon: The Book of the Pomegranate*, which associates it with Shekinah, the female aspect of Creation. Pomegranates feature prominently in many religions, including Islam, Judaism, Christianity, Buddhism, and Zoroastrianism. The fruit is the sigil of several British medical societies. The pomegranate symbolizes life, longevity, health, fecundity, knowledge, morality, immortality, spirituality, and divinity.[112]

NUTRIENT PROFILE

Pomegranate seed oil is unique due to its rich content of punicic acid, an omega-5 long-chain polyunsaturated fatty acid, and an isomer of alpha-linolenic acid. In several studies, punicic acid has demonstrated its potential as a chemopreventative agent for breast cancer.[114] Pomegranate seed oil may contain steroid hormones, including estrone, but the results are considered questionable;[115] it may contain only a trace of estrone.[116]

Pomegranate Seed Oil		
	Cold-Pressed[117, 118, 119]	**CO2 Extract**[120, 121, 122]
Saturated fatty acids		
Palmitic acid (C16:0)	3.19 - 3.54%	3.21 - 3.84%
Stearic acid (C18:0)	2.82 - 3.28%	2.1 - 3.19%
Monounsaturated fatty acids		
Oleic acid (C18:1 n-9)	5.7 - 6.38%	5.90 - 8.61%
Polyunsaturated fatty acids		
Linoleic acid (C18:2 n-6)	6.49 - 8.36%	6.00 - 11.85%
Punicic acid (C18:3 n-5)	**56.97 - 79.0%**	**66 - 73%**
Other conjugated linolenic acid isomers (CLnA) (C18:3)	6 - 22%	1 - 22%
Unsaponifiable fraction		
Sterols	**Total:** 4864 - 5938 mg/kg Beta-sitosterol (2999 - 3600 mg/kg), campesterol (474 - 589 mg/kg), stigmasterol (30 - 127 mg/kg)	**Total:** 0.46 - 0.98% Rich in Beta-sitosterol
Tocopherols	**Total:** 680 - 4950 mg/kg Gamma-tocopherol (1532 - 3361 mg/kg), delta-tocopherol (80 - 172 mg/kg), alpha-tocopherol (38 - 86 mg/kg)	**Total:** 2957.3 mg/kg Gamma-tocopherol (2774.1 mg/kg), delta-tocopherol (131.4 mg/kg), alpha-tocopherol (51.8 mg/kg)
Squalene	828 - 1449 mg/kg	0.085 - 0.13%

*Conjugated Linolenic Acids (CLnA) are all positional and geometric fatty acid isomers comprised of 18 carbons with 3 double bonds (octadecatrienoic acids). These molecules differ in the position of the double bonds (positional) and the double bonds' cis and trans configurations (geometric). Punicic, alpha-linolenic, and gamma-linolenic acids are the best known of the CLnA isomers.

Formulating with Pomegranate Seed Oil

Sensory info: Light red to yellow, light; mild, slightly nutty aroma

Absorption rate: Dry – readily absorbs into the skin

Dilution Cold-Pressed: Use at a 10 - 15% percent with other carrier oils. Can use in higher concentrations as needed.

Dilution CO2 Extract: Use at a 1 - 15% percent with other carrier oils. Can use in higher concentrations as needed.

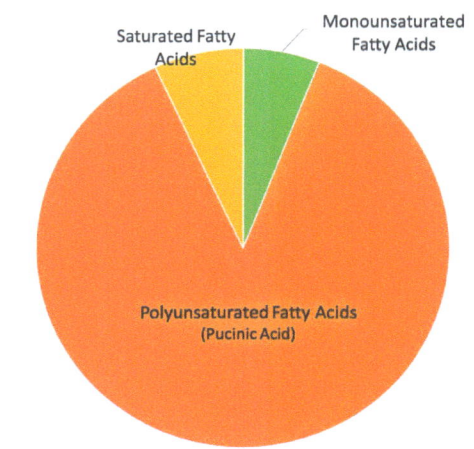

Note: It is best to add pomegranate seed oil only to a cool phase or near the end of skincare product preparation. Heat can damage its health benefits.

Antioxidant use: Recommend a 0.5% mixed tocopherols or rosemary CO_2 extract antioxidant to support shelf life and stability when using pomegranate seed oil in a formulation.

Therapeutic actions: anti-inflammatory, cellular regeneration, antioxidant, emollient

Therapeutic applications:
Pomegranate seed oil is an excellent anti-inflammatory[123] carrier oil, indicated for dermal inflammations such as acne, sunburn, psoriasis, and rosacea. Pomegranate seed oil supports cellular regeneration (specifically in the epidermis)[124] and combats free radicals (antioxidant activity). It may also be used to improve skin elasticity, revitalize premature aging or sun-damaged skin, and serve as a beneficial emollient for dry, irritated skin.

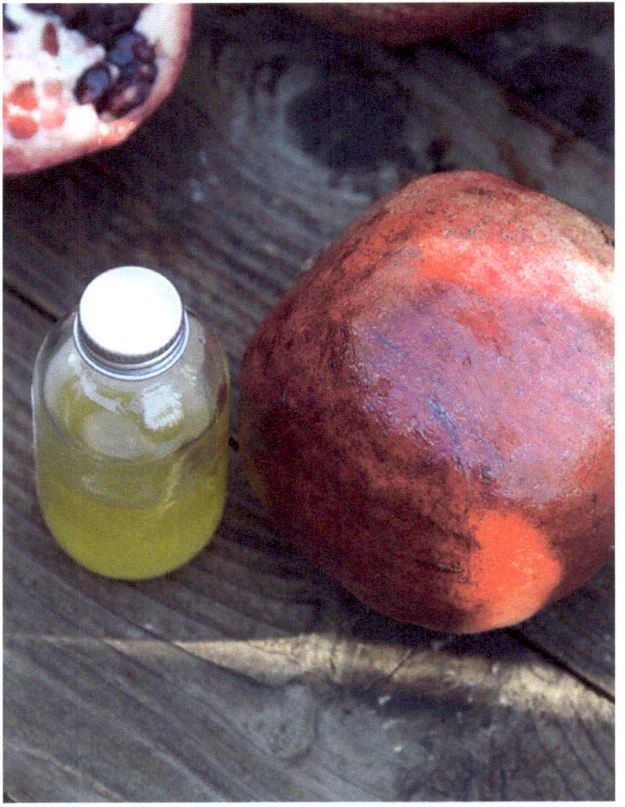

Pumpkin
Cucurbita maxima

Common name: Pumpkin
Scientific name: *Cucurbita maxima* Duchesne
Botanical family: Cucurbitaceae
Conservation status: Least concern[125]

Description: Pumpkins, a variety of winter squash in the Cucurbitaceae family, are best known for their mature, edible fruits, which usually grow on annual vines. The fruits are often large, around 9-18 pounds, but there is significant variability in size from small, weighing only a few pounds, to varieties of *C. maxima*, which can weigh more than 75 pounds. The fruits mature in early fall and are yellowish to orange, spherical or elliptical, with smooth, furrowed rinds.[126]

Ethnobotany: *Cucurbita* spp. have a long and widespread history of use as food and medicine. People worldwide have used the fruit, seeds, and leaves to relieve various internal and external ailments. For example, indigenous North Americans used pumpkin seeds to treat intestinal worms, high blood pressure, urinary maladies, kidney stones, and prostate disorders. In southeastern Europe, pumpkin seeds have been used to relieve irritable bladder issues and prostate enlargement, and Italians have applied the seed oil topically for healing wounds.[127]

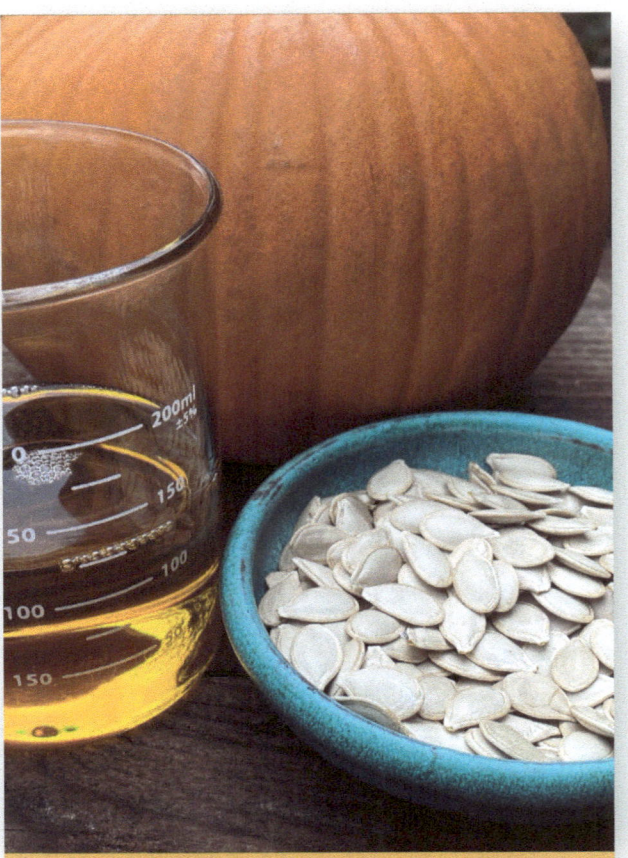

EXTRACTION INFORMATION

Country of origin: China
Part of plant: Seed
Oil content: 34 - 44%
Extraction method: Expeller pressing, Cold pressing, SFE CO2

MANUFACTURING INFORMATION

CAS number: 8016-49-7
EC number: 289-741-0
INCI name: Cold-pressed oil: Cucurbita Pepo (Pumpkin) Seed Oil
CosIng (functions): Skin conditioning, Skin conditioning - emollient

SHELF LIFE

12 months[128]

NUTRIENT PROFILE

Pumpkin Seed Oil[129, 130, 131]	
SATURATED FATTY ACIDS	
Palmitic acid (C16:0)	11 - 17.4.0%
Stearic acid (C18:0)	5.27 - 7.3%
MONOUNSATURATED FATTY ACIDS	
Oleic acid (C18:1 n-9)	27.52 - 38.0%
POLYUNSATURATED FATTY ACIDS	
Linoleic acid (C18:2 n-6)	53.19 - 65.0%
Alpha-linolenic acid (C18:3 n-3)	Tr - 1.27%
UNSAPONIFIABLE FRACTION approx. 2.8-3.8%	
Sterols 1894.8 - 8052 mg/kg	Sitosterol (506.4 - 1163.3 mg/kg), delta-5,24-stigmastadienol (272.5 - 799 mg/kg), delta-7-avenasterol (63 - 757 mg/kg), stigmasterol (8.2 - 31.7 mg/kg)
Tocopherols 2069 - 4264 mg/kg	Gamma-tocopherol (334.54 - 1136.6 mg/kg), alpha-tocopherol (84.9 - 1280 mg/kg), delta-tocopherol (70.2 - 177 mg/kg)
Squalene	5913 - 6325 mg/kg
Pigments	Carotenoids (5.4 - 6 mg/kg), chlorophyll (0.46 - 1.37 mg/kg)

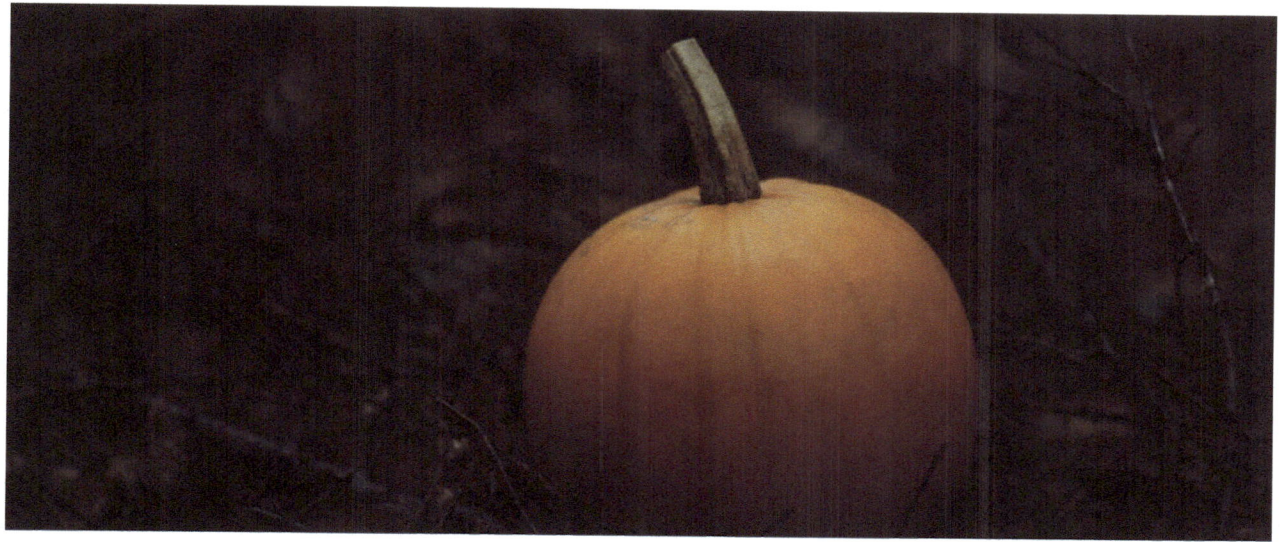

Formulating with Pumpkin Seed Oil

Sensory info: Dark green to brown color
Absorption rate: Dry – readily absorbs into the skin
Dilution: Use at 20 - 50% in a blend of other carrier oils

Note: It is best to add pumpkin seed oil only to a cool phase or near the end of skincare product preparation. Heat can damage its health benefits.

Antioxidant use: Recommend a 0.5% mixed tocopherols or rosemary CO2 extract antioxidant to support shelf life and stability when using pumpkin seed oil in a formulation.

Therapeutic actions: anti-inflammatory, wound healing, emollient, skin conditioning

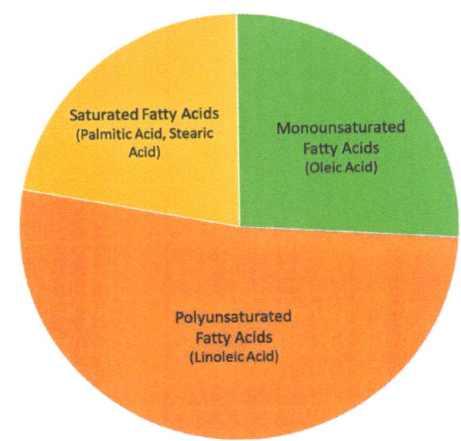

Therapeutic applications:
Studies on the internal use of pumpkin seed oil have shown positive results combatting depression, pattern baldness in men, lowering cholesterol, improving urinary tract health, and decreasing the symptoms of menopause.[132, 133]

One small clinical study, which, unfortunately, does not offer a good description of the methods used, showed a decrease in the number of acne blemishes and scarring after topical applications of pumpkin seed oil.[134] Pumpkin seed oil's effectiveness against acne may be due to its anti-inflammatory activity and wound healing support. At least one *in vivo* study has demonstrated topical application of a pumpkin seed oil blend can significantly decrease inflammation.[135] It can be effective in various wound healing applications, especially in the case of burns.[136]

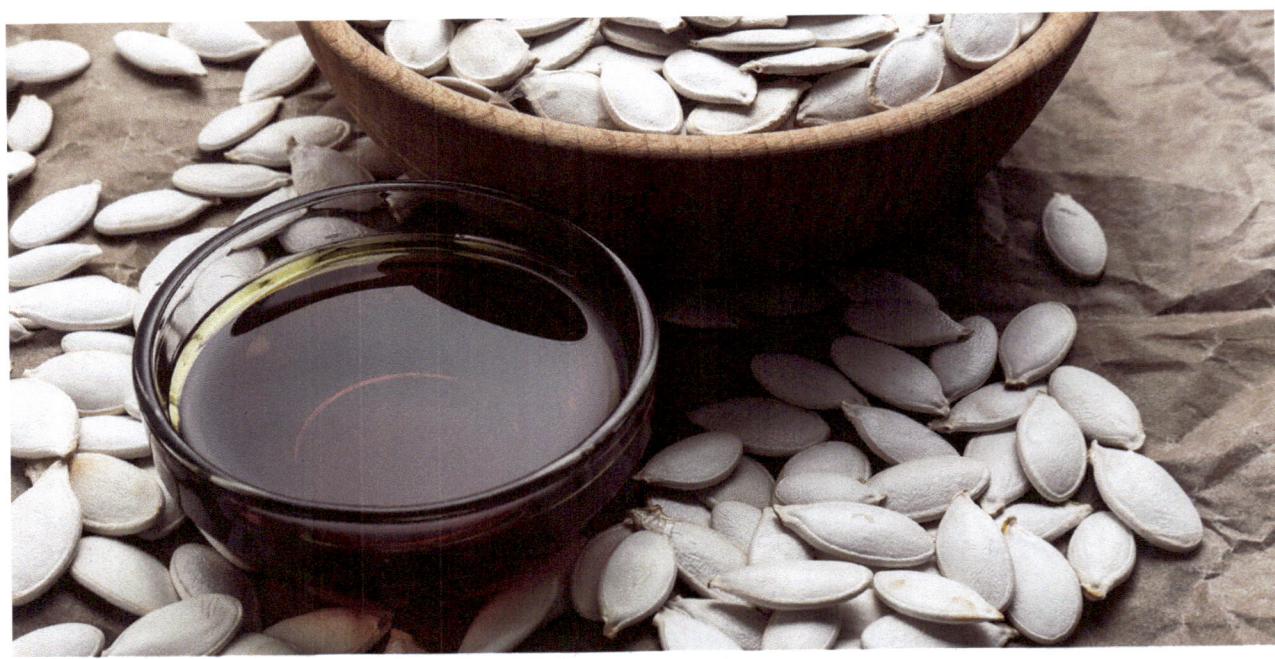

Raspberry
Rubus idaeus

Common names: Raspberry
Scientific name: *Rubus idaeus* L.
Botanical family: Rosaceae
Conservation status: Not assessed

Description: Red raspberry is a thicket-forming deciduous shrub in the Rosaceae family, growing wild in open woods, ravines, heaths, stream banks, bluffs, and wooded mountain slopes. There are two prominent varieties of *Rubus idaeus*: *R. idaeus* var. *idaeus*, the European raspberry native to Eurasia, and *R. idaeus* var. *strigosa*, the American red raspberry native to North America, where its range extends from Alaska and Canada south to California, Oklahoma, and North Carolina.

Red raspberry typically grows 3-9 ft. tall, with prickly cane-like stems. Leaves are alternate and commonly divided into 3 - 5 leaflets. These are arranged pinnately, pedately, or palmately (less common). First-year stems bear only leaves; in the second-year lateral branches produce leaves, flowers, and fruits. Flowers are white, sometimes pink or rosy-purple, usually borne in clusters, racemes, or panicles, although occasionally they are solitary. Each flower has five petals, five sepals, five bracts, many stamens, and a cluster of pistils positioned on its cone-shaped receptacle. Red raspberry blooms in spring, followed by fruits that ripen in summer. Contrary to their name, these fruits are not technically berries. Instead, they are aggregations of tiny drupelets that, once picked, resemble a hollow cone.

The genus name *Rubus* is the Latin name for "brambles" (both blackberry and raspberry), and the specific epithet means "of Mt. Ida," an allusion to the notion that raspberries were first discovered on the Greek Mt. Ida.[137]

Ethnobotany: Raspberry fruits are valued as a food, and raspberry leaf has a history of medicinal usage. In Europe, raspberry leaf has been used to treat menstrual disorders, stimulate and facilitate labor, and ease

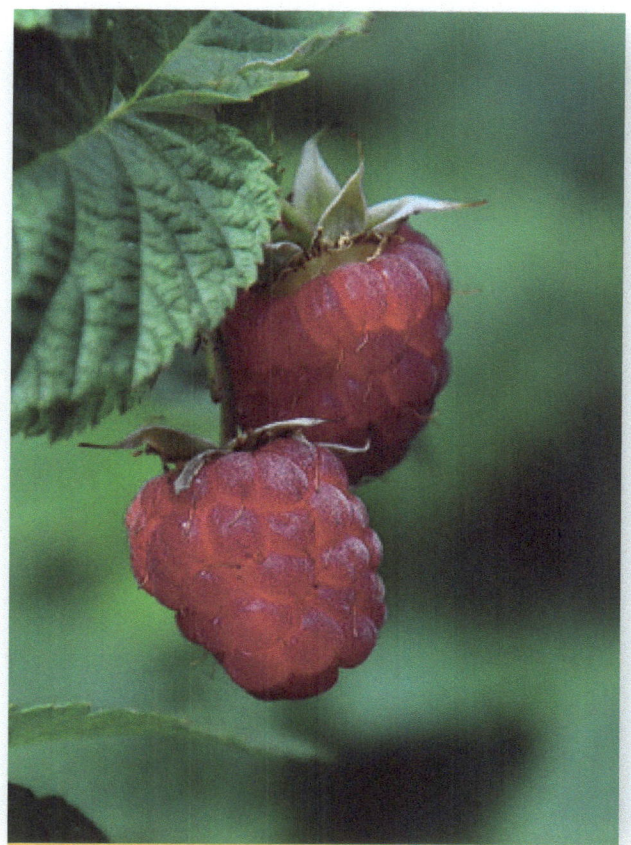

EXTRACTION INFORMATION

Country of origin: Chile, Poland
Part of plant: Seed
Extraction method: Cold pressing, Supercritical CO2 extract
Oil yield (SFE CO2): 20 - 23%
Color: Light yellow

MANUFACTURING INFORMATION

CAS number: 381718-28-1
EC number: 284-554-0
INCI name:
  Cold-pressed oil: Rubus Idaeus (Raspberry) Seed Oil
  CO2 extract: Rubus Idaeus (Raspberry) Seed Extract
CosIng (functions): Skin conditioning, Emollient

SHELF LIFE

6 - 12 months
* Store in the refrigerator.

gastrointestinal tract ailments, including diarrhea. Raspberry leaf tea has been used to treat conjunctivitis and chronic skin conditions and as an astringent gargle.[138]

NUTRIENT PROFILE

Raspberry seed oil is rich in linoleic acid and alpha-linolenic acid.

Raspberry Seed Oil		
	Cold-Pressed[139, 140, 141]	**CO2 Extract**[142, 143, 144, 145]
SATURATED FATTY ACIDS		
Palmitic acid (C16:0)	2.43 - 4.19%	2.2 - 2.74%
Stearic acid (C18:0)	0.90 - 1.19%	0.76 - 0.94%
MONOUNSATURATED FATTY ACIDS		
Oleic acid (C18:1 n-9)	10.0-13.0%	11.80 - 13.3%
POLYUNSATURATED FATTY ACIDS		
Linoleic acid (C18:2 n-6)	49.0 - 55.0%	48.0 - 59%
Alpha-linolenic acid (C18:3 n-3)	24 - 33.0%	24.0 - 29.0%
UNSAPONIFIABLE FRACTION (COLD-PRESSED)		
Sterols 5384.1 mg/kg	Sitosterol (3309.2 - 3374.6 mg/kg), 24-methylene-cycloartenol (505.7 - 540.9 mg/kg), cycloartenol (428.6 - 4 71 mg/kg), sitostanol (346.2 - 383 mg/kg), campesterol (234.5 - 274.9 mg/kg), citrostadienol (142.8 - 150.2 mg/kg), delta-7-stigmasterol (89.1 - 100.3 mg/kg), avenasterol (77.9 - 82.7 mg/kg), delta-7-avenasterol (61.4 - 71.8 mg/kg)	
Tocopherols 2951.9 - 3019.2 mg/kg	Gamma-tocopherol (1323 - 2720 mg/kg), alpha-tocopherol (461 - 710 mg/kg), delta-tocopherol (71 - 321.7 mg/kg)	
Squalene	84 mg/kg	
Note: Many suppliers add 0.1% organic rosemary CO2 as an antioxidant to stabilize the CO2 extract.		

Formulating with Raspberry Seed Oil

Sensory info: sweet, light raspberry aroma
Absorption rate: Dry – readily absorbs into skin
Dilution for Cold-pressed and CO2 extract: Can be used 1 - 5% in a blend of other carrier oils. Increase concentration as desired.

Note: It is best to add red raspberry seed oil only to a cool phase or near the end of skincare product preparation. Heat can damage its health benefits.

Antioxidant use: Recommend a 0.5% mixed tocopherols or rosemary CO2 extract antioxidant to support shelf life and stability when using red raspberry seed oil in a formulation.

Therapeutic actions: antioxidant, anti-inflammatory

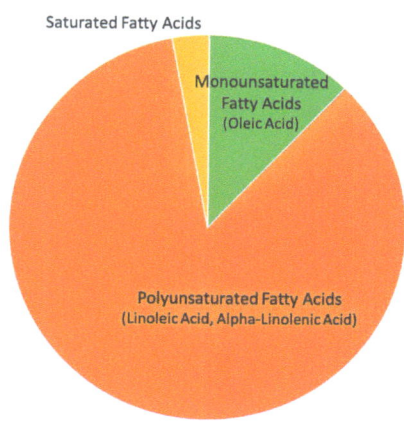

Therapeutic applications:
Raspberry seed oil, CO2 and cold-pressed, is an excellent enhancer carrier oil that benefits the skin by improving hydration, reducing TEWL, and softening the skin. Raspberry seed oil also has antioxidant and anti-inflammatory activity due to its content of tocopherols and phytosterols. Raspberry seed oil strengthens the lipid layer of the epidermis and improves the functioning of the sebaceous glands. It is also mildly photoprotective, demonstrating, *in vitro*, both UV scattering and UV absorbance properties.[146]

Raspberry seed oil is beneficial for inflamed skin conditions, tissue regeneration (scars, skin burns, etc.), premature aging, dry skin, preventative aging (antioxidant), acne, and oily skin. It is an appropriate ingredient in facial oils and serums.

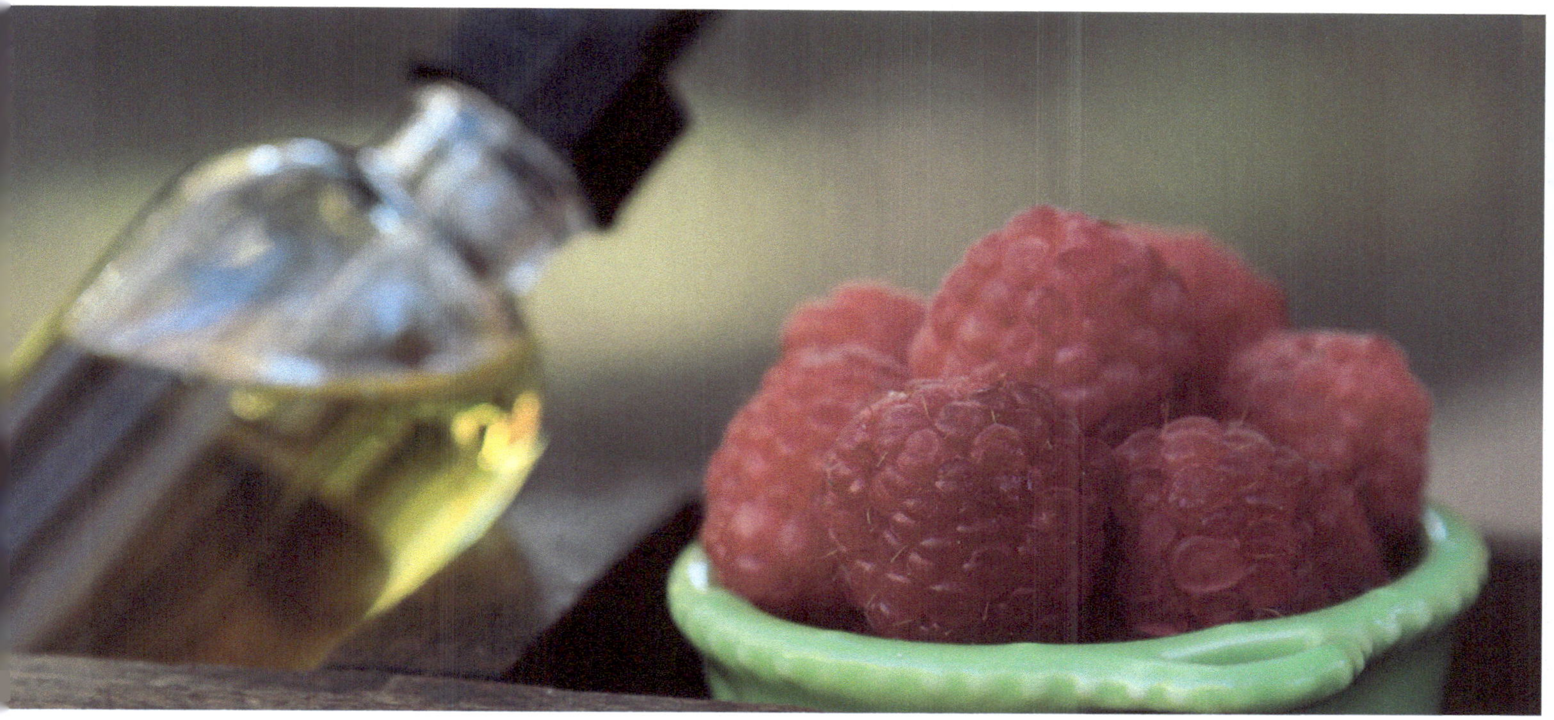

Rose
Rosa spp.

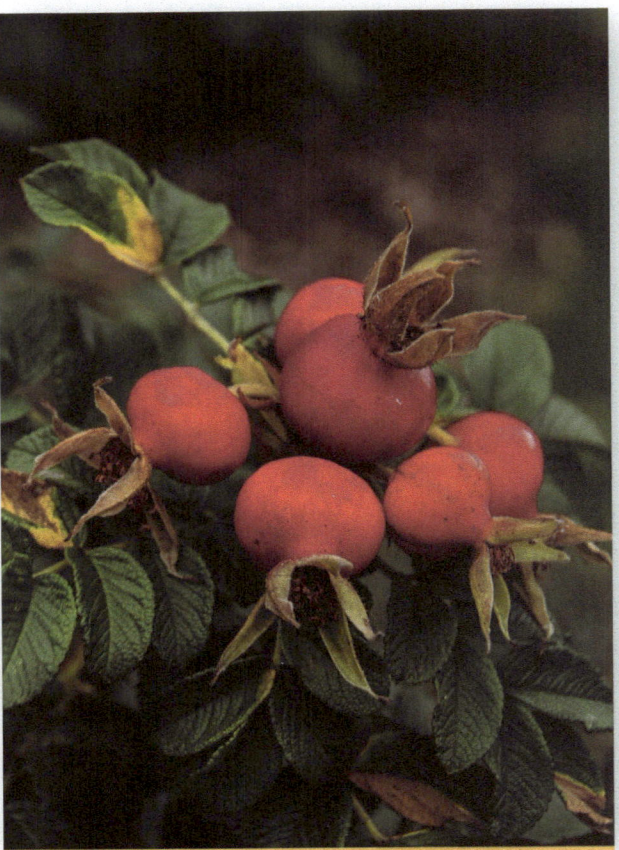

Common names: Rosehip, sweet briar rose, eglantine rose
Scientific name: *Rosa rubiginosa* L.
Synonym: *Rosa eglanteria* L.
Botanical family: Rosaceae
Conservation status: Not yet assessed

Common name: Dog rose
Scientific name: *Rosa canina* L.

Description: The *Rosa* genus contains over 100 species of perennial shrubs in the Rosaceae family that typically grow in temperate regions of the Northern Hemisphere. The majority of rose species are native to Asia, with some endemic to North America, Europe, and Northwest Africa. Roses readily hybridize, leading to some taxonomic confusion.

Rose plants are erect, climbing, or trailing shrubs with thorny stems. Leaves are both alternate and pinnately compound, with serrated oval leaflets. The flowers of wild roses are characterized by five petals, whereas cultivated roses feature multiple sets of petals. The flowers display a wide range of sizes, from 1.25-17.5 cm in diameter. The fleshy fruit, known as a hip, is the floral cup or cup-shaped tube formed by the union of the plant's calyx, corolla, and stamens. These are typically red to orange in color when ripe.

Rosa rubiginosa, commonly known as sweet briar or eglantine rose, is a European rose species that escaped gardens and naturalized in pastures and along roadsides. It is widely known in the Americas, where it also flourished. *R. rubiginosa* features dark green aromatic foliage redolent of apples. The hips, oranged-red and abundant, ripen in fall and typically persist well into winter. The specific epithet *rubiginosa* is from Latin, meaning "rusty."[147]

Rosa canina, known as the dog rose, got its name from Pliny the Elder (23 – 79 BC), who recommended the root to treat dog bites. Dog rose is endemic to Europe, and sailors consumed its hips to ward off scurvy. Due

EXTRACTION INFORMATION[151, 152]

Rosa rubiginosa
Country of origin: South Africa, Chile, Europe
Part of plant: Seed
Oil yield: 30 - 40%
Extraction method: Cold pressing

Rosa canina
Country of origin: South Africa, Chile, Europe
Extraction method: SFE CO_2
Oil yield (SFE CO_2): 5.72 - 16.5%
Extraction: Cold pressing
Oil yield (Cold pressing): 5 - 18%

MANUFACTURING INFORMATION

CAS number: 92347-25-6
EC number: 296-213-3
INCI name: Cold-pressed oil: Rosa Rubiginosa Seed Oil **CO_2 extract:** Rosa Rubiginosa Seed Extract
CosIng (functions): Skin conditioning – Emollient

to the high vitamin C content, *R. canina* was valued as a dietary supplement and spread worldwide. During WWII, the British government organized massive harvests of *R. canina* as a crucial source of vitamin C for the malnourished populace. The seed oil of *R. canina* is rich in flavonoids, and many countries use it in preparations to protect the skin from UV-B damage.[148]

Ethnobotany: One finds rosehips in preserves, beverages, soups, syrups, desserts, and wine. They are used for their flavor and their high vitamin C content.[149] In northeastern Portugal, the fruit is eaten raw. Decoctions or brandy macerations are employed as a tonic and used to treat internal and cutaneous ailments. In rural communities in the Cantabria region of northern Spain, rosehips are ingredients in cakes and spirits.

In traditional medicine, rosehips were valued for their astringency and used to relieve diarrhea, dysentery, thirst, cough, and hemoptysis (spitting up blood). 17th-century English herbalist, Nicholas Culpeper, recommended a conserve of ripe rosehips to relieve diarrhea and promote healthy digestion. He recommended dried, powdered hips to break up stones, promote urination, and relieve colic.[150]

Two Species: Equal Nourishment

Rosehip seed oil has recently become a popular ingredient in creams, lotions, facial oils, and massage oils. The oil is valued for being a gentle, "dry" emollient that does not leave a greasy residue on the skin. Rosehip seed oil is typically extracted by cold pressing the seeds or using a supercritical carbon dioxide extraction process. *Rosa canina* is the most common rose species used in CO2 extractions, while *Rosa rubiginosa* is typically cold-pressed. Both species have similar lipid profiles and can be used interchangeably. The CO2 extract may also come from the fruit pulp and the seed. The chemical profile of the fruit pulp is almost identical to the seed alone.

Picture on previous page: *Rosa rubiginosa*
Picture on right: *Rosa canina*

CAS number: 84696-47-9 (Rosa canina extract, including seed oil)
EC number: 283-652-0
INCI name:
  Cold-pressed oil: Rosa Canina Seed Oil
  CO2 extract: Rosa Canina Seed Extract
CosIng (functions): Skin conditioning – emollient

SHELF LIFE

- **Cold-pressed:** 6-12 months
- **CO2 extract:** 6-12 months

* Store in the refrigerator.

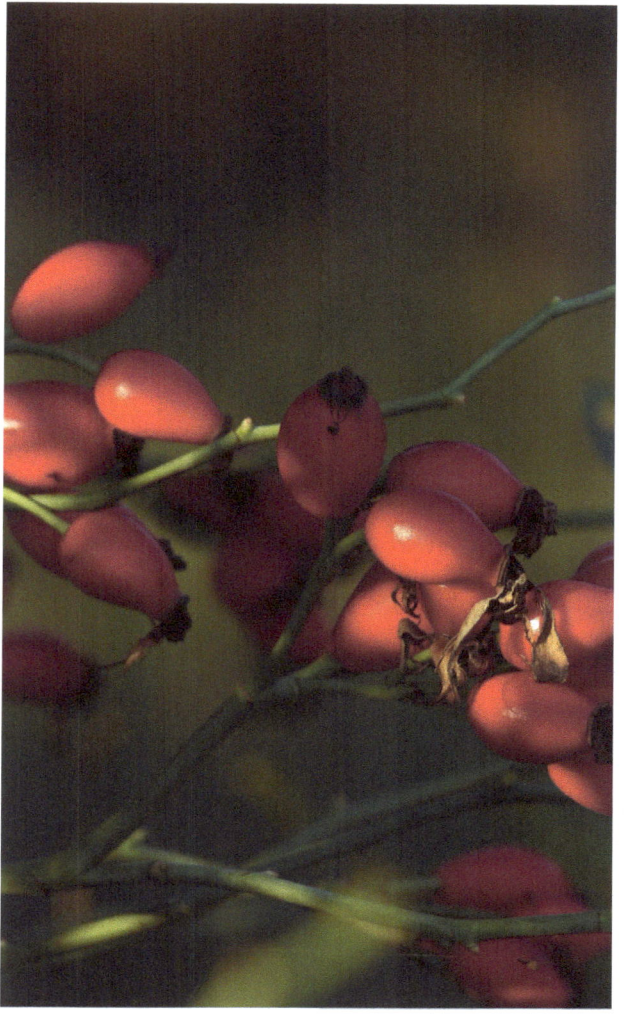

NUTRIENT PROFILE

Rosehip seed oil is rich in the essential fatty acids and sterols.

\multicolumn{3}{c}{**Rosehip (*R. rubignosa* and *R. canina*) Seed Oil**}		
\multicolumn{3}{c}{*R. canina* and *R. rubiginosa* have very similar profiles combined here.}		
Fatty acid composition	**Cold-Pressed**[151,153,154,155,156]	**CO2 Extract**[157,158,159]
SATURATED FATTY ACIDS		
Palmitic acid (C16:0)	3.6 - 4.8%	2 - 6%
Stearic acid (C18:0)	1.8 - 3%	<5%
MONOUNSATURATED FATTY ACIDS		
Oleic acid (C18:1 n-9)	14 - 17%	12 - 22%
POLYUNSATURATED FATTY ACIDS		
Linoleic acid (C18:2 n-6)	43 - 51.7%	41 - 59%
Alpha-linolenic acid (C18:3 n-3)	21 - 34%	20 - 35%
UNSAPONIFIABLE FRACTION (COLD-PRESSED)		
Sterols 4835.1 - 5837.3 mg/kg	Beta-sitosterol (715.1 - 2251.4 mg/kg), delta-5-avenasterol (269 - 361 mg/kg), campesterol (85.2 - 197.1 mg/kg), delta-7-avenasterol (55.8 - 145.7 mg/kg), stigmasterol (5.2 - 94.8 mg/kg)	
Tocopherols 866.9 - 1159.9 mg/kg	Gamma-tocopherol (533 - 683.4 mg/kg), delta-tocopherol (237.4 - 311.9 mg/kg), alpha-tocopherol (81.0 - 164.6 mg/kg)	
Carotenoids	81 - 90 mg/kg	
Squalene	151.5 - 214.9 mg/kg	
All-*trans*-retinoic acid (natural precursor of Vitamin A)	0.375 mg/L oil	

Formulating with Rosehip Seed Oil

Sensory info: Rich golden to yellow, light; mild, slightly nutty aroma
Absorption rate: Dry – readily absorbs into the skin
Dilution Cold-Pressed: Use at a 10 - 25% percent with other carrier oils. Can use in higher concentrations as needed or desired.
Dilution CO2 Extract: Can be used 1 - 2.5% in a blend of other carrier oils.

Note: It is best to add rosehip seed oil only to a cool phase or near the end of skincare product preparation. Heat can damage its health benefits.

Antioxidant use: Recommend a 0.5% mixed tocopherols or rosemary CO2 extract antioxidant to support shelf life and stability when using rosehip seed oil in a formulation.

Therapeutic actions: tissue regeneration, wound healing, antioxidant, anti-inflammatory, addresses EFA deficiency, emollient

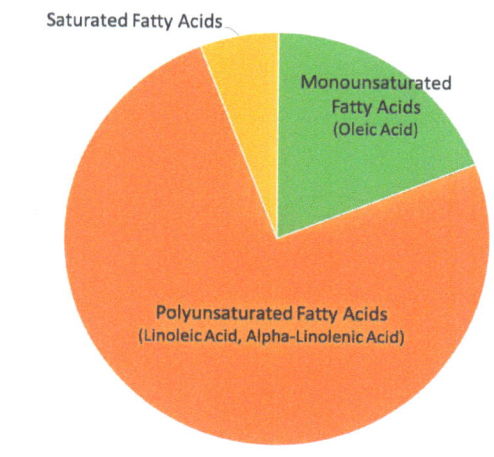

Therapeutic applications:
Rosehip seed oil is rich in linoleic and alpha-linolenic acids, which contribute to the oil's anti-inflammatory and cellular regeneration activity as well as its ability to prevent TEWL.[160] Rosehip seed oil is suitable to include in formulations to address EFA deficiency. Linoleic acid also strengthens collagen fibers, which may help with wound healing, skin burns, and premature aging.

As one of the best tissue regenerators, rosehip seed oil has shown an exceptional ability to reduce the hyperpigmentation and appearance of scars.[15] Rosehip seed oil is also indicated for reducing photoaging.[161]

Rosehip seed oil addresses inflamed skin conditions, so it is an appropriate ingredient for the treatment of eczema, trophic ulcers of the skin, cheilitis (inflammation of the lips or dry, chapped lips).[162]

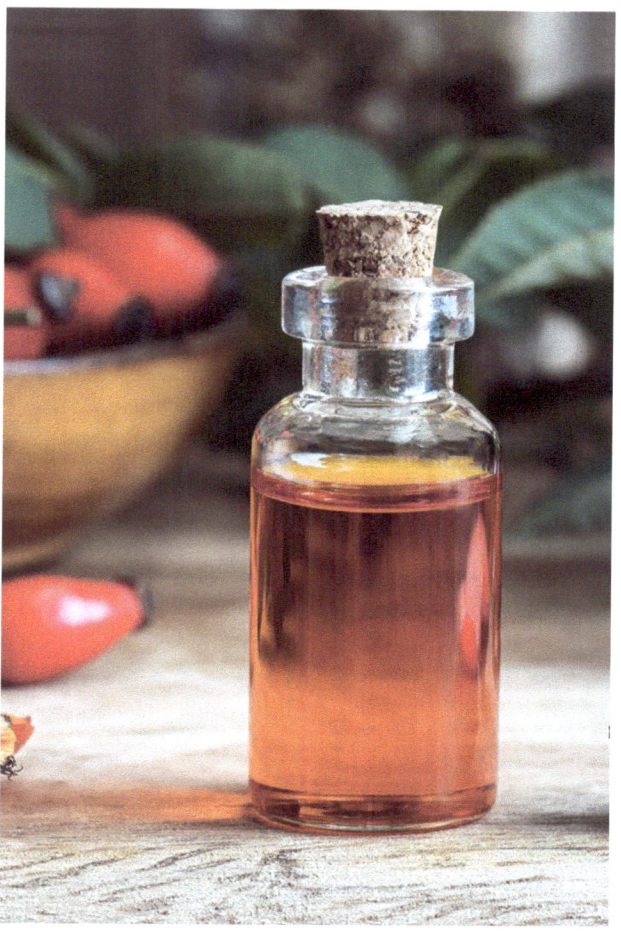

Sacha Inchi
Plukenetia volubilis

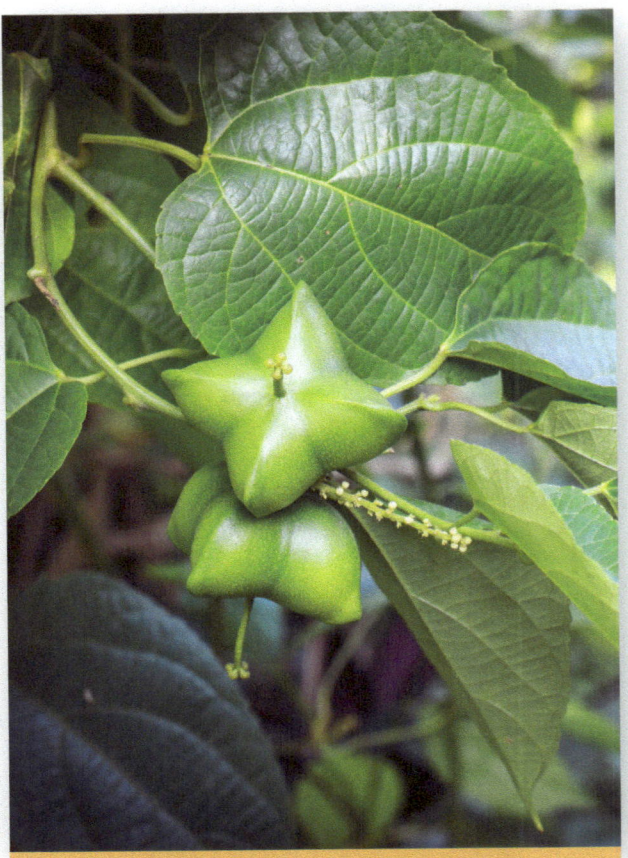

Common name: Sacha inchi, Incan-peanut, Inca nut, sacha peanut, mountain peanut
Scientific name: *Plukenetia volubilis* L.
Synonyms: *Fragariopsis paxii* Pittier, *Plukenetia macrostyle* Ule, *Plukenetia peruviana* Müll.Arg., *Sajorium volubile* (L.) Baill.[163, 164]
Botanical family: Euphorbiaceae
Conservation status: Not yet assessed

Description: Sacha inchi or Inca nut is native to South America and the Lesser Antilles, growing at higher altitudes in the tropical areas of Suriname, Venezuela, Bolivia, Colombia, Ecuador, Peru, and Brazil. Thailand cultivates the plant commercially. The species is divided into two groups with slightly different leaf blade, seed, and fruit morphologies; these may be identified as separate species in the future.

Sacha inchi's common name comes from the variations in the local Amazonian dialects. "*Sacha*" refers to "mountain" or "resembling," and "*inchi*" means "groundnut or peanut."

P. volubilis is a perennial, monecious, short, semi-woody, climbing shrub in the spurge family Euphorbiaceae. The palmate leaves are elongated triangles with three to five primary veins with two nectaries sitting at the base of each leaf blade. The pistillate and staminate flowers are separate. Pistillate flower inflorescences contain one or two flowers at the base of a stem, while the plant grows copious staminate flowers. The flowers are light yellow or cream-colored.

Wild plant ovaries have four carpels, while cultivated plants may have five or six carpels. The style grows four lobes at the top. The fruit is also divided into four parts, each containing one flattened, round seed, approximately 1.8 x 0.8 x 1.6 cm. The dried fruit looks like a star anise pod.

Ethnobotany: Archeologists have found depictions of *Plukenetia volubilis* on pottery in Incan tombs, suggesting that it was a well-known and prized plant over 3000 years ago. Today, local indigenous people

EXTRACTION INFORMATION

Country of origin: Peru (Colombia, Ecuador, Thailand, China, Myanmar, and Laos)
Part of plant: Seed
Oil content: 35 - 60%[164]
Extraction method: Expeller pressing

MANUFACTURING INFORMATION

CAS number: 68956-68-3
EC number: 282-015-4/273-313-5
INCI name: Plukenetia Volubilis (Sacha Inchi) Seed Oil
CosIng (functions): Humectant, Skin protecting, Emollient

SHELF LIFE

9 months - 24 months from extraction[166, 167]

from the region cook the leaves and seeds and use the oil they extract from the seeds in their food. They roast the seeds, eat the fresh leaves, and use the leaves for tea. They eat the roasted seeds individually or as ingredients in other dishes. Indigenous people also value ground *P. volubilis* seeds and seed oil for skincare, skin infection or injury, muscle pain, rheumatism, and bug bites.[165]

NUTRIENT PROFILE

Sacha inchi oil chemistry may vary noticeably from one batch to another, as there is significant genetic and morphological diversity in the plant populations. However, it is characteristic of authentic sacha inchi oil to have a linoleic to alpha-linolenic fatty acid ratio of approximately 1:1, a relatively low saturated fatty acid content (6 - 9%), beta-sitosterol comprising approximately half of the sterols, carotenoid content approximately 1 mg/kg, and a significant portion of gamma-tocopherol.

Sacha Inchi Oil[168, 169, 170, 171, 172]	
SATURATED FATTY ACIDS	
Palmitic acid (C16:0)	3.74-11%
Stearic acid (C18:0)	2-4%
MONOUNSATURATED FATTY ACIDS	
Oleic acid (C18:1 n-9)	9-23%
POLYUNSATURATED FATTY ACIDS	
Linoleic acid (C18:2 n-6)	21-53%
Alpha-linolenic acid (C18:3 n-3)	10-55%
UNSAPONIFIABLE FRACTION	
Sterols 1623-2899 mg/kg	Beta-sitosterol (736.2 - 1879 mg/kg), stigmasterol (220.2 - 764.5 mg/kg), campesterol (101.4-414.4 mg/kg), delta-5-avenasterol (41.3 - 213.7 mg/kg), delta-7-avenasterol (n.d. - 72.7 mg/kg)
Tocopherols 700-3300 mg/kg	Gamma-tocopherol (568 - 1879 mg/kg), delta-tocopherol (259 - 1387 mg/kg), alpha-tocopherol (0.8 - 194 mg/kg)
Carotenoids 0.31 - 2.94 mg/kg	Beta-carotene (0.7 - 0.9 mg/kg)

Formulating with Sacha Inchi Oil

Sensory info: clear, pale-to-dark yellow liquid; light texture; mild-to-moderate, nutty fragrance
Absorption rate: Light - absorbs quickly
Dilution: May be used up to 100%

Antioxidant use: Recommend a 0.5% mixed tocopherols or rosemary CO2 extract antioxidant to support shelf life and stability when using sacha inchi oil in a formulation.

Therapeutic actions: anti-inflammatory,[173] addresses EFA deficiency, antibacterial (*S. aureus*), antioxidant, skin repair

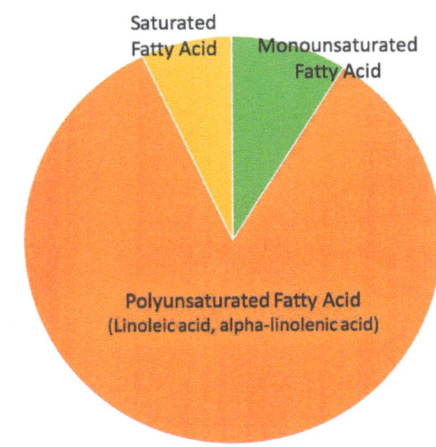

Therapeutic applications:
Sacha inchi oil has two characteristics that make it a highly prized oil. It has one of the highest proportions of essential fatty acids (EFA), approximately 80%. The EFAs are divided fairly evenly, with about half linoleic and half alpha-linolenic fatty acids. Sacha inchi oil also contains relatively high tocopherol, phenol, and carotenoid contents, providing the oil with considerable antioxidant capacity and oxidative stability to protect the high percentage of PUFAs.

The high proportion of antioxidants and PUFAs make sacha inchi oil an excellent choice for inflamed or UV-exposed skin. Sacha inchi oil is helpful for all skin types, but it is particularly effective for dry,[174] mature skin,[175] promoting an even skin tone while calming itch and irritation. It is a preferred ingredient in anti-aging products.

Sacha inchi oil is also an excellent ally for hair health. It can be included in products to discourage hair loss, and when blended in a hair conditioner, sacha inchi can help protect hair from breakage.

An *in vitro* study demonstrated that the application of sacha inchi oil to human skin blocked *Staphylococcus aureus* from sticking,[176] suggesting it might be appropriate for bacterial skin infections and acne.

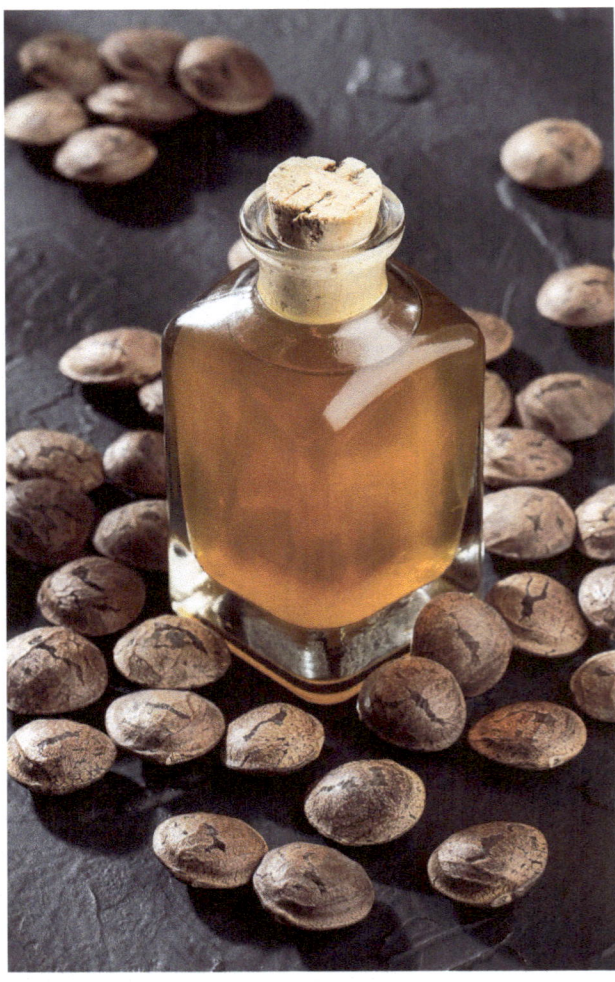

Sea Buckthorn
Hippophaë rhamnoides

Common name: Sea buckthorn, Siberian pineapple, sandthorn, sallowthorn, seaberry
Scientific name: *Hippophaë rhamnoides* L.
Synonym: *Elaeagnus rhamnoides* (L.) A. Nelson
Botanical family: Elaeagnaceae
Conservation status: Least concern, stable[177]

Description: Sea buckthorn is a thorny shrub in the Elaeagnaceae family. *Hippophae* species grow up to 7 meters tall, covered in a bark that may be smooth or cracked. Its long, lanceolate leaves are coated underneath with silvery hairs. The plant is dioecious, with green and brown flowers growing in racemes; male flowers are significantly larger than female flowers. The flowers produce oval, yellow or orange berries, 6 – 9 mm long, which ripen in September. Each orange berry contains a smooth, small stone covering an oily seed. The brown seeds are 2.8-4.2 mm long and have an oval shape with a shiny surface.

Sea buckthorn grows across much of the European and Asian continents, often in sandy soil and on or near mountains. *Hippophae* species are tolerant of drought, frost, and air pollution.

The genus name *Hippophae* arose in ancient Greece (*hippos* means "horse;" *phaos* is "shiny") due to the practice of feeding horses sea buckthorn fruits to render their coats lustrous and shiny. Sea buckthorn fruits are bitter and sour, with a fragrance akin to pineapple, and they are rich in vitamins C and A, as well as malic and citric acids.

Ethnobotany: Traditional systems of medicine have used *Hippophae* spp. to treat diarrhea, constipation, skin diseases, cough, jaundice, respiratory distress, high blood pressure, arthritis, and genital inflammation. Indian, Chinese, and Tibetan practitioners valued sea buckthorn fruits as a tonic for the gastrointestinal, respiratory, and circulatory systems, recording therapeutic effects in texts from the Tang (618-906 AD) and Qing dynasties (1644-1912) in China as well as in a Tibetan medicinal from early 900 AD. Russians used the berries and berry oil for treatments requiring

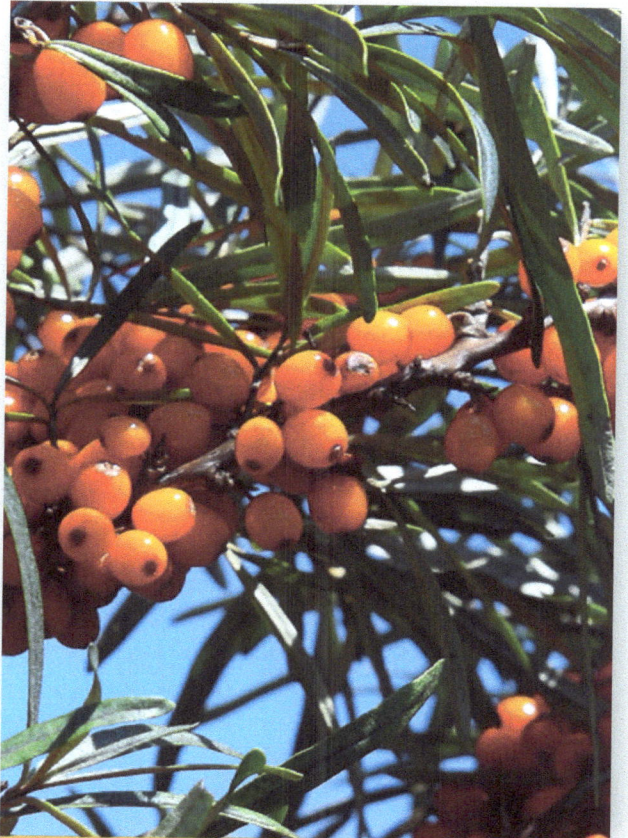

EXTRACTION INFORMATION

Note: Sea buckthorn oil has extracts from two different parts of the plant: seeds or fruit pulp.

Country of origin: South Africa, Chile, Europe

Part of plant: Seed
Extraction method: Cold pressing or CO2 extraction
Oil yield (Cold-Pressed): Dried seeds 7 - 15%, Fresh seeds 4 - 8%
Oil yield (SFE CO2): 8 - 20%

Part of plant: Fruit pulp
Extraction method: Cold pressing (screw press), SFE CO2, Aqueous extraction
Oil yield (Cold pressing): 8 - 12%
Oil yield (SFE CO2): Fresh pulp: 4 - 17%, dry pulp: 20 - 25%

skin regeneration, such as skin grafts, infections, burns, injuries, as well as digestive disorders, and uterine issues. More recently, sea buckthorn has become an important ingredient in cosmeceuticals for anti-aging and dry skin products.[178, 179]

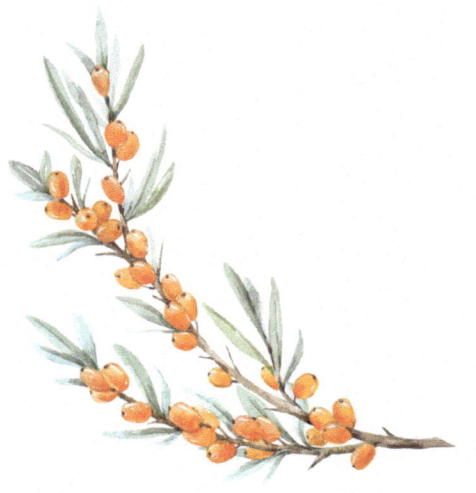

MANUFACTURING INFORMATION

CAS number: 225234-03-7
EC number: 607-094-8
INCI name:
    Cold-pressed oil: Hippophae Rhamnoides (Sea Buckthorn) Oil, Hippophae Rhamnoides Seed Oil, Hippophae Rhamnoides Fruit Oil
    CO_2 extract: Hippophae Rhamnoides (Sea Buckthorn) Extract, Hippophae Rhamnoides Seed Extract, Hippophae Rhamnoides Fruit Extract
CosIng (functions): Emollient, Skin conditioning

SHELF LIFE

- **Seeds:** 24 months (seeds)
- **Pulp:** 12 months (pulp)

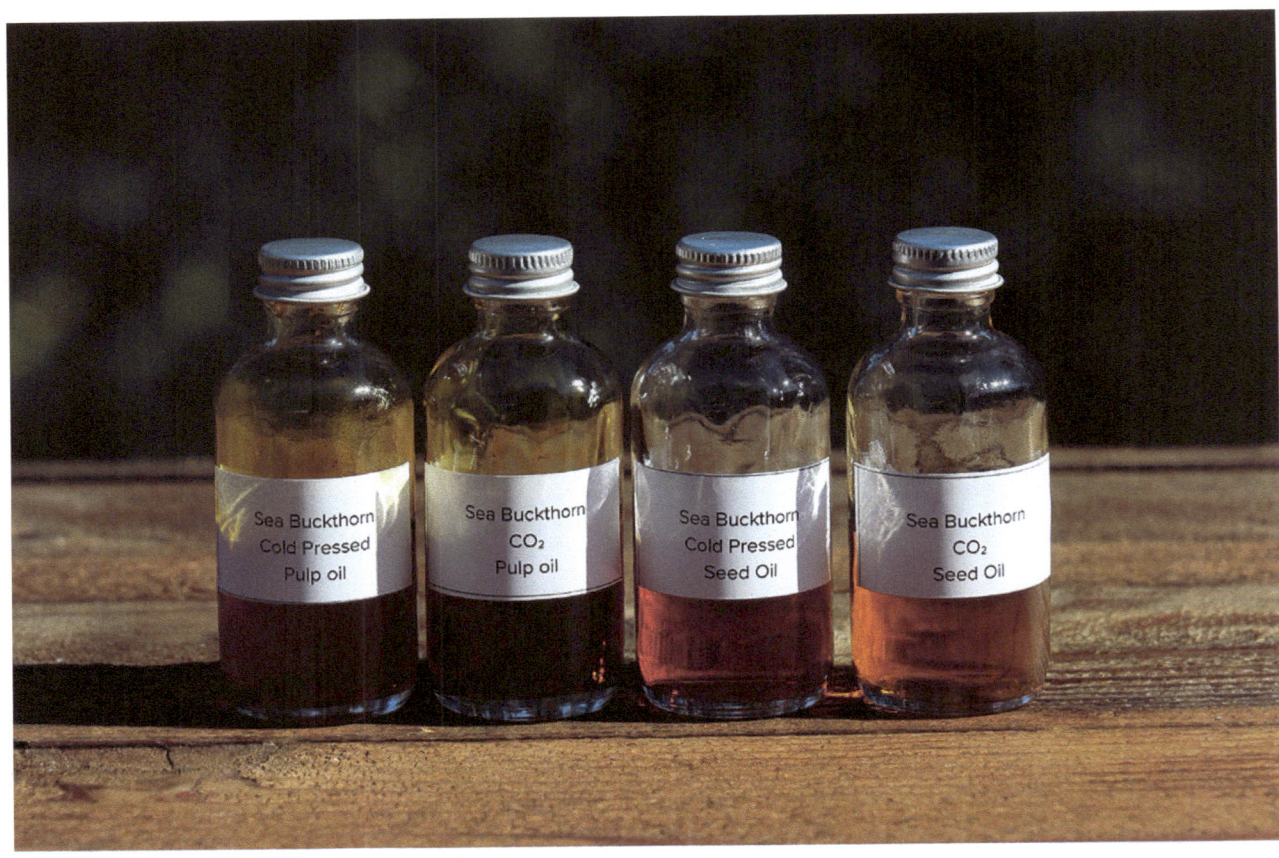

NUTRIENT PROFILE

Cold-pressed seed and pulp oils[14, 180, 181]
SFE CO2- extracted seed and pulp oils[180, 182, 183]

Sea buckthorn seed oil is rich in the essential fatty acids, carotenoids, and tocopherols.

Sea Buckthorn Seed Oil (dried seed)		
	CO2 Extract	Cold-Pressed
SATURATED FATTY ACIDS		
Palmitic acid (C16:0)	7.2 - 8.9%	6.5 - 6.9%
Stearic acid (C18:0)	1.9 - 2.4%	2.5%
MONOUNSATURATED FATTY ACIDS		
Oleic acid (C18:1 n-9)	13 - 20.3%	13%
POLYUNSATURATED FATTY ACIDS		
Linoleic acid (C18:2 n-6)	35.9 - 37.4%	35%
Alpha-linolenic acid (C18:3 n-3)	29.0 – 37.9%	38%
UNSAPONIFIABLE FRACTION		
Sterols[184]	Total: 1640 mg/kg Beta-sitosterol (647 - 787 mg/kg), delta-5-avenasterol (218 mg/kg), campesterol (198 - 240 mg/kg)	Total: 879 mg/kg Beta-sitosterol (465.9 -753 mg/kg), campesterol (87 – 287 mg/kg), delta-5-avenasterol (97.3 mg/kg)
Tocopherols	Total: 1700 - 4026 mg/kg Alpha-tocopherol (900 - 1967 mg/kg), gamma-tocopherol (800-1760 mg/kg), beta-tocopherol (112 - 121 mg/kg)	Total: 2736 - 2954 mg/kg Alpha-tocopherol (143.4 - 152.2 mg/kg), gamma-tocopherol (1231 - 1301 mg/kg), beta-tocopherol (81 mg/kg)
Carotenoids	277 - 545 mg/kg	151 - 154 mg/kg
NOTE: Sea buckthorn seed CO2 extract may contain 0.05% organic rosemary extract as an antioxidant.		

Formulating with Sea Buckthorn Seed Oil

Sensory info: Light orange-yellow to light red, sweet, nutty aroma
Absorption rate: Medium to dry - leaves a shine on the skin
Dilution: Can be used 1 - 5%

Note: It is best to add sea buckthorn oil only to a cool phase or near the end of skincare product preparation. Heat can damage its health benefits.

Therapeutic actions: anti-inflammatory, antioxidant, anticarcinogenic, antipruritic, cell regenerative, cytophylaxis, emollient, vulnerary

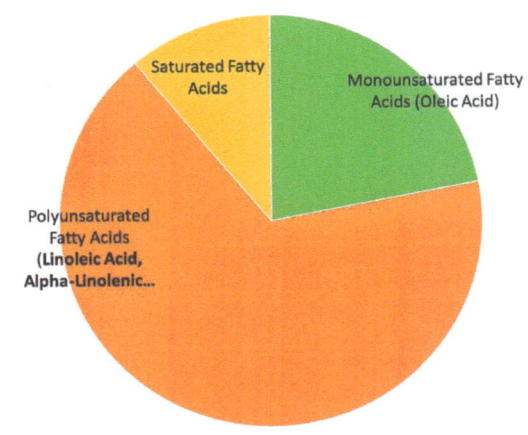

Therapeutic applications:
Sea buckthorn seed oil is widely used to promote skin recovery from various conditions, including eczema, burns, poorly healing wounds, skin damaged by the sun, and after radiation treatment.[186] It may strengthen the protective lipid barrier of the stratum corneum to guard against TEWL, making it suitable for dry, irritated, rough, flaking, or itchy skin. It may improve sebaceous gland functioning in oily or problematic skin types - unblocking pores and reducing the formation or number of blackheads.

It is appropriate to use sea buckthorn oil to promote tissue regeneration and counter inflammatory skin conditions in cosmetic products for cell anti-aging, microcirculation enhancement, antioxidant protection, epidermal regeneration, anti-inflammation, natural UV blocking, and sunscreen cosmetics.[187]

Other skin conditions that might benefit from sea buckthorn seed oil application are essential fatty acid deficiency, bedsores, slow-healing wounds, and burns, including sunburn.

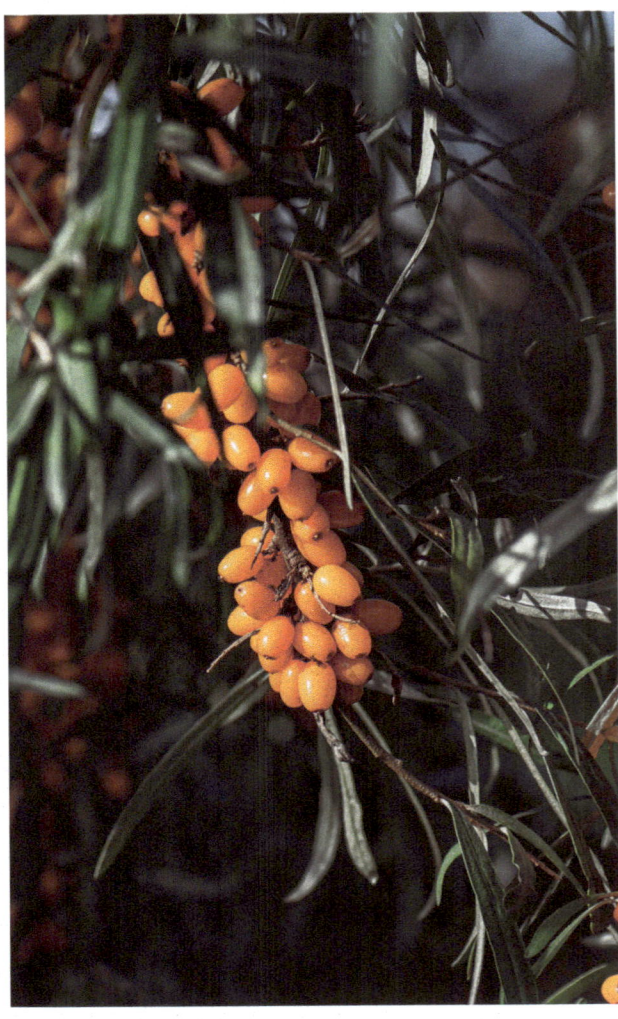

NUTRIENT PROFILE

Sea buckthorn pulp oil differs from sea buckthorn seed oil in its rich palmitic acid and palmitoleic acid content. The pulp oil also contains a remarkable percentage of carotenoids, making it a dark reddish-orange color.

	Sea Buckthorn Pulp Oil	
	CO2 Extract	Cold-Pressed
SATURATED FATTY ACIDS		
Palmitic acid (C16:0)	34.4 - 35.5%	28 - 40%
Stearic acid (C18:0)	1.1 - 1.33%	<2%
MONOUNSATURATED FATTY ACIDS		
Palmitoleic acid (C16:1 n-7)	20.26 - 36.3%	32 - 42%
Vaccenic acid (C18:1 n-7)	6.9%	
Oleic acid (C18:1 n-9)	3.5 - 31.91%	6 - 15% (includes vaccenic acid)
POLYUNSATURATED FATTY ACIDS		
Linoleic acid (C18:2 n-6)	7.09 - 12.4%	4 - 16%
Alpha-linolenic acid (C18:3 n-3)	1.2 - 3.18%	0.5 - 2.5%
Nervonic acid (C24:1 n-9)	0.8 - 1.1%	<1.5%
UNSAPONIFIABLE FRACTION[185]		
Sterols	Total: 6684 - 7711 mg/kg Beta-sitosterol (5125-5309 mg/kg), campesterol (109 mg/kg)	Total: 8494 - 8627 mg/kg Beta-sitosterol (6567 - 6629 mg/kg), delta-7 stigmasterol (1730 - 1782 mg/kg), campesterol (197-215 mg/kg)
Tocopherols	Total: 716.2 - 1700 mg/kg Alpha-tocopherol (359.9 - 1200 mg/kg), gamma-tocopherol (241.7 - 500) mg/kg	Total: 827.5 - 952.1 mg/kg Alpha-tocopherol (780 - 915 mg/kg), delta-tocopherol (36 - 46 mg/kg)
Carotenoids	1223 - 1484 mg/kg*	692 - 3420 mg/kg
Squalene		18.4 - 19.4 mg/kg

NOTE: Sea buckthorn seed CO2 extract may contain 0.05% organic rosemary extract as an antioxidant. *Rich carotenoid content is extracted with alcohol to increase the yield of carotenoids.

Formulating with Sea Buckthorn Pulp Oil

Sensory info: Rich reddish-orange color, sweet, nutty aroma

Absorption rate: Dry – readily absorbs into skin

Dilution: Can be used 1 - 2.5% in a blend of carrier oils. Oil may stain skin and clothing, especially at higher concentrations.

Note: It is best to add sea buckthorn oil only to a cool phase or near the end of skincare product preparation. Heat can damage its health benefits.

Antioxidant use: Recommend a 0.5% mixed tocopherols or rosemary CO2 extract antioxidant to support shelf life and stability when using sea buckthorn pulp oil in a formulation.

Therapeutic actions: analgesic, anti-inflammatory, antioxidant, anticarcinogenic, antipruritic, cell regenerative, cytophylaxis, emollient, gastroprotective, vulnerary

Therapeutic applications:

Topical use:[188, 189] Sea buckthorn pulp oil can strengthen the protective lipid barrier of the stratum corneum to guard against TEWL, making it suitable to address dry, irritated, rough, flaking, or itchy skin as well as sun-damaged skin. It is a suitable ingredient in anti-aging products. It can soothe inflammatory skin conditions like eczema, psoriasis, and atopic dermatitis. It can also relieve oral mucous membrane inflammation or damage and improve oral hygiene.[190]

Sea buckthorn may help with regenerative skincare needs, such as bedsores, wound healing, burns, and minimizing scars. It can also address skin infections and lighten areas of hyperpigmentation.

Internal use:[191, 192] Both traditional medicine and modern research have explored using sea buckthorn pulp oil internally as a treatment for a broad range of conditions from cardiovascular disease to dermatitis to arthritis to Sjögren's syndrome. It is a powerful internal antioxidant, can increase beneficial high-density lipoprotein (HDL) cholesterol levels in the blood, reduce symptoms of rheumatoid arthritis, support brain functions, and support bone health. It has demonstrated an ability to regulate immune function so that it may reduce the immune-suppressive effects of chemotherapy treatment.

The oil's unique profile makes sea buckthorn pulp oil a potent tool when dealing with mucous membrane issues. It can help with dry eyes and dry mouth, which commonly afflict people with Sjögren's syndrome. Digestive system mucous membrane issues, such as ulcers, damage from irradiation therapy, or inflammatory conditions, can benefit from orally ingested sea buckthorn pulp oil. It has also demonstrated its ability to address issues presenting in other mucous membranes in the urogenital system, such as vaginal or cervical inflammations and vaginal atrophy.[193]

Internal use preparations with sea buckthorn pulp oil may include mouthwash, pessaries, suppositories, sprays, capsules, and drinks. It can be used with children and the elderly with no known contraindications or cautions.

Tamanu
Calophyllum inophyllum

Common names: Tamanu, kamani, Alexandrian laurel, Pannay tree, Borneo mahogany, sweet scented calophyllum
Scientific name: *Calophyllum inophyllum* L.
Botanical family: Calophyllaceae syn. Clusiaceae syn. Guttiferae
Conservation status: Least concern, stable[194]

Description: Tamanu (*Calophyllum inophyllum*), a member of the Calophyllaceae family, is an evergreen tree native to tropical Asia, where it grows above the high-tide line on rocky and sandy seashores of the Indian and Pacific Oceans. Alternatively, wild populations also grow in inland sandy valleys at up to 200-meter elevations and on coral reefs surrounding the volcanic South Pacific islands. The tree tolerates exposure, brackish groundwater, and salt-laden winds; it is a markedly xerophytic plant.

C. inophyllum is slow-growing, typically reaching 25 meters and occasionally up to 35 meters tall. The tree has a thick and twisted or leaning trunk, elliptical leaves, fragrant white flowers, and large round drupes, containing one yellow seed in each drupe. The tree primarily relies on the ocean to disperse its fruits, which float when ripe, but fruit bats are also instrumental in dispersing the fruit.

Ethnobotany: Tamanu serves many diverse purposes, including food, medicine, building material, eco remediation, and ornamental. The pulp of immature fruits is considered edible, but toxic compounds may be present in mature fruits. The seed oil, once refined, is edible.[195]

In Indonesia, the tamanu tree provides a pharmacy of medicines. A tea made from the leaves is applied to relieve hives, skin infections, skin irritations, and the bark juice is used as a purgative. The cold-pressed seed oil is used in wound healing (especially suppurating wounds and burns), treating skin fungal and viral infections, acne, psoriasis, eczema, easing arthritis, treating gonorrhea, and leprosy-induced neuropathy.[196]

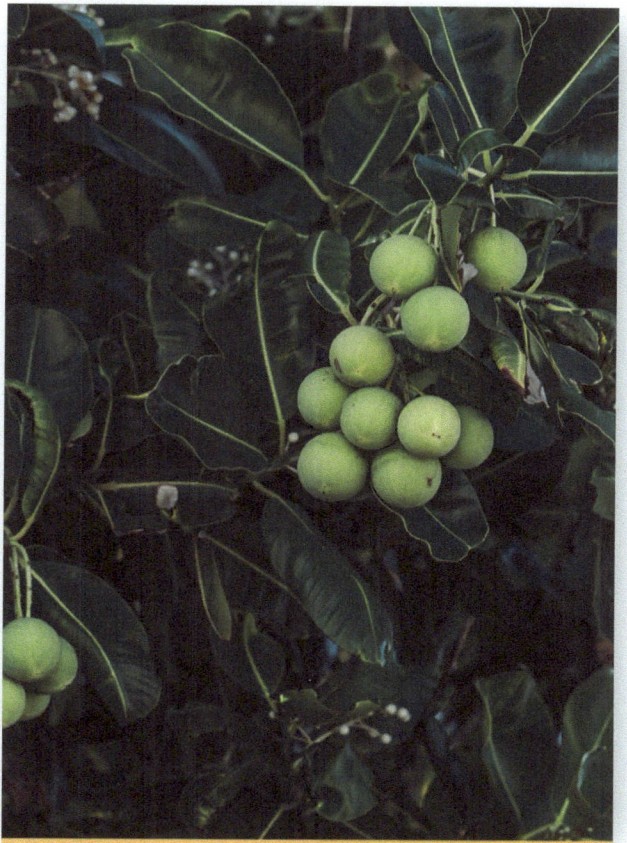

EXTRACTION INFORMATION

Country of origin: Madagascar, Tahiti, Hawaii
Part of plant: Seed
Oil yield: 40 - 60%[198]
Extraction method: Cold pressing

MANUFACTURING INFORMATION

CAS number: 223748-12-7
EC number: 273-313-5
INCI name: Calophyllum Inophyllum (Tamanu) seed Oil
CosIng (functions): Antimicrobial, Antioxidant, Hair Conditioning, Oral Care, Skin Conditioning, UV Absorber
Additional commercial oil name: Foraha oil

SHELF LIFE

48 months (4 years)

Ironically, Samoans consider the plant poisonous and tip their arrows in the sap to poison their enemies. Before Christianity's impact, Polynesians held tamanu trees as sacred, believing the gods would hide in the tamanu trees to watch human sacrifices. They would carve tamanu wood to produce idols for worship.[197]

NUTRIENT PROFILE

Tamanu oil offers a balance of oleic, linoleic, and stearic acid.

Tamanu Oil[199, 200]	
SATURATED FATTY ACIDS	
Palmitic acid (C16:0)	13.7 – 16.6%
Stearic acid (C18:0)	**14.3 – 29.14%**
MONOUNSATURATED FATTY ACIDS	
Oleic acid (C18:1 n-9)	28 - 39.24%
POLYUNSATURATED FATTY ACIDS	
Linoleic acid (C18:2 n-6)	23.9 - 31.24%
UNSAPONIFIABLE FRACTION	
Sterols 1310 mg/kg	Beta-sitosterol (564.6 mg/kg), stigmasterol (469 mg/kg), campesterol (188.6 mg/kg)
Tocopherols (includes tocotrienols) 370 mg/kg	Gamma-tocopherol (36 mg/kg), delta-tocopherol (16 mg/kg), alpha-tocopherol (15 mg/kg)

Formulating with Tamanu Oil

Sensory info: Rich, powerful, curry-like, slightly warming aroma; Light to dark green.

Absorption rate: Dry – readily absorbs into the skin. Leaves a slightly tacky feeling on the skin when applied at 100%.

Dilution: Usually 10 - 25% combined with other carriers. Can be used at 100%.

Therapeutic actions: wound healing, skin-regenerating, antioxidant, anti-inflammatory, antifungal, antiviral, antibacterial (Gram-positive bacteria)

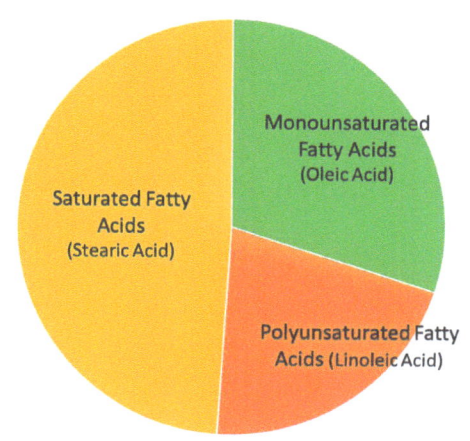

Therapeutic applications:
Tamanu is highly prized for its wide range of applications, from wound healing to relieving pain and supporting skin health. Indeed, modern research (*in vitro* and *in vivo*) provides evidence of tamanu oil's many therapeutic qualities, including its antioxidant and UV-protective properties.[201, 202] The antioxidant activity of tamanu oil helps protect the skin from free radicals and photodamage.

Of particular interest may be tamanu oil's demonstrated (*in vitro* and *in vivo*) anti-inflammatory,[203,204] antimicrobial,[205] and wound healing properties. Tamanu is especially effective against those Gram-positive bacteria that infect the skin. These properties make it especially suitable to address acne and infected wounds.[206] Well-known aromatherapist Kurt Schnaubelt popularized the application of tamanu oil in the treatment of shingles due to its anti-inflammatory, antiviral, and analgesic activity.[207]

We now have evidence to support the indigenous population's use of tamanu oil for skin healing., as it promotes the formation of new tissue and accelerates healing and growth of healthy skin.[208] A component of tamanu oil, calophyllolide, may contribute to its anti-inflammatory and wound healing activity.[209] Dermal application of tamanu oil may improve the appearance of scar tissue.[15] These qualities also make tamanu a potentially effective choice to combat atopic dermatitis.[210]

Tamanu oil is indicated for cuts, scrapes, burns, insect bites or stings, abrasions, acne, acne scars, psoriasis, diabetic sores, anal fissures, sunburn, dry or scaly skin, blisters, eczema, herpes sores, fungal skin infections, and to reduce foot or body odor. It may also be indicated for sciatica, neuralgia, and rheumatism.[231] In Ayurveda, tamanu oil addresses Kapha and Pitta imbalances. Historical use and current research show that tamanu oil and extracts from other *Calophyllum* species address a broad range of health issues.[212, 213]

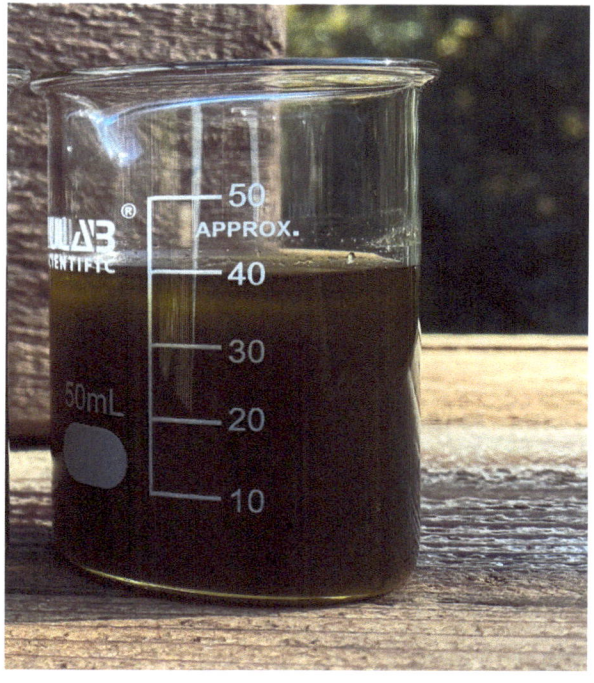

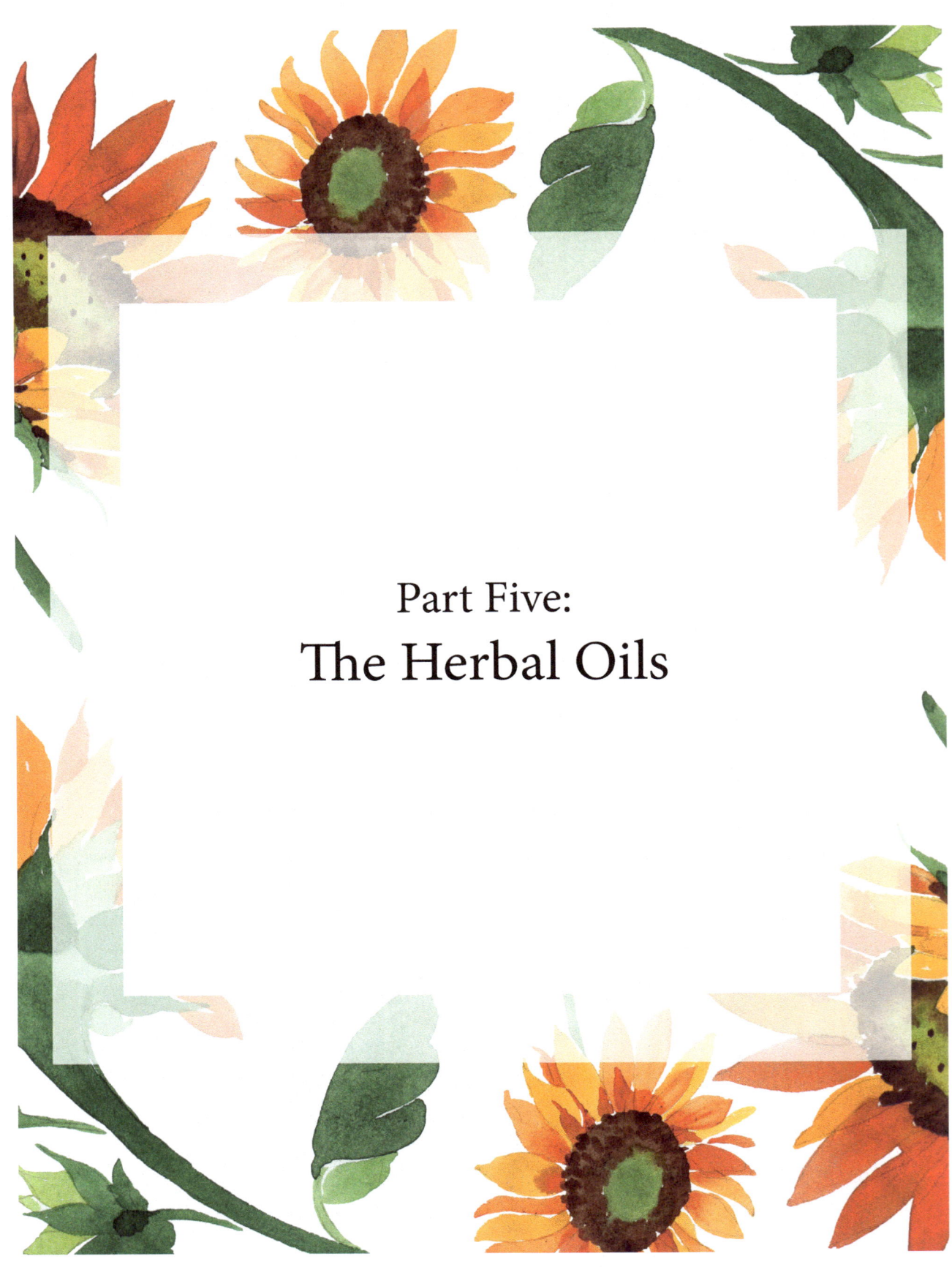

Part Five:
The Herbal Oils

The Herbal Oils

An herbal oil is a maceration (soaking) of medicinal plant material in a vegetable oil that extracts the fat-soluble substances of the plant. Lipophilic medicinal phytochemicals are fatty acids, triglycerides, resins, and oleoresins. Other constituents extracted in lipids are terpenes, triterpenoids, and steroidal alkaloids.[1]

Dilution of Herbal Oils

We typically classify herbal oils as enhancer carrier oils. The standard dilution for an herbal oil is between 10 to 25% of your total formulation, depending on the type of product and the goals of the formula. Most herbal oils can also be used at 100%.

CO_2 Extracts of the Herbal Oil Palette

Some CO_2 extracts belong in the herbal oil palette, including common herbs such as arnica and calendula. The CO_2 extracts of these medicinal plants contain the lipid-soluble components considered to be responsible for their therapeutic actions. The dilution rate for these extracts is in the range of 0.5-3%.

Storage of Herbal Oils

Herbal oils and CO_2 extracts should be stored in amber bottles, away from direct sunlight, and in a cool environment. Protect them from exposure to light, air, moisture, and pests. Avoid extreme temperatures and keep tightly sealed.

How to Make an Herbal Oil

Making herbal oils is a wonderful way to interact with medicinal plant material, and we highly recommend making at least a few of your own.

Folk method

Fill a clean sterilized jar with dried plant material, leaving a couple of inches of space at the top of the jar. Cover the plant material with the carrier oil of your choice. Secure the lid on the jar and shake for a few minutes to ensure all plant material is covered in oil. After 24 hours, open the jar and add more of your chosen carrier oil to ensure all plant matter is still covered in oil. Leave the jar on a sunny windowsill for 4-8 weeks. You may place the jar in a paper bag to protect it from direct sunlight, except when making St. John's wort oil, which requires direct sun exposure to develop its therapeutic chemistry. Be sure to shake the jar at least once a day during this time. After 4-8 weeks, strain the oil through cheesecloth to remove all plant material from the oil. Store the herbal oil in a clean, sterilized amber or clear glass jar.

Double-boiler method

We can increase extraction by adding heat to the equation. Place the herbs in a mason jar, cover them with oil, and seal the jar. A productive ratio to use is 1 part herb (grams) to 5 parts oil (milliliters). For example, cover 100 g of herb with 500 ml of oil. Line the bottom of a large pot with mason jar rings or bands, place the jar of oil on top of the rings, and add water until it is well below the lid of the jar. You do not want the water to cover the lid as you risk water entering your oil. Set the pot on the stove on low heat, keeping the oil preferably below 160 degrees Fahrenheit. Leave to simmer for 8-12 hours. Add warm water, as needed, to keep much of the jar submerged.

Dried vs. Fresh Herbs

We generally use dried herbs for infused oils because water in our oil will cause it to spoil, but you can use fresh herbs that have a low water content. When using fresh plants, first air dry the herbs for 24 - 48 hours to remove significant moisture from the plant material. Too much moisture left in the plant may introduce bacteria/fungi into the final product, spoiling the oil.

The following herbs must be fresh when infusing in oil:

- Mullein flowers
- Cottonwood
- St. John's wort
- Garlic

Additionally, you could remove any residual water from your final product. Once your oil is done infusing, you put the jar in the freezer upside down and allow the infusion to freeze. The oil will move upward, while the

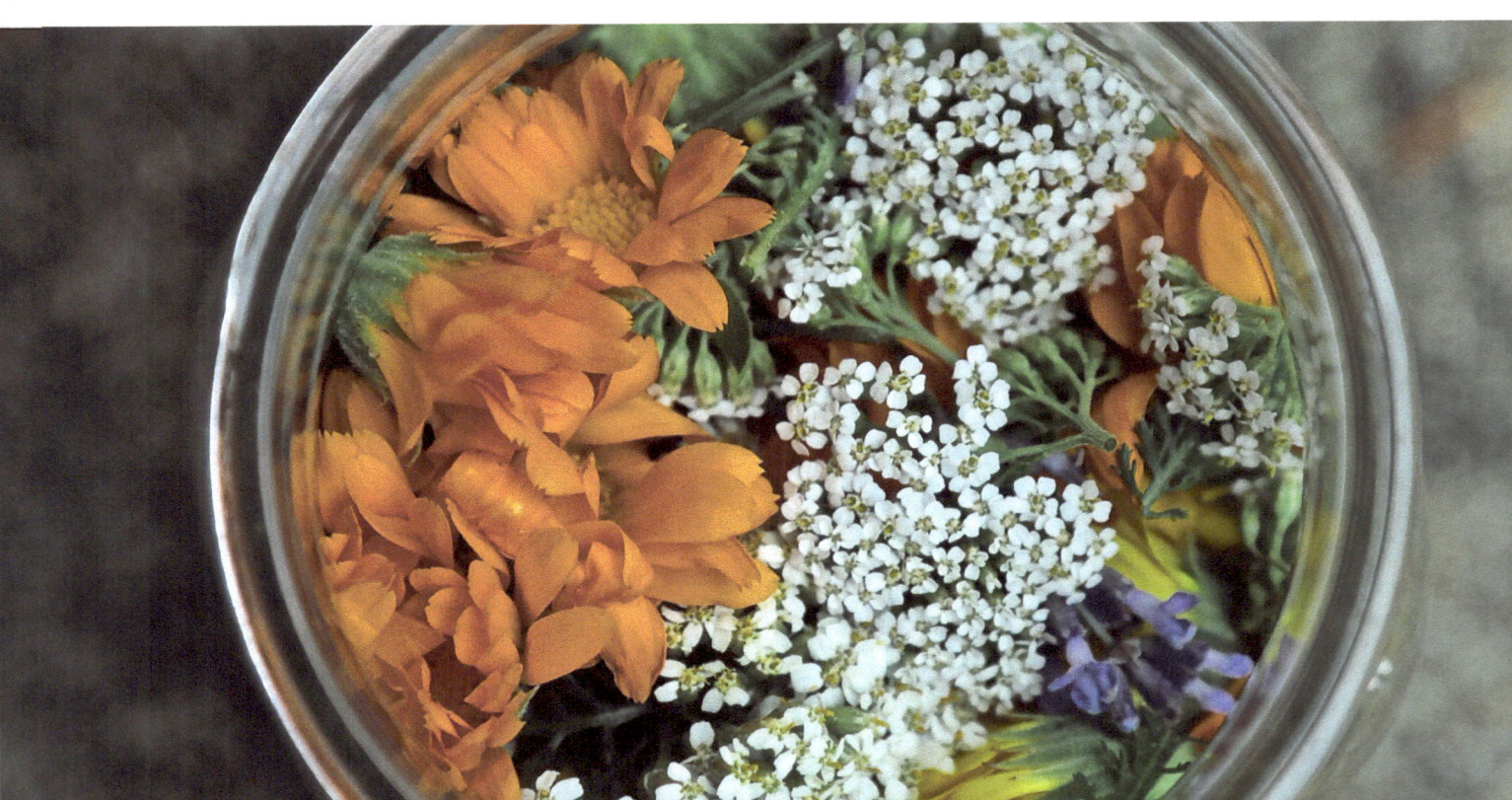

water will be frozen on the bottom (near the lid). You can then scrape off the water content, preserving your oil for many days to come, or generally, six months.

Blending herbal oils

Taking individual herbal oils and combining them as part of a carrier oil base can multiply the therapeutic benefits each oil demonstrates. A popular combination is equal parts arnica, calendula, and St. John's wort, which is effective for pain, inflammation, and bruising. A small clinical study (24 patients) demonstrated that a 70% St. John's wort – 30% calendula herbal oil blend helped cesarean section incisions close more quickly.[2]

A mixture of herbal oils can address multiple facets of a condition or provide a wider variety of chemical constituents to target one specific concern.

Shelf life of herbal oils

When stored properly, the average shelf life of herbal oils is 2 - 3 years.

Shelf life of CO2 extracts

The average shelf life of CO_2 extracts in the herbal palette is 3- 5 years when stored properly.

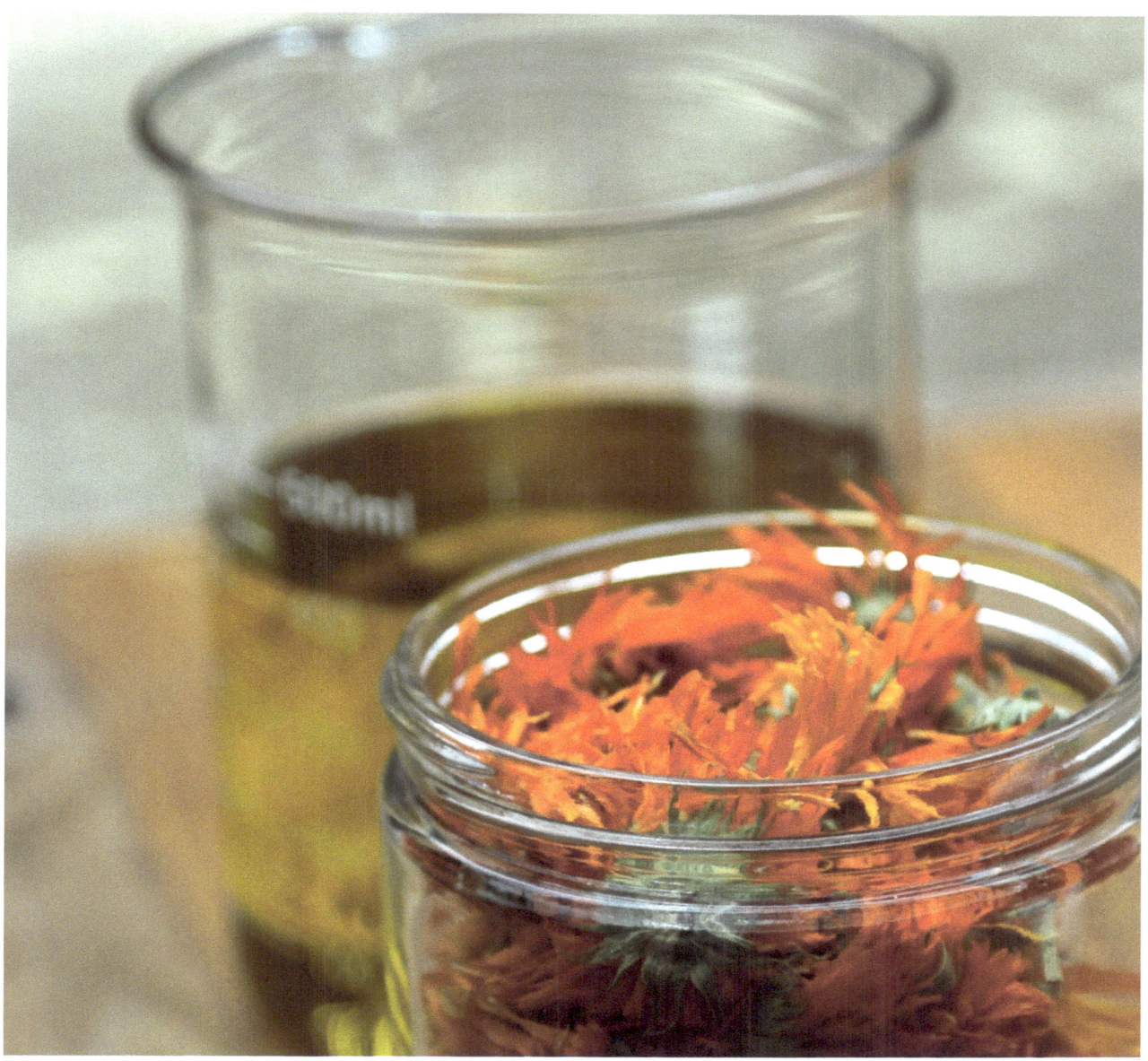

Arnica
Arnica montana

Common names: Arnica, leopard's bane
Scientific name: *Arnica montana* L.
Botanical family: Asteraceae
Conservation status: Least concern but declining[3]
United Plant Savers: Several *Arnica* species in the United States are on the "To watch" list[4]

Description: *Arnica montana* is an herbaceous perennial of the Asteraceae family endemic to Europe. *Arnica* spp. feature a basal rosette with dark green elliptical-to-oblanceolate leaves and a 1- to 2-ft. tall hairy stalk. Flowers are daisy-like, bright yellow-orange, and bloom in July and August. Each plant has 1 - 7 flower heads, which are typically harvested for medicinal preparations. Sometimes the dark brown cylindrical rhizomes are also used.

The genus *Arnica* contains some 40 species, of which *Arnica montana* is best known. Arnica prefers to grow at an altitude of 500–2500 meters in less fertile meadows and the acidic soils of alpine meadows and peat bog heathlands.[5]

Ethnobotany: In folk usage, the flower tincture was added to foot baths to relieve sore feet and rubbed into the scalp to increase hair growth. A poultice of the root was applied to tumors. Arnica was taken internally as a cardiotonic, central nervous system stimulant, expectorant, nervine, sedative, and to treat liver, stomach, and intestinal cancers.[6,7] For centuries, homeopathic arnica has been used to treat wounds, contusions, rheumatism, inflammation, and over 60 different health imbalances.[5]

Sustainability concerns:
Romania is the most significant producer of commercial arnica, over half of which is harvested from the wild. Unsustainable harvesting threatens the natural populations of *A. montana* in southern and eastern Europe. In northern Europe, the plant is threatened by changes in land use, including the conversion of meadows to farmland, which reduces habitat for *A. montana*.[8] Many affected countries currently prohibit

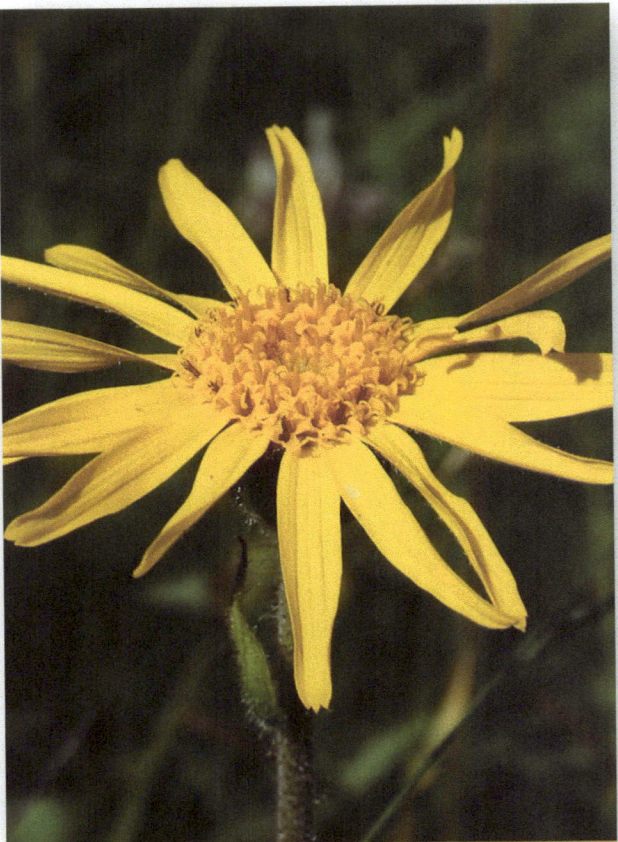

EXTRACTION INFORMATION

Herbal Oil
Part of plant used: Dried flowers, dried aerial parts
Oil used for extraction: Extra virgin olive oil or another suitable carrier oil
Extraction method: Maceration

CO2 Extract
Country of origin: Europe
Part of plant used: Dried flowers, dried aerial parts
Extraction method: SFE CO2

MANUFACTURING INFORMATION

Herbal Oil
CAS number: 68990-11-4
EC number: 273-579-2
INCI name: Name of extracting oil, Arnica Montana Flower Extract
　　Example: Helianthus Annuus (Sunflower) Seed Oil, Arnica Montana Flower Extract
CosIng (functions): Fragrance, Perfuming, Skin Conditioning

harvesting the plant from the wild populations.[5]

PHYTOCHEMISTRY

Arnica is comprised of 150 therapeutically active constituents.[5] The lipophilic components include the volatile fractions (0.2-0.5%), fatty acids, and sesquiterpene lactones (0.2–0.8%).[1] The primary sesquiterpene lactones are helenalin, 11 alpha,13-dihydrohelenalin, and their ester derivatives.[9] The sesquiterpene lactones are considered to be the main active components mediating the potent anti-inflammatory[10, 11, 12, 13] and pain-reducing activity of arnica oil.[5] Sesquiterpene lactones are oil-soluble terpenoids and will be extracted in an infused oil of arnica.

CO2 Extract
CAS number: 68990-11-4
EC number: 273-579-2
INCI name: Arnica Montana Flower Extract
CosIng (functions): Fragrance, Perfuming, Skin Conditioning

SHELF LIFE

- **Herbal oil:** 2-3 years
- **CO2 extract:** 3-5 years

Arnica CO2 Extract Chemistry

Arnica Flower CO2 Extract is a standardized extract containing 3.5-5.5% sesquiterpene lactones, triterpenediol esters, and approximately 0.2-0.5% volatile constituents, with a small amount of waxes and resins. Some suppliers may also include 0.05% rosemary CO2 extract antioxidant.

Arnica CO2 Total Extract Chemistry[14, 15]	
Triterpenediol esters (faradiol)	3 - 7%
Sesquiterpene lactones	3.5 - 5.5%
Helenalin	less than 0.02%
11 alpha, 13-dihydrohelenalin	tr. - 0.04
Helenalin esters	3.8%
Dihydrohelenalin esters	0.53%
Volatile oil components	0.2 - 0.5%

The volatile oil components in arnica flowers can vary widely depending on their source. Commercial arnica essential oil from Croatia, used in the flavoring industry, is known for its rich beta-caryophyllene (70%) and eugenol (10%) contents. Serbian arnica volatile oil content is rich in beta-caryophyllene (34.6%), germacrene D (12-16%), trans-b-ionone (3.9-4.3%), and decanal (2.7-5.3%).[12]

SAFETY INFORMATION

Do Not Apply to Open Wounds or Broken Skin. Arnica is considered to be toxic internally. Avoid all use if the client has allergies to other species within the Asteraceae family, e.g., ragweed, German chamomile, daisy. Extended herbal oil use may cause eczema.[16] Do not use arnica internally except in its homeopathic form.

Formulating with Arnica Herbal Oil and CO2 Extract

Herbal Oil
Sensory info: Light yellow-green
Dilution: Can be used 10-25% in a blend of other carrier oils.

CO2 Extract
Sensory info: Orange-yellow to brown; semi-viscous at room temperature; sweet, hay-like, slight caramel aroma
Dilution: Can be used at 0.5-1.5% as a part of the total carrier oil base.

Therapeutic actions: analgesic, anti-arthritic, antibacterial, anti-inflammatory[17], anti-hematoma, antimicrobial

According to Moore, in his book *Medicinal Plants of the Pacific Northwest*:

> Arnica works by stimulating and dilating blood vessels, particularly the specialized capillaries that control whether blood is piped into the small peripheral capillary beds or is shunted over to small veins, bypassing more widespread blood dispersal. Good, diffused blood transport and circulation into injured, bruised, or inflamed tissues helps speed up the resolution and removal of waste products.[18]

Therapeutic applications:

- Bruises, hematomas, contusions, traumatic injuries
- Arthritis, bursitis, or myalgia
- Sprains and strains; Hyperextensions
- Stiffness and swelling associated with trauma
- Joint stiffness
- Counterirritant to treat rheumatism (rheumatic muscle and joint problems)
- First degree burns, including sunburns
- Superficial inflammation of the skin
- Varicose veins

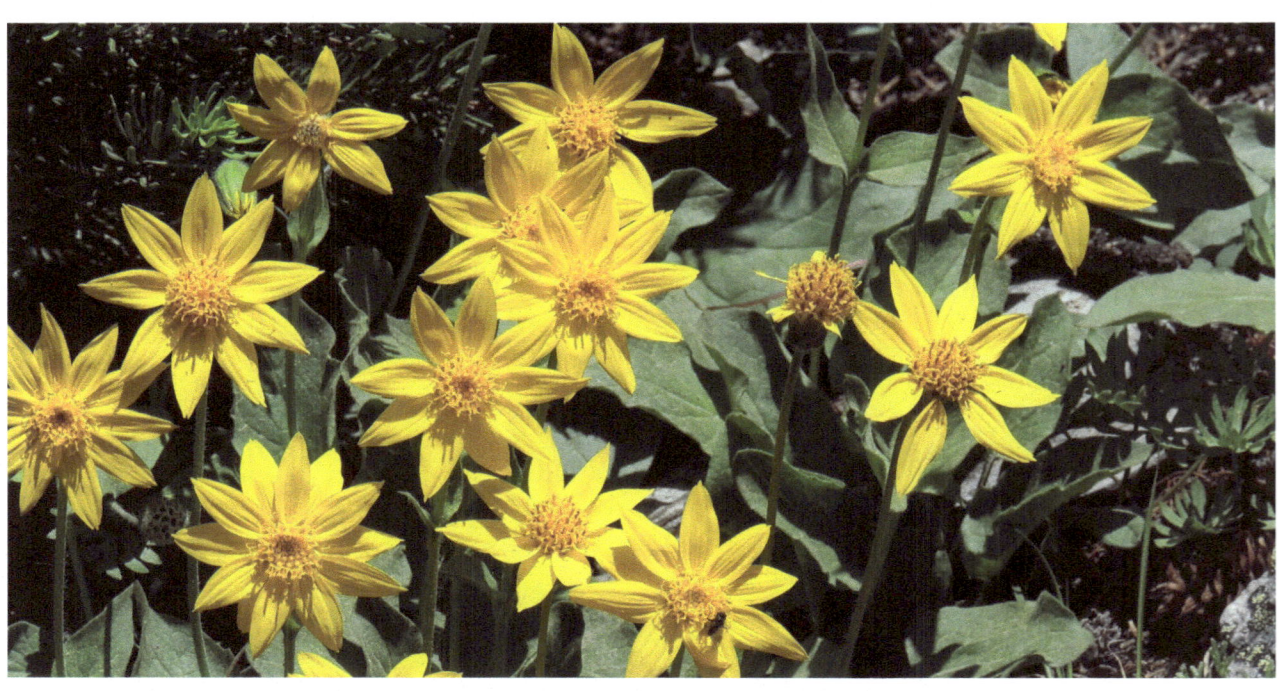

Calendula
Calendula officinalis

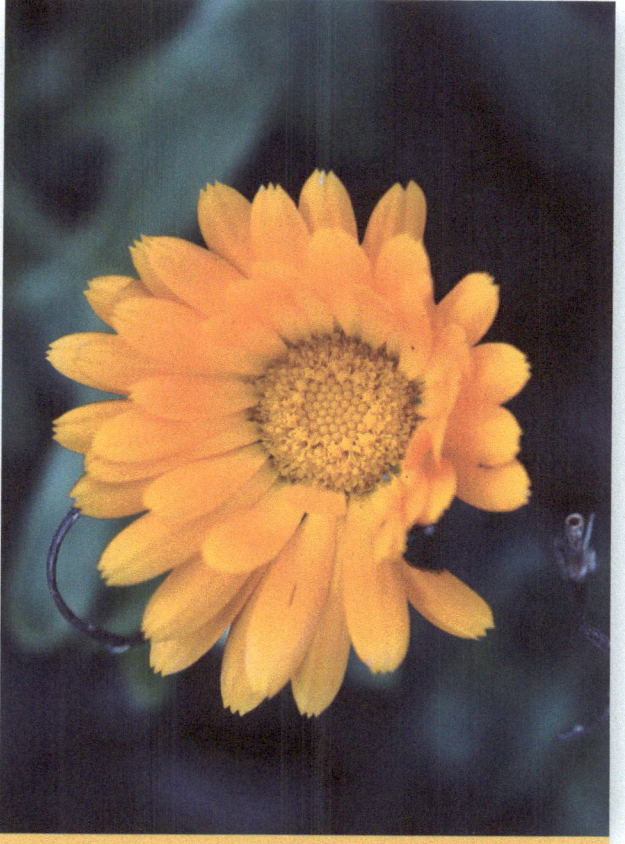

Common names: Calendula, pot marigold
Scientific name: *Calendula officinalis* L.
Botanical family: Asteraceae
Conservation status: This species not assessed

Description: *Calendula officinalis* is an annual herb in the Asteraceae family native to the Mediterranean and Egypt. It is widely cultivated in temperate regions around the world. Calendula features waxy, smooth, or glandular stems and simple, somewhat toothed leaves arranged alternately along the stems. Flower heads are composite and vary in color from bright yellow to deep orange. The fruit is a curved achene (dry one-seeded fruit).[19] Calendula typically grows 1-2 feet tall and just as wide. Leaves are aromatic, lanceolate/oblong-obovate, green in color, and grow up to 6 inches long. Calendula flourishes in moderately fertile, well-drained soil in full sun.

The genus name *Calendula* is derived from the Latin name *calendae*, meaning "first day of the month."[20]

Ethnobotany: Calendula, an Old-World potherb and garden plant, was popular in England. The bitter flowers and leaves are edible and used for culinary and medicinal purposes.[21]

Calendula officinalis has traditionally been used to treat skin tumors, dermatological lesions, ulcers, swellings, skin and mucous membrane inflammation, dysmenorrhea, and nervous disorders. Calendula was used during the United States Civil War to treat wounds and as a remedy for measles, smallpox, and jaundice. It is a prominent ingredient in cosmetic formulations, including creams, lotions, and shampoos in modern times.[22]

EXTRACTION INFORMATION

Herbal Oil
Part of plant used: Dried whole flowers
Oil used for extraction: Extra virgin olive oil or another suitable carrier oil
Extraction method: Maceration

Calendula CO2 Extract
Country of origin: Germany, Egypt
Part of plant used: Dried flowers (petals and calyx)
Extraction method: SFE CO2
Oil yield (SFE CO2): 5%
Shelf life: 5 years, recommended using within 2 years

PHYTOCHEMISTRY

Calendula contains a wide range of lipid, water, and alcohol soluble components. The lipophilic components that may be found in the herbal oil include waxes, fatty acids and fatty acid esters, steroids, tocopherols, non-polar carotenoids, mono-, sesqui-, and triterpenoid esters, and triterpene mono-alcohols and diols. A small percentage of carotenoids, polar triterpenoid triols, and phenolic acids may also be extracted.[23]

The main components of lipophilic extracts of *Calendula officinalis* flowers are the triterpendiol esters, also called the faradiol esters. Triterpendiol esters, which are considered to be the major anti-inflammatory components of calendula, include faradiol 3-O-laurate, faradiol palmitate, and faradiol myristate.[24, 25]

Calendula CO2 Extract Chemistry

The core components of calendula CO2 extract include faradiol esters, taraxasterol, and volatile oil components. The presence of carotenoids gives the extract its light orange color.

MANUFACTURING INFORMATION

Herbal Oil
CAS number: 84776-23-8 / 70892-20-5
EC number: 283-949-5
INCI name: Name of extracting oil, Calendula Officinalis Flower Extract
   Example: Olea Europaea (Olive) Fruit Oil, Calendula Officinalis Flower Extract
CosIng (functions): Fragrance, Perfuming, Skin Conditioning

CO2 Extract
CAS number: 84776-23-8 / 70892-20-5
EC number: 283-949-5
INCI name: Calendula Officinalis Flower Extract
CosIng (functions): Fragrance, Perfuming, Skin Conditioning

SHELF LIFE

- **Herbal oil:** 2-3 years
- **CO2 extract:** 3-5 years

Calendula CO2 Total Extract[26]	
Faradiol esters	17 - 25%
Sum of taraxasterol and amyrin	4.8 - 10.7%
Sum of sterols	1.3 - 1.5%
Volatile oil consists of mainly sesquiterpenoids (alpha-cadinol, isomers of cadinene, alpha-copaene, germacrene D, alpha-elemene, and others)[28]	1.5 - 1.7%
Carotenoids (calculated as beta-carotene[29])	0.85 - 1.2%
The CO2 extract includes cuticular waxes, which are partially responsible for the thick viscosity of the CO2 extract.	

Component notes:

- Taraxasterol, a pentacyclic-triterpene, exhibits anti-inflammatory activity.[29, 30]
- Alpha-amyrin and beta-amyrin exhibit anxiolytic, sedative, antidepressant, anti-inflammatory, and analgesic properties.[31, 37]
- **Note:** Calendula essential oil is not commercially produced. The flowers yield approximately 0.3% of essential oil.

SAFETY INFORMATION

Calendula does not contain sesquiterpene lactones, a potential cause of allergies found in other Asteraceae species. Calendula has no known safety concerns.

Formulating with Calendula Herbal Oil and CO2 Extract

Herbal Oil
Sensory info: Light to rich orange-yellow, sweet hay-like aroma
Dilution: Use at a 10 - 25% percent with other carrier oils. Can use 100%.

CO2 Extract
Sensory info: Rich dark orange; viscous almost to the point of being solid; very light, dry, sweet grass to hay-like aroma.
Dilution: Use 1-3% as a part of the total carrier oil base.
Note on CO2 extract: Calendula CO2 extract can be challenging to work with due to its viscosity; therefore, it is commonly sold already diluted in a carrier oil, typically at 10%.

Therapeutic actions: anti-inflammatory,[32, 33] antimicrobial (antiviral, antibacterial, antifungal), antioxidant,[34, 35] vulnerary[36]

Therapeutic applications:

- Wound healing/Tissue repair
- Inflamed skin conditions
- Cracked skin conditions
- Cracked nipples due to breastfeeding (nontoxic to baby)
- Burns
- Insect bites
- Allergic contact dermatitis, vitiligo, rosacea, melasma, psoriasis, and cutaneous toxicities resulting from cancer treatment[34]
- Damaged tissue, skin rashes, ulcers
- Inflammation of the oral mucosa
- Contusions

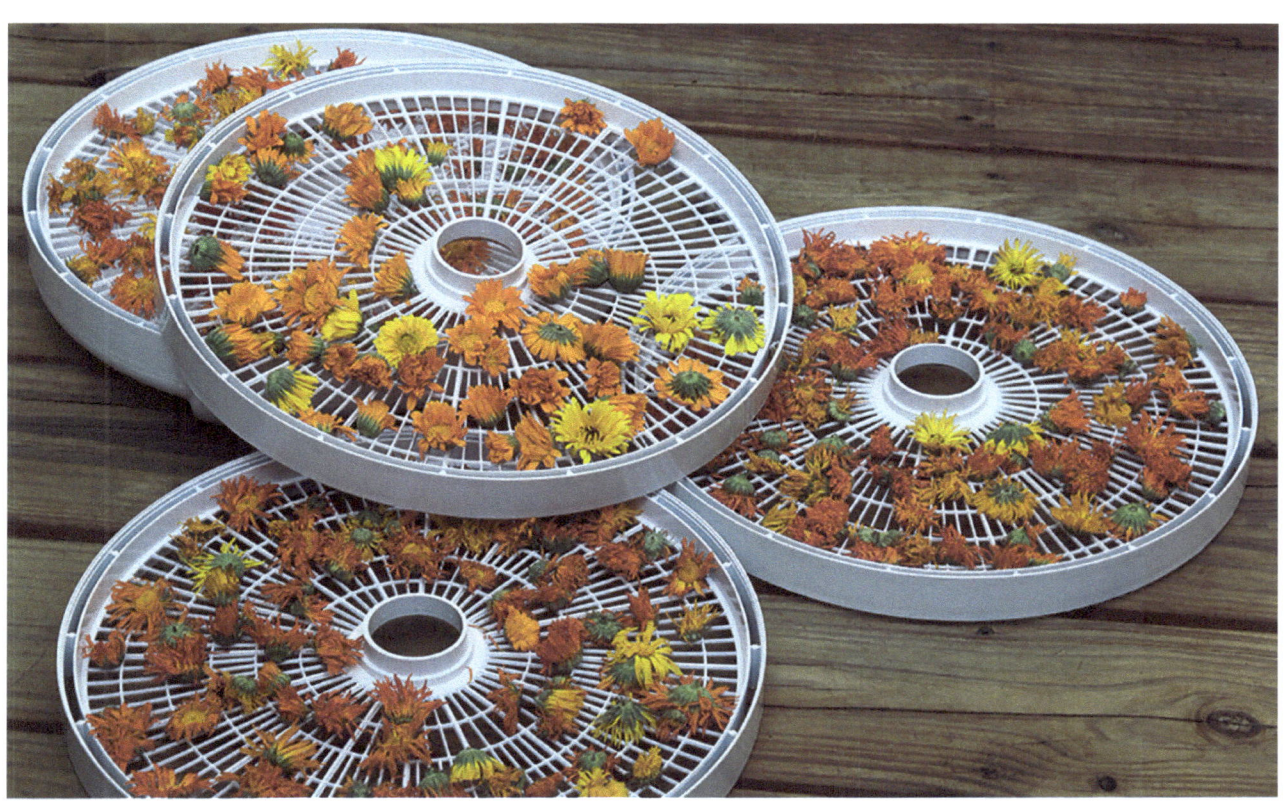

Carrot
Daucus carota var. *sativus*

Common names: Carrot, common cultivated carrot
Scientific name: *Daucus carota* L. var. *sativus* Hoffm.
Botanical family: Apiaceae
Conservation status: Least concern

Description: *Daucus carota* subsp. *sativus*, known as cultivated or domesticated carrot, is a root vegetable in the Apiaceae family indigenous to Afghanistan. The cultivated carrot was developed from the weedy wild carrot (*Daucus carota* subsp. *carota*, commonly known as Queen Anne's lace), which is native to Europe and Asia and naturalized throughout North America. Cultivated carrots typically grow 3-36" tall, depending on variety, and feature edible tapered taproots, typically orange in color. Foliage is finely divided, with a lacy appearance. Carrots are biennial and produce umbels of tiny white flowers in their second year.

Cultivated carrots grow best in loose, fertile, well-drained soil free of rocks or clumps that might inhibit root development. *D. carota* prefers full sun but tolerates light shade.[38] Domesticated carrot and wild carrot are the same species (*Daucus carota*) and readily hybridize, but the roots of these two variants are distinct. Wild carrot roots are white and woody with lateral offshoots, whereas domesticated carrots have large, smooth, pigmented, edible roots. Cultivated carrots are a popular root vegetable, valued for their high concentrations of carotenoids and tocopherols. The nutritional content of cultivated carrots is a direct result of selective plant breeding over the course of the past 400 years.[39]

In addition to its culinary applications, cultivated carrot is a common ingredient in body care products. Carrot oil is typically prepared by extracting the constituents of cultivated carrot root with a carrier oil. Carrot oil is distinct from carrot seed essential oil, which is an aromatic oil customarily steam distilled from wild carrot seeds.

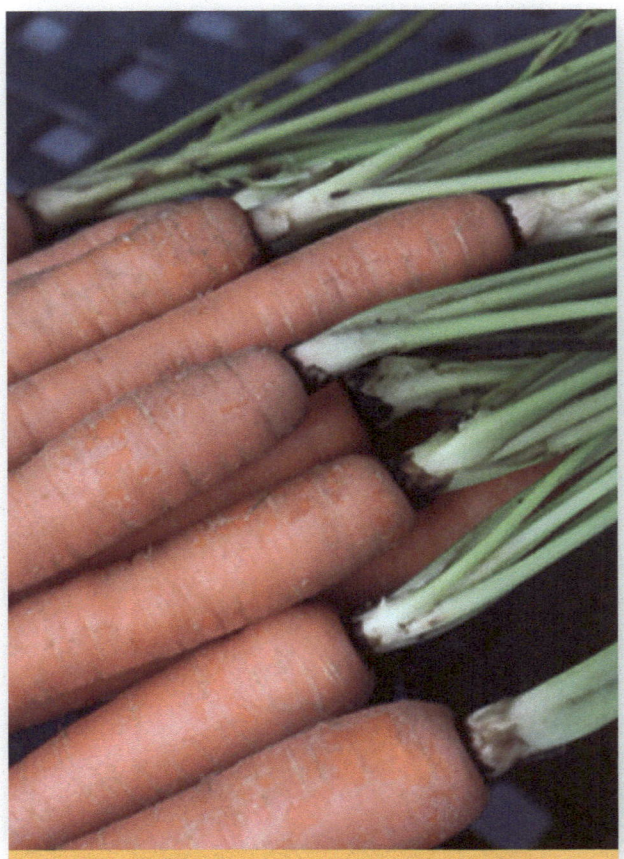

EXTRACTION INFORMATION

Part of plant used: Root
Oil used for extraction: Extra virgin olive oil or another suitable carrier oil
Extraction method: Maceration

MANUFACTURING INFORMATION

CAS number: 84929-61-3
EC number: 284-545-1
INCI name: Name of extracting oil, Daucus Carota Root Extract
    Example: Helianthus Annuus (Sunflower) Seed Oil, Daucus Carota Root Extract
INCI name: Daucus Carota Sativa Root
CosIng (functions): Skin conditioning

SHELF LIFE

2-3 years

PHYTOCHEMISTRY

Carrot herbal oil is rich in the fat-soluble sterol beta-carotene, which is the most well-known pro-vitamin A carotenoid.[40] Beta-carotene is the component responsible for giving carrot-infused oil its rich red/orange color as well as its therapeutic benefits. It is a potent oxygen radical scavenger.[41] Beta-carotene acts as a photoprotective agent in the skin,[42] as it functions as a cellular screen against sunlight-induced free radical change.[43]

Formulating with Carrot Herbal Oil

Sensory info: Orange to light reddish color due to beta-carotene content
Dilution: Can be used 5-25% in a blend of other carrier oils.

Therapeutic actions: Antioxidant, photoprotective

Therapeutic applications:

- Wound healing
- Burns
- Mature/aging skin
- Impetigo
- Dermatitis, eczema
- Improve the appearance of scar tissue
- Dry skin
- Rashes, itching

To make carrot infused oil

Carrots hold between 90-92% water and when infusing herbal oils, water is a source of potential bacterial growth. Therefore, it is important to dehydrate or dry the carrots prior to infusing.

1. Peel and thinly slice or shred the carrots.
2. Blanch the sliced or shredded carrots. Blanching is beneficial for enhancing the quality of the herbal oil.
3. Spread the carrots on a tray for the dehydrator.
4. Dehydrate at 125F for 8-12 hours. Shredded carrots may take less time.
5. Once the carrots are dehydrated, fill a sterilized, glass jar with the dehydrated carrots.
6. Cover with extra virgin olive oil or other appropriate carrier oil.
7. Macerate for 4-8 weeks.
8. Strain the oil through cheesecloth.

The carrot infused oil is now ready for use!

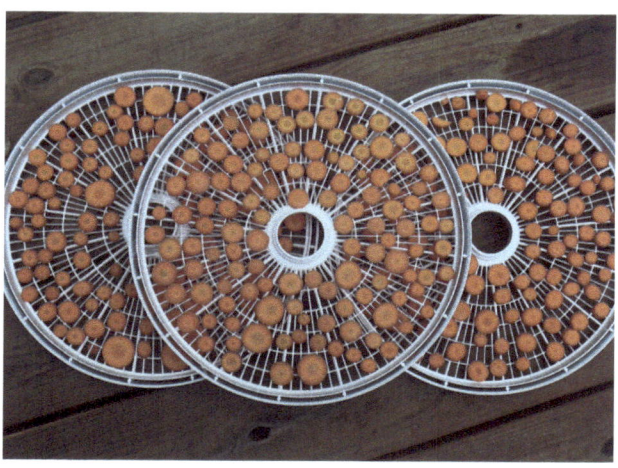

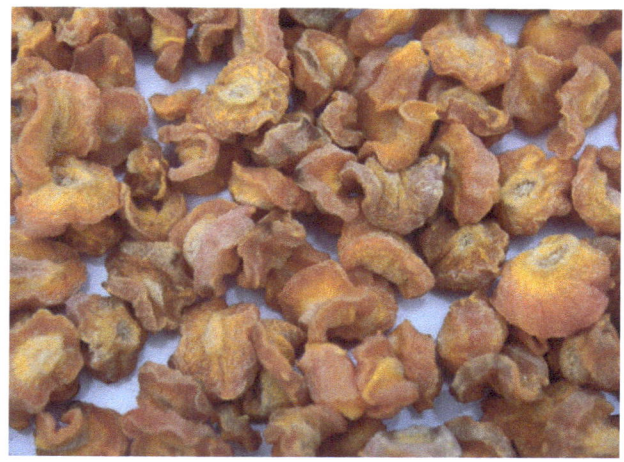

Chickweed
Stellaria media

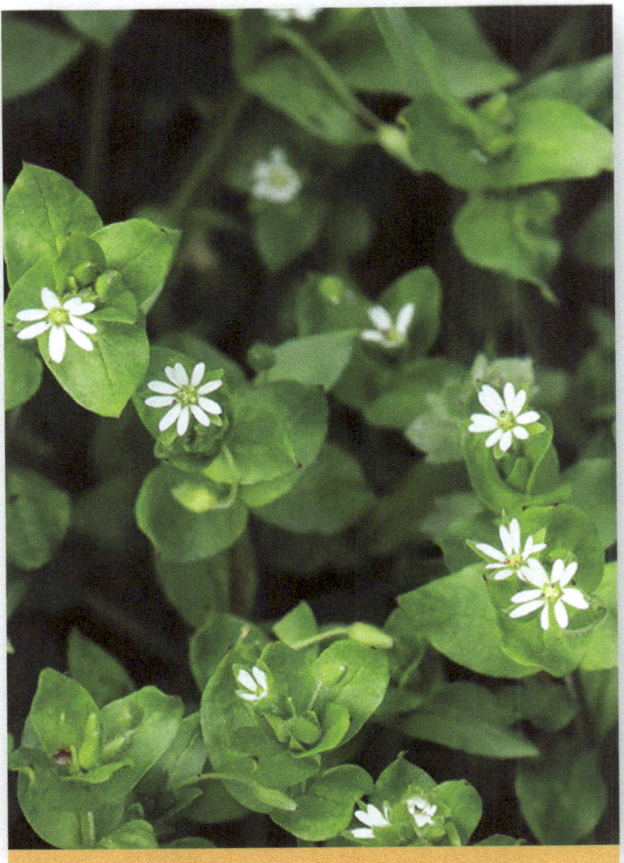

Common names: Chickweed, starweed
Scientific name: *Stellaria media* (L.) Vill.
Botanical family: Caryophyllaceae
Conservation status: Least concern

Description: Chickweed, a member of the Caryophyllaceae family, is a prolific perennial plant found widely throughout North America, Europe, Asia, and Africa. A common spring herb, chickweed thrives in cool, moist climates. Chickweed has willowy soft, fleshy stems, oval leaves, and tiny, white, star-shaped flowers with deep-lobed petals.[44]

Ethnobotany: Chickweed has a long and widespread history of use in folk medicine for treating various ailments such as skin disorders, dermal infections, hemorrhoids, obesity, diabetes, inflammation, gastric ulcers, and stomach cramps. The dried leaves have been used in pills, powders, or decoctions for various ailments, while the fresh leaves have been pulverized to be used as a plaster for skin ailments, dislocated bones, or swellings. In Chinese medicine, chickweed has been used in the treatment of skin diseases such as dermatitis due to its ability to reduce and soothe inflammation. In India, chickweed leaves are made into a tea to treat wounds, stop bleeding, and apply to tumors.[44, 45] In traditional Western herbal medicine, chickweed is a highly prized spring herb as a nutritive tonic and for its demulcent, diuretic, wound healing, and anti-inflammatory activities.[46]

EXTRACTION INFORMATION

Part of plant used: Dried aerial part
Oil used for extraction: Extra virgin olive oil or another suitable carrier oil
Extraction method: Maceration

MANUFACTURING INFORMATION

CAS number: 90131-34-3
EC number: 290-345-5
INCI name: Name of extracting oil, Stellaria media (Chickweed) extract
    Example: Helianthus Annuus (Sunflower) Seed Oil, Stellaria media (Chickweed) extract
CosIng (functions): Skin Conditioning

SHELF LIFE

2-3 years

PHYTOCHEMISTRY

Chickweed contains coumarins, phytosterols, flavonoids (mainly apigenin C-glycosides and rutin), organic acids, vitamin C, and triterpene saponins. Vitamin C is a water-soluble vitamin and hence will not be found in the herbal oil. However, the lipid-soluble triterpene saponins are the active constituents that provide chickweed oil's itch-relieving properties.[9,47]

Formulating with Chickweed Herbal Oil

Sensory info: Light green
Dilution: Can be used 5-25% in a blend of other carrier oils.

Therapeutic actions: relieve skin itchiness and irritation

Therapeutic applications:

- Inflamed skin conditions
- Sunburn
- Rashes or skin irritations (such as bug bites)
- Itchiness
- Nodular growths on the skin
- Eczema

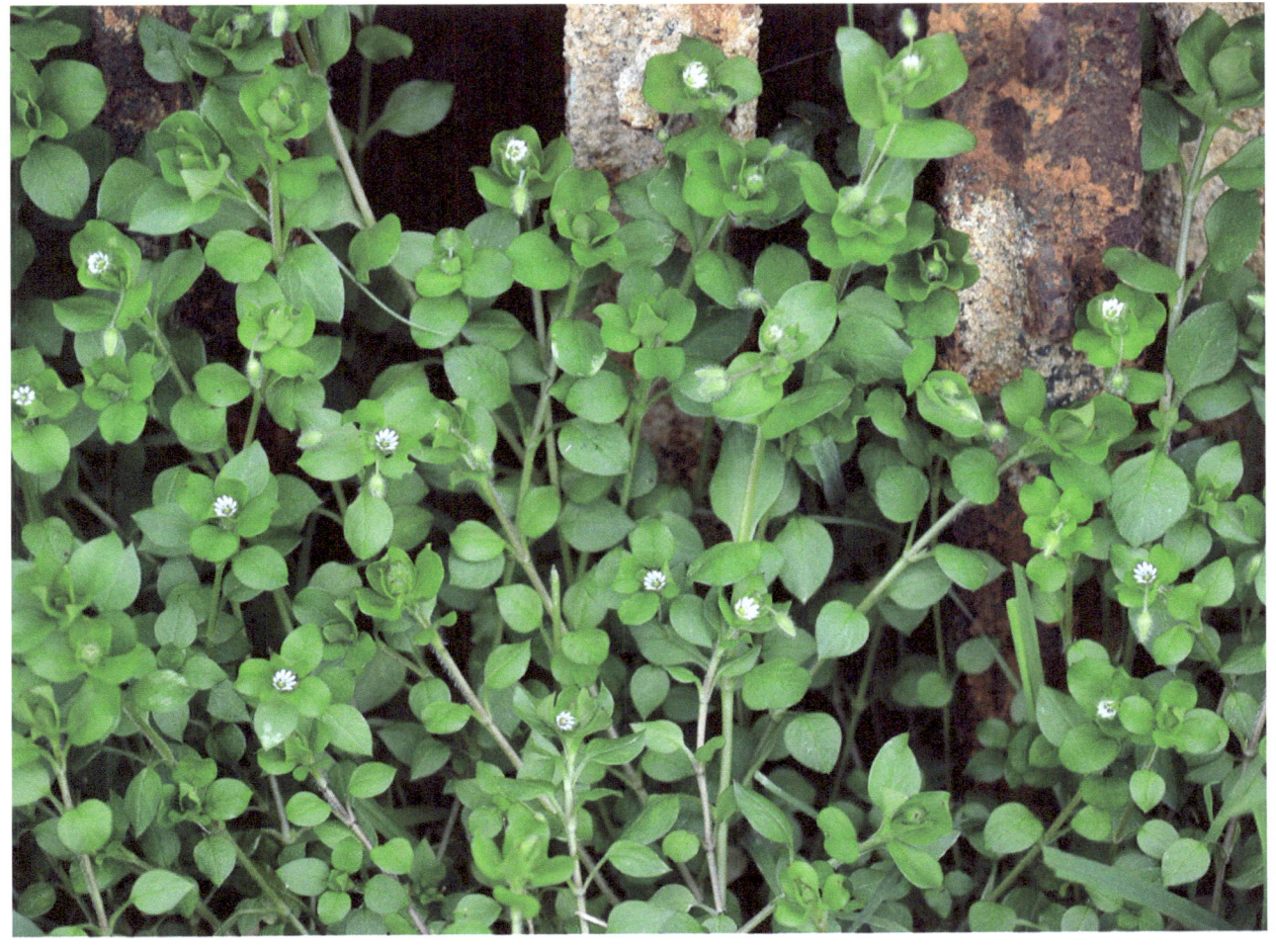

Comfrey
Symphytum officinale

Common name: Comfrey, knitbone
Scientific name: *Symphytum officinale* L.
Botanical family: Boraginaceae
Conservation status: Least concern, stable[48]

Description: Comfrey is a large, coarse, clumping perennial shrub in the Boraginaceae family native to Eurasia. The plant grows 3 feet tall and 2.5 feet wide, with tuberous roots. Leaves are large, pointed, hairy, ovate-lanceolate, dark green in color, and up to 8 inches long. Upper leaves are decurrent and smaller than basal leaves. Mature stems are winged. Flowers are tubular, white to pink to purple, and arranged in drooping clusters that bloom from mid-spring to early summer.

Symphytum grows best in medium moisture, organically-rich well-drained soils in full sun to partial shade.

Ethnobotany: Comfrey has been cultivated since 400 BC for medicinal purposes. The leaves and roots were used in traditional medicine as poultices to relieve external inflammations, rashes, swellings, cuts, bruises, sprains, and broken bones. Comfrey has been taken internally to treat ulcers and colitis. The young leaves and stems have been cooked and eaten as a vegetable, while the leaves were used in herbal teas.

The genus name *Symphytum* arises from the Greek *symphyo*, meaning "to grow together," and *phyton* for "plant," as comfrey was a well-known wound healer. The common name purportedly derives from the Latin *con firma*, meaning "with strength," an allusion to comfrey's value in tissue repair.[49]

Comfrey oil and ointments are used topically to treat wounds, bruises, pulled muscles and ligaments, fractures, sprains, strains, and osteoarthritis. Symphytum officinale roots and leaves contain allantoin, a compound that encourages the growth of new skin cells and other substances. Comfrey also contains hepatotoxic pyrrolizidine alkaloids and should be used internally only under the supervision

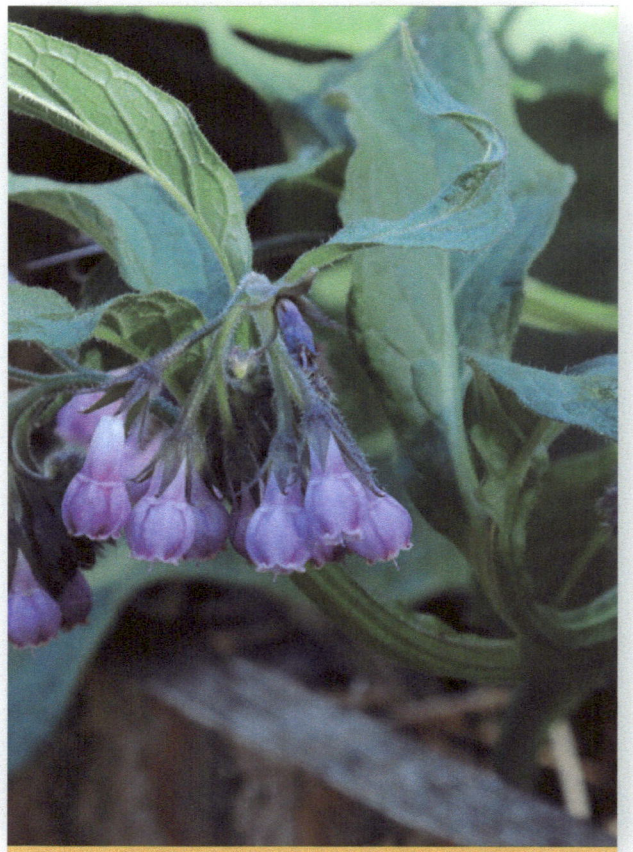

EXTRACTION INFORMATION

Part of plant used: Dried root or leaf
Oil used for extraction: Extra virgin olive oil or another suitable carrier oil
Extraction method: Maceration

MANUFACTURING INFORMATION

CAS number: 84696-05-9
EINECS number: 283-625-3

Comfrey Leaf
INCI name: Name of extracting oil, Symphytum Officinalis Leaf Extract
    Example: Olea Europaea (Olive) Fruit Oil, Symphytum Officinalis Leaf Extract
CosIng function (leaf): Fragrance, Perfuming, Tonic

of a trained herbalist. Due to its capacity to cause liver damage and death, comfrey products are sold in the US only in creams and ointments for topical application. Likewise, the UK, Australia, Canada, and Germany banned the sale of oral products containing comfrey.[50]

PHYTOCHEMISTRY

Comfrey root contains allantoin at an average level of 0.8 % and mucilage in the form of fructans. These two components are active skin-healing constituents through their ability to increase cellular proliferation. While they are mainly water-soluble, we still find the oil extraction of comfrey root to be an effective topical application to increase skin regeneration and reduce skin irritation. Other active constituents found in comfrey root are triterpenes, tannins, and organic acids, such as rosmarinic acid.[9]

SAFETY INFORMATION

Avoid application of comfrey herbal oil on deep cuts or puncture wounds as this may cause the skin to heal over the deeper wound.

The potential for toxicity of comfrey root comes from the presence of pyrrolizidine alkaloids (PAs) and their N-oxides, which include symphytine, intermedine, and echimidine in concentrations of up to 0.4%. The leaf also contains PAs but in much lower concentrations. Pyrrolizidine alkaloids are highly water-soluble and minimally extracted in oil. Infused oils containing comfrey root and leaf should contain low quantities of PAs. While they should not be applied topically to broken skin as a safety measure, toxicity from PAs from an herbal oil is a very low risk.[51]

Pregnancy and breastfeeding: Use only for the short term, especially on areas with broken skin.[52]

Comfrey Root
INCI name: Name of extracting oil, Symphytum Officinalis Root Extract
    Example: Helianthus Annuus Seed Oil, Symphytum officinalis Root Extract
CosIng function (root): Anti-seborrheic, Skin conditioning, Soothing

SHELF LIFE

2-3 years

Formulating with Comfrey Herbal Oil

Sensory info: Light yellow
Dilution: Can be used 5-15% in a blend of other carrier oils.

Therapeutic actions: skin regeneration, reduce skin irritation

Therapeutic applications:

- Cuts, scrapes
- Wound healing
- Slow-healing wounds
- Bruises
- Sprained muscles and/or ligaments

Cottonwood
Populus balsamifera

Common names: Cottonwood, balsam poplar, bam tree, hackmatack, tacamahaca
Scientific name: *Populus balsamifera* L.
Botanical family: Salicaceae
Conservation status: Least Concern[53]

Description: Balsam poplar, cottonwood, is a large, fragrant tree in the Salicaceae family native to North America. *P. balsamifera* grows 20-60 feet tall with dark grey furrowed bark and a narrow, open crown of upright branches. The trunk is straight, the branches sturdy and erect, and the leaves are dark green, shiny on top, and silvery or brown underneath. Catkins emerge prior to the leaves. Seeds are cottony and windblown; the resinous buds emit a powerful balsam aroma.

P. balsamifera grows in the deep moist sandy soils of river bottomlands, stream banks, and along the borders of lakes and swamps.

Ethnobotany: Indigenous North Americans valued the balsam poplar both as food and medicine. The mucilaginous inner bark was harvested in the spring, dried, ground, and used as a thickener in soups or added to cereals in breadmaking. The bitter catkins were eaten raw or cooked. As a medicine, balsam poplar was valued for its ability to address lung and skin maladies. The resin of the bud was taken internally as a tea to treat cough and lung ailments, while steam from a preparation of the buds in hot water could be inhaled as a nasal decongestant. The bud resin was applied topically as an antiseptic styptic or salve and as a wash for sores, wounds, sprains, and rheumatism. Due to the inner bark's mucilaginous quality, a tea from the inner bark was used in traditional medicine as an eyewash. The outer bark was used in the treatment of rheumatism, fever, and menstrual cramps due to its possible pain-relieving and fever-reducing activity.[54, 55]

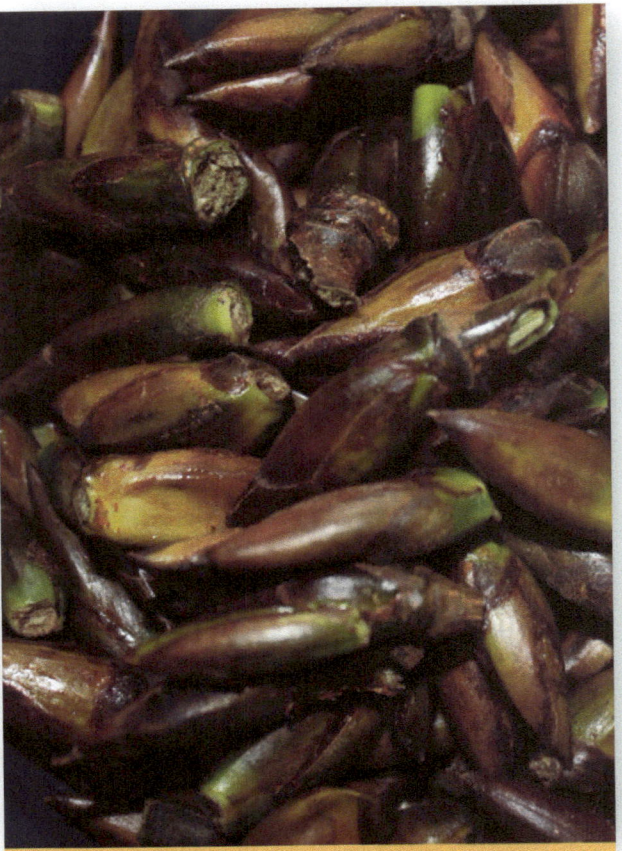

EXTRACTION INFORMATION

Part of plant used: Leaf bud
Oil used for extraction: Extra virgin olive oil or another suitable carrier oil
Extraction method: Maceration using heat
Note: Fresh buds need to be dried overnight until tacky to the touch to ensure moisture has evaporated off, particularly in moist climates.

MANUFACTURING INFORMATION

CAS number: 91721-76-5
EC number: 294-377-0
INCI name: Name of extracting oil, Populus Balsamifera (bud) Extract
   Example: Helianthus Annuus (Sunflower) Seed Oil, Populus Balsamifera (bud) Extract
CosIng (functions): N/A
Additional commercial name: Balm of Gilead oil - Not to be confused with the balm of Gilead plant (*Commiphora gileadensis*) or the perfume of the same name.

SHELF LIFE
3-4 years

PHYTOCHEMISTRY

Cottonwood buds are rich in a lipophilic, balsamic resin. The buds contain a volatile yellow oil comprised principally of humulene, gallic acid, malic acid, salicin, populin, mannitol, chrysin, tectochrysin, arachidonic acid, trichocarpin, and bisabolol.[56]

Formulating with Cottonwood Herbal Oil

Sensory info: Rich golden color; powerful, sweet, warm aroma

Dilution: Can be used 5-15% in a blend of other carrier oils.

Therapeutic actions: Cottonwood buds exhibit anti-inflammatory, analgesic, and antiseptic activity.[57] It has an affinity for the musculoskeletal system as an analgesic and anti-inflammatory herbal oil.

Therapeutic applications:

- Arthritic joints
- Sprains, strains, hyperextensions
- Pain caused by inflammation
- Pain and swelling

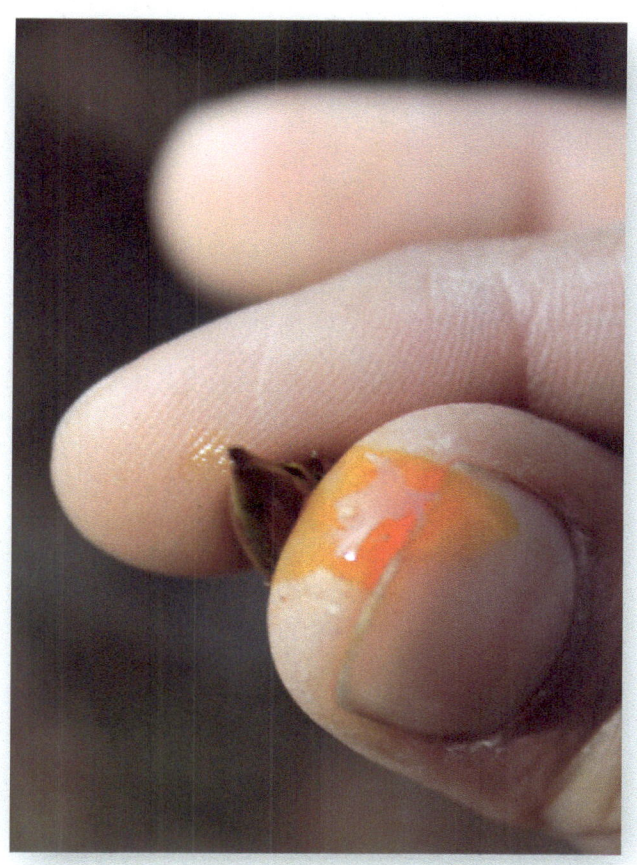

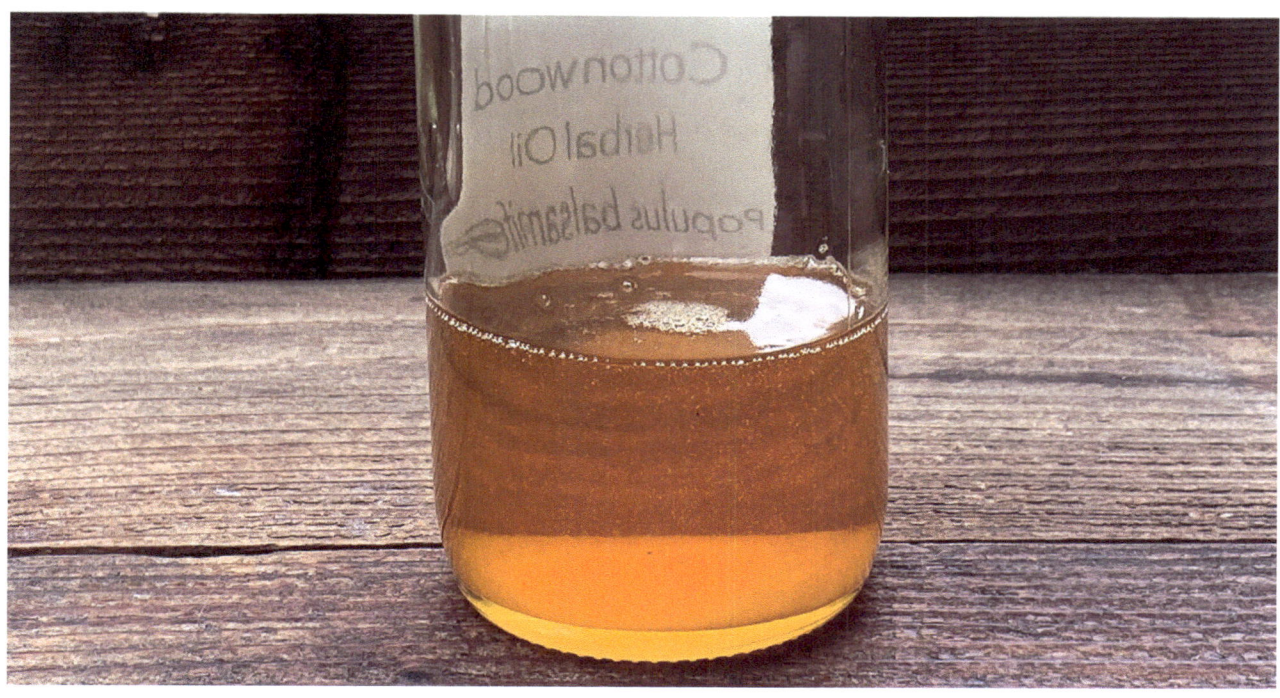

St. John's Wort
Hypericum perforatum

Common name: St. John's wort
Scientific name: *Hypericum perforatum* L.
Botanical family: Hypericaceae or Clusiaceae
Conservation status: Not yet assessed

Description: St. John's wort is an herbaceous perennial in the Hypericaceae family native to Northern Africa, Western Asia, and Europe. *H. perforatum* is a freely branching shrubby herb that grows 40 - 80 cm tall. Branches and stems are densely covered in oblong leaves 1 - 3 cm long and 0.3 - 1.0 cm wide. The leaves are punctuated by minute, translucent perforations visible when held up to the light, hence the species name *perforatum*. Mature plants produce dozens of five-petaled yellow flowers that exude a blood-red pigment when crushed. In late summer, the flowers produce capsules containing many diminutive dark brown seeds. St. John's wort has spread throughout temperate regions of the world, where it grows wild in open, disturbed areas.

Ethnobotany: St. John's wort was thought to be a plant of mystical protection, capable of warding off demons and evil spirits. Indeed, the genus name *Hypericum* originated from the Greek name for the plant, *hyperikon*, which stems from *hyper*, meaning "over," and *eikon*, which refers to an image or apparition. The common name St. John's wort arises from the practice of harvesting the plant at the height of its flowering on Saint John's Day (June 24). Olive oil infusions of the flowering tops turn a brilliant carmine after several weeks; according to early Christian legends, the plant releases its blood-red oil on August 29, the day of St. John's beheading.

Hypericum perforatum has been valued for its medicinal properties for over 2000 years. Greek physicians of the 1st century used the plant in wound healing, as a diuretic, to treat menstrual disorders, eradicate intestinal worms, and heal snakebites.

H. perforatum was a popular remedy throughout the Middle Ages, used to treat wounds and alleviate pain.

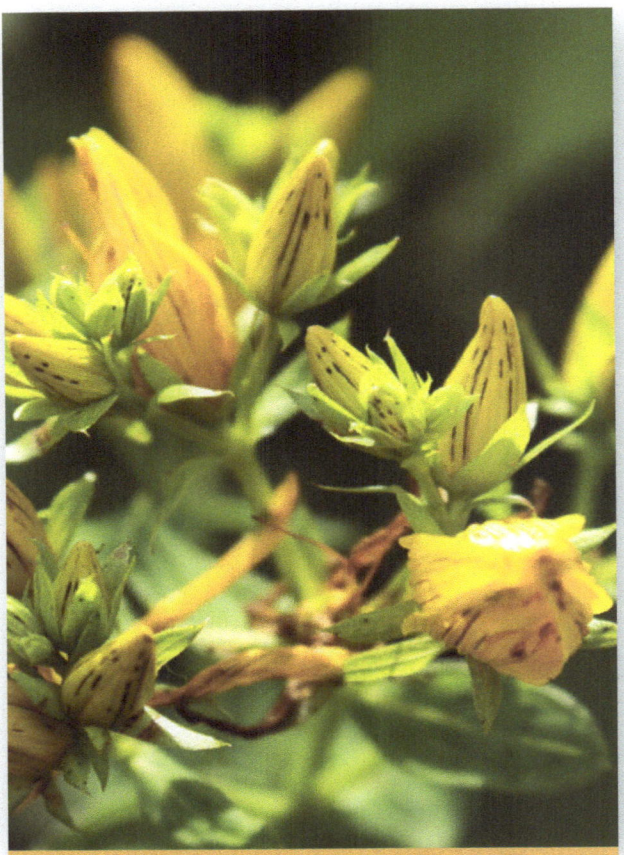

EXTRACTION INFORMATION

Part of plant used: Fresh flower bud
Oil used for extraction: Extra virgin olive oil or another suitable carrier oil
Extraction method: Solar Maceration
Note: St. John's wort oil maceration requires fresh plant material and sun exposure. The sunlight catalyzes the chemical reactions that develop many of the oil's therapeutic constituents.

MANUFACTURING INFORMATION

CAS number: 84082-80-4
EC number: 282-026-4
INCI name: Name of extracting oil, Hypericum Perforatum Flower/Leaf/Stem Extract
    Example: Olea Europaea (Olive) Fruit Oil, Hypericum Perforatum Flower/Leaf/Stem Extract
CAS number: 68917-49-7
INCI name: Hypericum Perforatum Oil
CosIng (functions): Skin Conditioning – emollient

SHELF LIFE

24-36 months

Sixteenth-century physician Paracelsus recommended it as a remedy for depression, melancholy, and overexcitation. In the 18th and 19th centuries, St. John's wort was used widely across Europe in the forms of teas and tinctures to treat anxiety, depression, insomnia, water retention, and gastritis. Preparations of the flowering tops in vegetable oils were used topically to treat hemorrhoids, sores, cuts, burns, and abrasions, especially those involving nerve damage.[58]

PHYTOCHEMISTRY

Hypericum perforatum is rich in naphthodianthrones, phloroglucinols, and flavonoids (such as phenylpropanes, flavonol glycosides, and biflavones), as well as volatile constituents.[59] The naphthodianthrone component, hypericin, is responsible for the red-colored oil the fresh buds exude as well as for the therapeutic activity of St. John's wort tincture. However, hypericin is not found in lipophilic extractions; therefore, the red color of St. John's wort herbal oil is thought to be due to a degradation product of hypericin upon exposure to sunlight.[59]

Lipophilic compounds found in St. John's wort herbal oil include phloroglucinol components, hyperforin, adhyperforin, and their derivatives. St. John's wort olive oil macerations contain 4.2% hyperforin and 0.8% adhyperforin,[60, 61] whereas the CO_2 extract may contain up to 27.02% hyperforin and 5.23% adhyperforin.[73] Hyperforin is considered to be responsible for the oil's therapeutic activity.[60] Both hyperforin and adhyperforin exhibit powerful anti-inflammatory activity.[63] It should be noted that hyperforin is unstable with light and heat and is susceptible to oxidation into furohyperforin within weeks of finished extraction and will not be found in aged St. John's wort herbal oils.[63]

St. John's wort flowers contain 0.05% to 0.92% volatile fraction.[59] The volatile components vary widely depending on the country of origin. In general, the essential oil is rich in monoterpenes and sesquiterpenes, primarily alpha- and beta-pinene, beta-caryophyllene, 2-methyl octane, spathulenol, germacrene D, and caryophyllene oxide.[64, 65]

SAFETY INFORMATION

The infused oil of St. John's wort does not contain hypericin, which may be responsible for the photosensitizing activity of some *Hypericum* extracts. The infused oil is safe for external applications.[62]

Formulating with St. John's wort Herbal Oil

Sensory info: Rich deep red color
Dilution: Can be used 5-25% in a blend of other carrier oils.

Therapeutic actions: analgesic, antibacterial[66], anti-inflammatory, antioxidant, vulnerary

Therapeutic applications:

- Insect bites
- Burns, including sunburns
- Bruises
- Herpes lesions
- Myalgia (muscle pain)
- Dermal inflammation
- Atopic dermatitis (mild to moderate)[67]
- Sprains and bruises (not as potent as arnica)
- Damaged tissue, slow healing wounds or ulcers

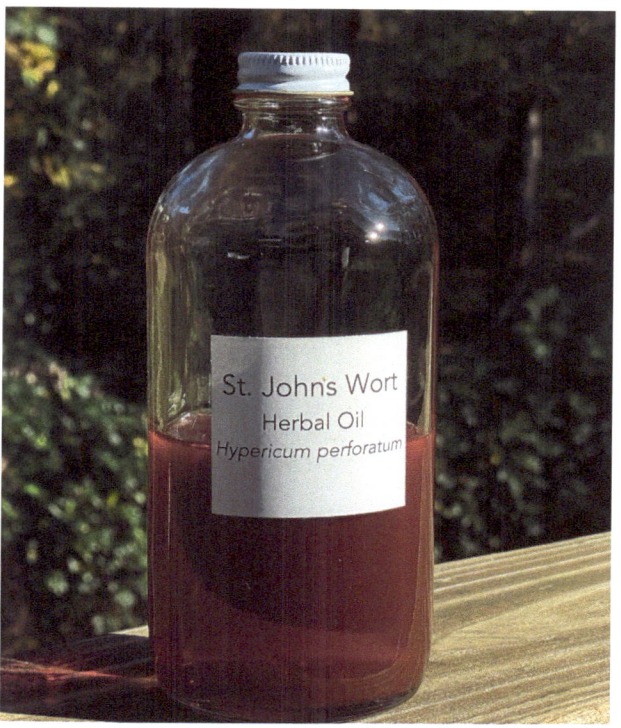

Part Six:
The Butters

The Butters

There are many natural butters on the market, and there will undoubtedly be new ones as the market continues to grow with increased interest in natural butters and oils. Natural butters are solid or semi-solid, although we call a few of them, like coconut, "oil" instead of "butter." Some butters, like mango and shea nut, are popular and well-known. Others, like cupucaçu and kombo butter, are less familiar but have many desirable therapeutic qualities.

Should we use hydrogenated butters?

Whether or not to use hydrogenated butters is a personal choice, but we recommend against it. If hydrogenated fats are unhealthy for us physiologically, they cannot possibly be good for our skin. There are quite a few hydrogenated butters made from plants that do not naturally produce a butter, including aloe butter, apricot butter, avocado butter, coffee bean butter, hemp seed butter, and olive butter. There are also nut butters, such as sweet almond and macadamia, where an oil may be hydrogenated or blended with a hydrogenated butter. As with oils, be sure to check on the manufacturing process with butters before purchasing.

Benefits of Butters

- Emollient
- Anti-inflammatory
- Antioxidant
- Humectant properties (e.g., cupuaçu butter)
- Excellent for psoriasis, eczema, atopic dermatitis, dry itchy conditions, and sunburn
- Supports the health of the skin's barrier function
- Build viscosity (thickness) of cream or lotion formulations
- Moisturizing (by slowing TEWL)

Storage of Butters

Store in cool/dark location. Protect from exposure to light, air, moisture, and pests. Do not expose to extreme temperatures and keep tightly sealed.

Products that use butters

- Body balms
- Creams and lotions
- Deodorants
- Lip balms
- Lotion bars
- Whipped butters

Classification of Butters

Hard Butters	Semi-hard Butters	Soft Butters
Cocoa butter Cupuaçu butter	Kokum butter Mango butter Kpangnan butter Shea butter	Babassu oil Coconut oil Kombo butter Palm kernel oil

Melting Points of Carrier Oil Butters

Butter	Melting temp.°F (°C) (Approx.)
Babassu oil	76 – 79 (24 – 26 C)
Cocoa butter	93 – 100 (34 - 38 C)
Coconut oil	76 - 78 (24 – 25 C)
Cupuaçu butter	84 - 93 (29 - 34 C)
Kokum butter	102 – 103 (39 – 40 C)
Kombo butter	102 - 109 (39 – 43 C)
Kpangnan butter	95 – 104 (35 – 40 C)
Mango butter	86 – 99 (30 - 36 C)
Palm kernel oil	68 - 75 (20 - 24 C)
Shea butter	90 – 104 (32 - 40 C)

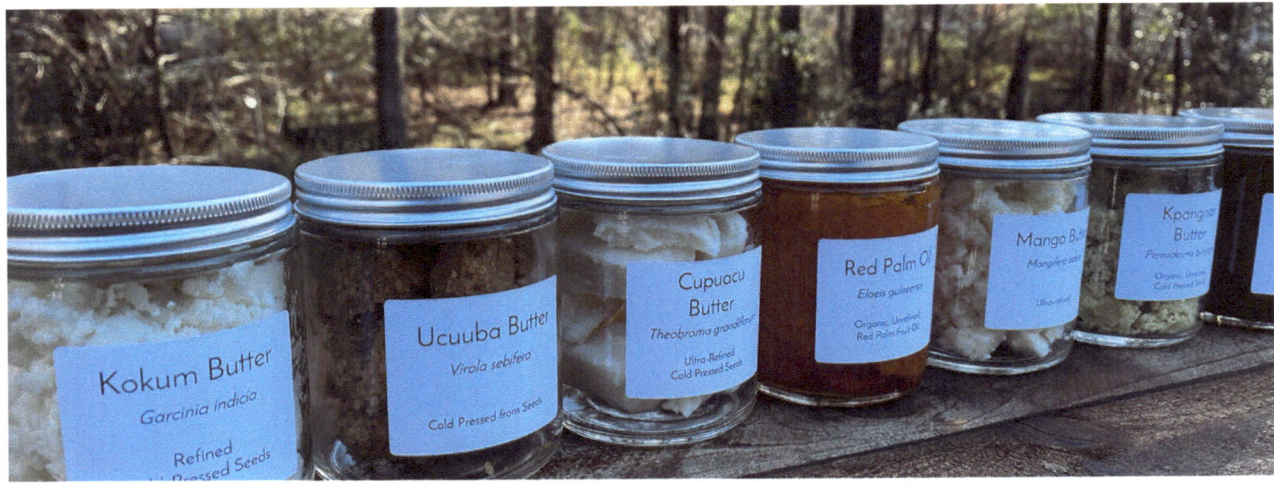

Formulating with Butters

To make a body balm or butter, melt and combine the ingredients in the following order:

1. Wax ingredients – both solid and liquid (beeswax, carnauba wax, candelilla wax, jojoba oil, and meadowfoam oil)
2. Hard butters (cocoa butter, cupuaçu butter)
3. Medium-hard butter ingredients except for shea butter
4. Soft butters
5. Liquid carrier oils
6. Remove from heat.
7. Add shea butter and stir until melted.
8. Add essential oils, antioxidants, and any other special extracts.

To make products with wax, use the following ratios (approximate):

Product	Carrier Oils (incl. liquid wax)	Solid Wax
Hard salve	55 - 70%	30 - 45%
Balm (Hard to soft – lotion bar, lip balm, deodorant)	75 - 80%	20 - 25%
Body butter	75 - 90%	10 – 25%
Soft body butter	85 – 90%	10 – 15%

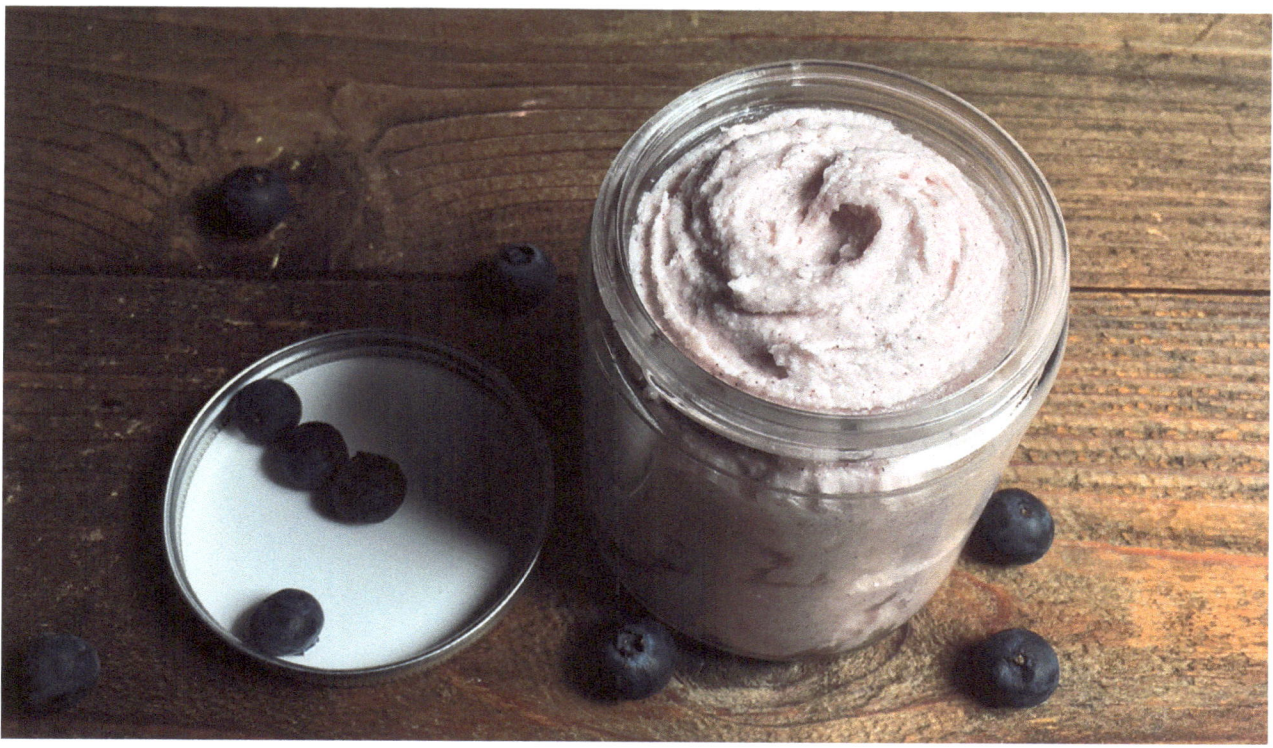

Babassu

Attalea speciosa

Common name: Babassu, babaçu, cusi, babassu palm
Scientific name: *Attalea speciosa* Mart. Ex Spreng.
Synonym: *Orbignya oleifera* Burret, *Orbignya phalerata* Mart.
Botanical family: Arecaceae
Conservation status: Least concern[1]

Description: *Attalea speciosa* is a monoecious, evergreen species belonging to the Palm family. The tree grows 20-30 m tall and displays a broad canopy of large, pinnate leaves. The flowers develop in long (up to 1.5 m) inflorescences. The numerous oblong babassu fruits look like small coconuts, about 6 cm in diameter.[2] Each kernel contains one or two seeds with a white, oily endosperm. The babassu palm begins to produce fruit when 7-10 years old and can continue producing fruit for up to 35 years.

Ethnobotany: The babassu palm provides a livelihood for over 300,000 people, including many women, called babassu nut breakers, across northeastern Brazil. The indigenous people of Maranhão, Brazil, have used various parts of the babassu tree, including the leaves, roots, and fruits, for food, handicrafts, construction, cosmetics, religious, and medicinal purposes. They use the oil to treat inflamed skin diseases, wounds, fungal infections, hemorrhoids, constipation, leukorrhea, vulvovaginitis, and joint and muscular inflammation.[3,4,5,6]

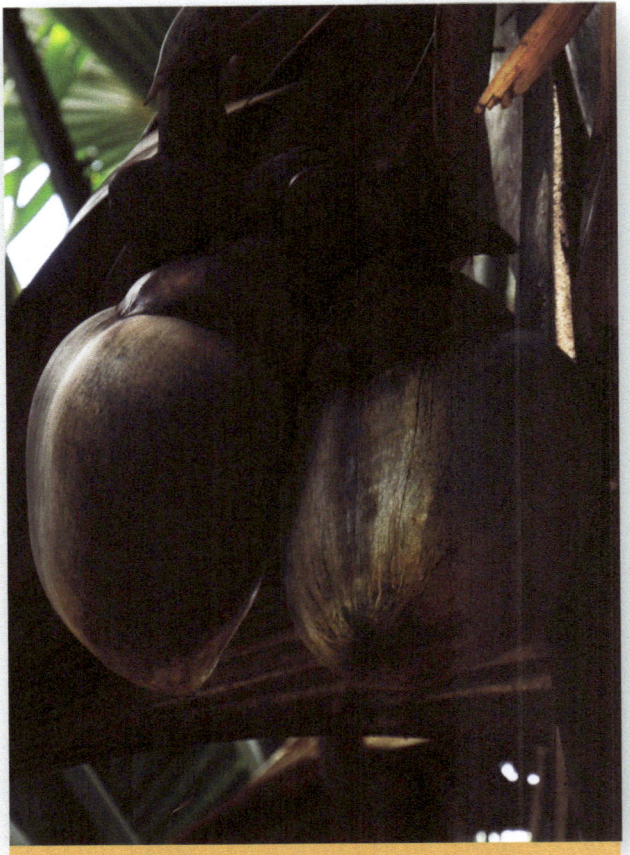

EXTRACTION INFORMATION

Country of origin: Brazil
Part of plant: Seed
Oil content: 65-68%
Extraction method: Cold pressing, Expeller pressing

MANUFACTURING INFORMATION

CAS number: 91078-92-1
EC number: 293-376-2
INCI name: Attalea Speciosa Seed Butter, Orbignya Oleifera Seed Oil
CosIng (functions): Skin conditioning, Skin conditioning - emollient

SHELF LIFE

2 years

NUTRIENT PROFILE

Babassu oil is a rich source of saturated fatty acids, especially lauric acid.

Babassu Butter[4, 7, 8]	
SATURATED FATTY ACIDS	
Caprylic acid (C8:0)	2.6 - 7.3%
Capric acid (C10:0)	1.2 - 7.6%
Lauric acid (C12:0)	**40 - 55%**
Myristic acid (C14:0)	**11 - 27%**
Palmitic acid (C16:0)	5.2 - 11%
Stearic acid (C18:0)	1.8 - 7.4%
MONOUNSATURATED FATTY ACIDS	
Oleic acid (C18:1 n-9)	9 - 20%
POLYUNSATURATED FATTY ACIDS	
Linoleic acid (C18:2 n-6)	1.4 - 6.6%
UNSAPONIFIABLE FRACTION	
Sterols 500 – 800 mg/kg	Beta-sitosterol (241 - 431.2 mg/kg), delta-5-avenasterol (84.5 - 163.2 mg/kg), campesterol (88.5 – 149.6 mg/kg), stigmasterol (43.5 - 73.6 mg/kg), cholesterol (6 - 13.6 mg/kg), delta-7-avenasterol (2 - 8 mg/kg), brassicasterol (n.d. - 2.4 mg/kg)
Tocopherols 60 – 65 mg/kg	Beta-tocopherol (n.d. - 35.8 mg/kg), alpha-tocopherol (n.d. - 16.9 mg/kg), gamma-tocopherol (n.d. - 16.7 mg/kg)

Formulating with Babassu Oil

Sensory info: Lightweight white solid, melts quickly on the skin due to low melting point, non-greasy

Babassu oil can replace coconut oil or palm kernel oil in body butters, whipped butters, lip and body balms, and creams.

Therapeutic actions: non-comedogenic emollient, anti-inflammatory[4, 9] and wound healing properties[4]

Therapeutic applications:
- Acne-prone skin[10]
- Itchy skin
- Eczema
- Contact dermatitis
- Hives
- Seborrheic dermatitis
- Psoriasis
- Hair care

Considered cooling in Ayurvedic medicine and is indicated for Pitta skin conditions

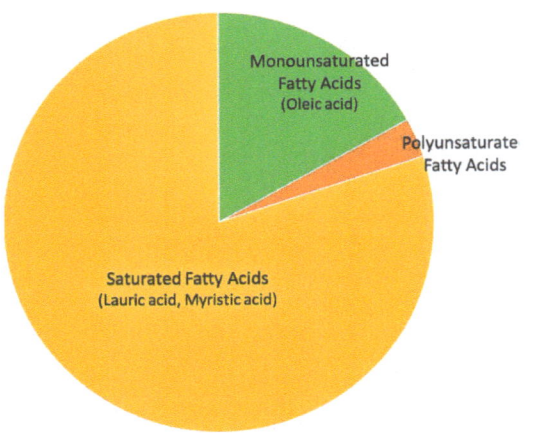

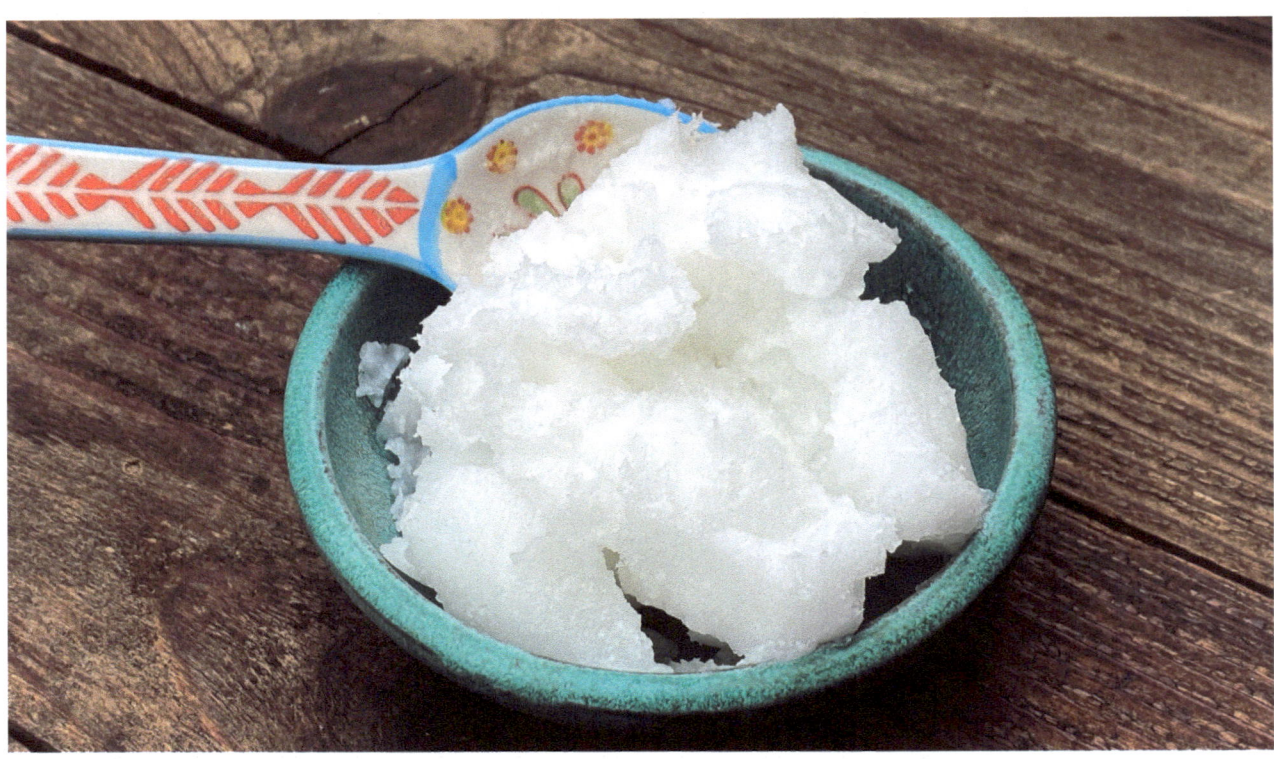

Cocoa
Theobroma cacao

Common name: Cocoa, cacao
Scientific name: *Theobroma cacao* L.
Botanical family: Malvaceae
Conservation status: Not yet assessed

Description: *Theobroma cacao* grows in the understory of tropical rainforest regions of Central and South America. In the wild, the evergreen tree typically grows 20-30 feet tall, with bright green leaves 4-8 inches long, which are oval and glossy. The fragrant flowers are small and pink and grow directly on the trunk and branches all year. Ten-ribbed seedpods may be yellow to yellow-brown, green, or red when ripe and grow up to 12 inches long and 3 inches in diameter. Each pod contains 20-50 flat seeds surrounded by a creamy-white, edible pulp that tastes sweet.

The *T. cacao* tree is widely cultivated for its seeds in lowland tropical regions worldwide. The seeds must go through several processing steps, including fermentation, drying, and roasting, before they become the chocolate we value so highly. These processed seeds, known as cocoa beans, must be cracked open to separate the nibs from the shell. The nibs are ground into a thick paste known as cocoa liquor, which is used to make chocolate. This paste can also be pressed to extract the fat, cocoa butter, a common ingredient in soaps, cosmetics, and medicines. The non-fatty portion that remains is ground to form cocoa powder. Cocoa seeds contain the alkaloid theobromine, a stimulant reminiscent of caffeine.[11]

Ethnobotany: *Theobroma cacao* trees have a long history of cultivation in Mexico, Central America, and South America. Various components of the tree provided food, medicine, currency, offerings and tributes for gods and royalty, fiber for cloth, thread, paper, and as material for construction. The Aztecs of Mexico made a bitter drink from the seeds; indeed, the name chocolate may be derived from the Aztec word *xocolatl*, which means "bitter water," although there is some debate about this claim. Both Columbus (1502) and Cortez (1520) brought cocoa seeds back to Spain,

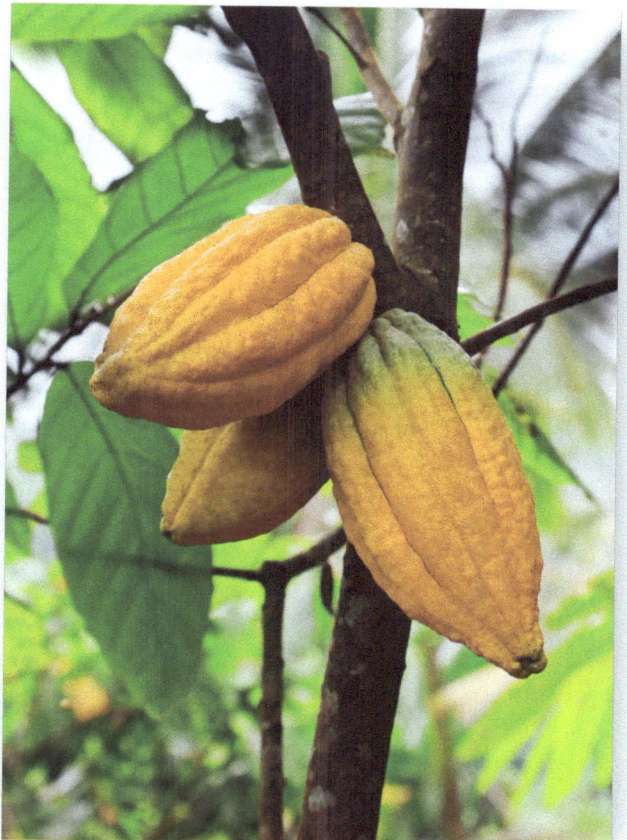

EXTRACTION INFORMATION

Country of origin: Cote d'Ivoire, Ghana, Indonesia, Nigeria, Cameroon, Mexica, Costa Rica
Part of plant: Seed (nibs)
Oil content: 55%
Extraction method: Cold pressing, Expeller pressing

MANUFACTURING INFORMATION

CAS number: 8002-31-1
EC number: 616-793-7
INCI name: Theobroma Cacao Seed Butter
CosIng (functions): Fragrance, Skin conditioning, Skin conditioning – emollient, Skin protecting

SHELF LIFE

24-48 months

though they did not gain immediate popularity.

The genus name *Theobroma* was coined by Linnaeus from the Latin theos, meaning "god," and *broma* meaning "food," so the name literally means "food of the gods." The specific epithet cacao comes from the Aztec name for the tree.[12]

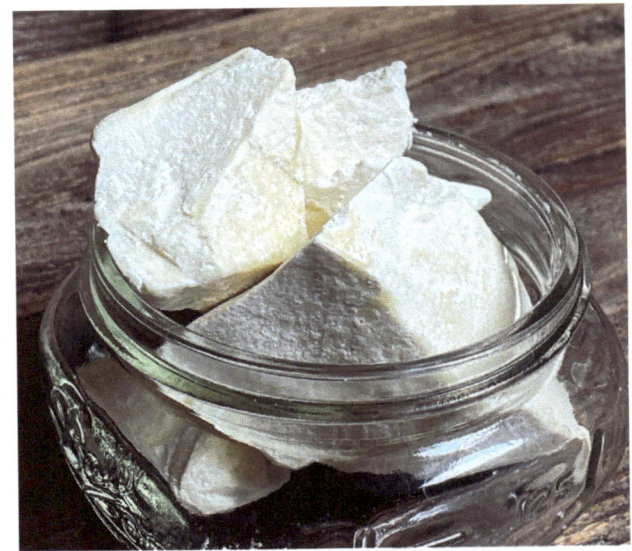

Cocoa butter has been used to soothe and soften damaged or chapped skin, relieve bruising, and treat burns. It is a common ingredient in skin creams and as a suppository base. As a medicinal food, chocolate is valued as a bitter stimulant diuretic that lowers blood pressure. The seeds were used in Central America and the Caribbean as a heart and kidney tonic, and an infusion of baked seed membranes was a remedy for anemia.[11]

NUTRIENT PROFILE

Cocoa or Cacao Butter[13, 14, 15]	
Saturated fatty acids	
Myristic acid (C14:0)	0 - 4.0%
Palmitic acid (C16:0)	**23.0 - 33.7%**
Stearic acid (C18:0)	**32.86 - 40.2%**
Monounsaturated fatty acids	
Palmitoleic acid (C16:1 n-7)	0 - 4.0%
Oleic acid (C18:1 n-9)	**26.30 - 35%**
Polyunsaturated fatty acids	
Linoleic acid (C18:2 n-6)	1.09 - 3.6%
Unsaponifiable fraction	
Sterols 4960 - 6441 mg/kg	Stigmasterol (1645 - 2795 mg/kg), beta-sitosterol (1911 - 2030 mg/kg), campesterol (1404 - 1721 mg/kg)[16]
Tocopherols 100 - 300 mg/kg	Gamma-tocopherol (3.4 - 246.9 mg/kg), alpha-tocopherol (1.10 - 9.00 mg/kg), delta-tocopherol (2.6 - 5 mg/kg)

Formulating with Cocoa Butter

Sensory info: Pale yellow color, brittle, melts readily at body temperature; cocoa / chocolate-like aroma. Stays solid at room temperature.

Therapeutic actions: emollient, occlusive, antioxidant

Indicated for:
- Dry, sore, chapped skin conditions,
- Chapped lips
- Rough skin
- Wrinkles
- Mature skin

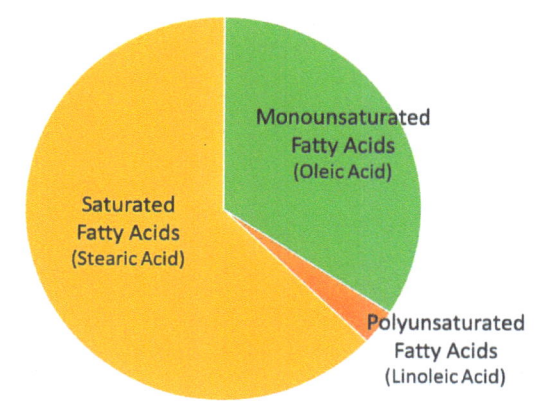

Notes: Cocoa butter is used to make suppositories for herbal and aromatic medicine.

Special Considerations

Heating and Melting
Due to the nature of cocoa butter and its differing melting and cooling curves, chill formulations that contain more than 20% cocoa butter quickly. Put the formulation into the refrigerator or freezer for at least 15-20 minutes. This rapid cooling will also prevent cocoa butter from producing "bloom," which looks like a dusty white coating. One of the reasons it is best to keep dark chocolate in the freezer is it prevents bloom from forming.

Overheating or heating cocoa butter for too long results in a change in its structure, so that its melting point is below room temperature.

Dilution: Cocoa butter will harden any product, so if you are formulating a softer product, use 40% or less, usually 20-35% in a body butter formulation. If you want to make a stick or solid bar using cocoa butter, you can include 50% or more.

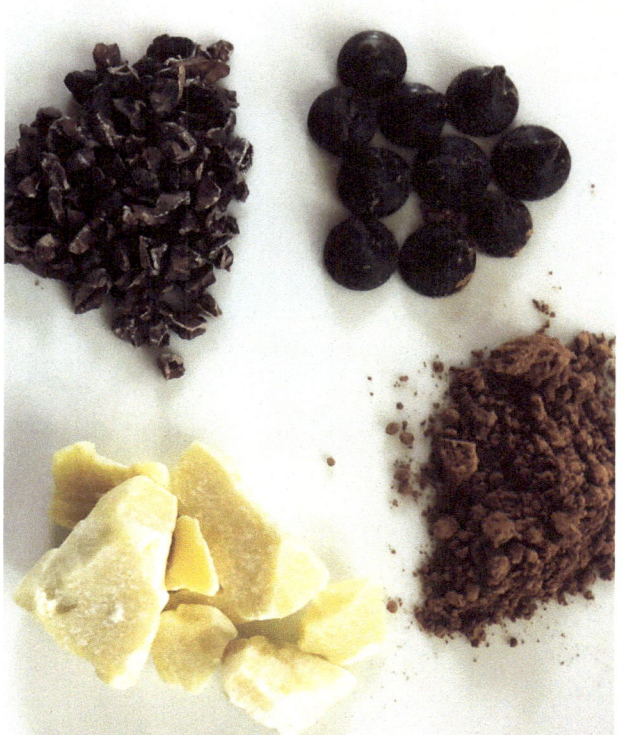

Coconut
Cocos nucifera

Common names: Coconut
Scientific name: *Cocos nucifera* L.
Botanical family: Arecaceae syn. Palmaceae
Conservation status: Not yet assessed

Description: Coconut, a single-trunked palm tree, which typically grows to a height of 50-100 feet tall, is native to the tropical islands of the western Pacific. The coconut's branchless, smooth, light-grey trunk rises from a swollen base to a majestic crown of pinnate, downward-arching green fronds, which can be up to 15-20 feet in length. Fragrant, yellow flowers grow in elongated 4-foot-long clusters, appearing only in tropical climates and blooming throughout the year.[17]

Coconut fruit, a drupe, comprises three layers: an outer epicarp, a mesocarp, and an inner endocarp. The epicarp and the heavy fibrous mesocarp have many industrial applications. The woody endocarp is hard and dark brown. Inside, the endosperm comprises two parts- a liquid portion and a solid portion. The liquid part, known as "coconut water," is a thick, sweet, and slightly acidic liquid albumen, which, as the coconut fruit matures, develops into solid white albumen, which we call the "meat" of the coconut.[18]

Interestingly enough, palm "trees," including the coconut palm, are not trees at all, despite their appearance; instead, they are classified as "grass." Coconut palms are also unusual in that their trunks curve into the wind and not away from it.[19]

The genus name *Cocos* comes from Portuguese slang for "head or face;" the specific epithet *nucifera* means "nut-bearing."[17]

Ethnobotany: *C. nucifera* is the most naturally widespread fruit plant on the planet and has a long history of people using every part of the coconut plant, in addition to eating the food the coconut fruit provides. The trunk is used in construction, the fronds in basket weaving and thatching, the endosperm in cosmetics and medicine, and the flower stalk sap in

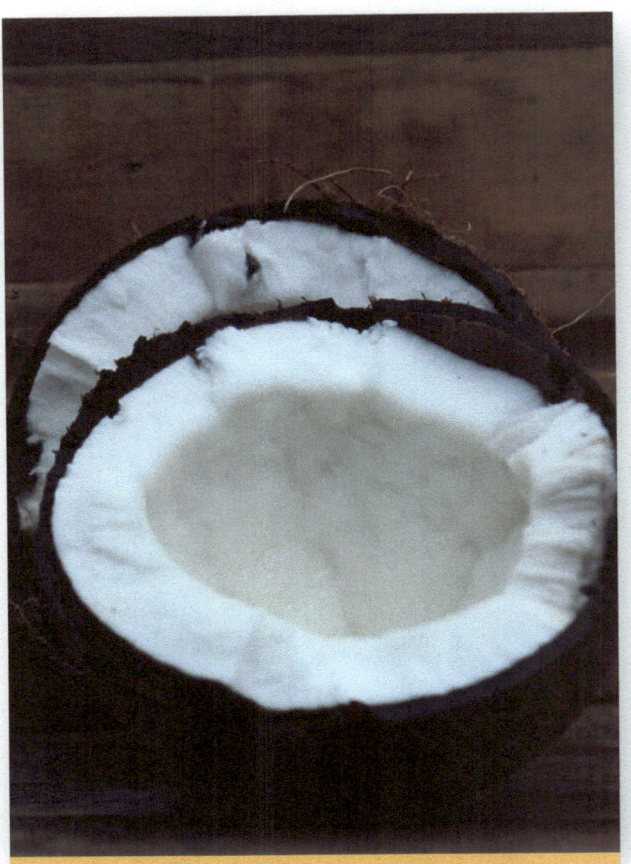

EXTRACTION INFORMATION

Country of origin: Indonesia, Hawaii, Philippines
Part of the plant: kernel / meat of mature coconuts
Oil content: 30-60%
Extraction method: Centrifuge, Expeller pressing, Cold pressing

MANUFACTURING INFORMATION

CAS number: 8001-31-8
EC number: 232-282-8
INCI name: Cocos Nucifera (Coconut) oil
CosIng (functions): Fragrance, Hair conditioning, Perfuming, Skin conditioning

SHELF LIFE

24 months

palm sugar manufacture.[20]

In areas where coconuts grow, traditional medicine also uses all parts of the coconut plant. In Brazil, people use a tea made from husk fibers to treat diarrhea; Guatemalans use a similar tea to reduce fever, relieve renal inflammation, and in a topical ointment for dermatitis, abscesses, and wounds. Ghanaians use the milk derived from coconut meat to alleviate diarrhea. The people of Papua New Guinea treat diarrhea and stomachache by chewing the leaves and young plants. Fijians apply coconut oil to prevent hair loss and drink coconut water to treat renal disease. Haitians drink a decoction of the dry pericarp to promote menstruation and apply coconut oil to burns. In Trinidad, a bark decoction is used to treat sexually transmitted diseases. In India, people may treat menstrual disorders with infusions of coconut flowers. Indonesians apply the oil to wounds, drink coconut milk as a contraceptive, and use a root extract to relieve fever and diarrhea.[18]

NUTRIENT PROFILE

Coconut oil belongs to a unique group of vegetable oils called lauric oils and is predominantly composed of saturated fatty acids (about 75-90%). It contains only about 0.5% of unsaponifiable components.

Coconut Oil[7, 21, 22, 23]	
SATURATED FATTY ACIDS	
Caproic acid (C6:0)	0.4 - 0.7%
Caprylic acid (C8:0)	4.6 - 10.0%
Capric acid (C10:0)	5.0 - 8.0%
Lauric acid (C12:0)	**45.1 - 53.2%**
Myristic acid (C14:0)	16.8 - 21%
Palmitic acid (C16:0)	7.5 - 10.2%
Stearic acid (C18:0)	2.0 - 4.0%
MONOUNSATURATED FATTY ACIDS	
Oleic acid (C18:1 n-9)	5.0 - 10%
POLYUNSATURATED FATTY ACIDS	
Linoleic acid (C18:2 n-6)	1.0 - 2.5%
UNSAPONIFIABLE FRACTION	
Sterols 400 - 1200 mg/kg	Beta-sitosterol (130 - 608 mg/kg), delta-5-avenasterol (80 - 488 mg/kg), stigmasterol (45 - 187 mg/kg), campesterol (24 - 134 mg/kg), cholesterol (n.d. - 36 mg/kg), delta-7-stigmastenol (n.d. - 36 mg/kg), delta-7-avenasterol (n.d. - 36 mg/kg), brassicasterol (n.d. - 3.6 mg/kg)
Tocopherols 35 - 58 mg/kg	Alpha-tocopherol (n.d. - 17 mg/kg), gamma-tocopherol (n.d. - 14 mg/kg), beta-tocopherol (n.d. - 11 mg/kg)

Formulating with Coconut Oil

Sensory info: Colorless at or above 30 degrees C (86 degrees F). White when solid. It has a sweet coconut aroma that may range from mild to intense, depending on the process used for extraction.

Therapeutic actions: emollient, slightly occlusive, prevents transepidermal water loss (TEWL), anti-inflammatory, antimicrobial[24]

Therapeutic applications:

- Dry skin
- Dry and damaged hair
- Mild skin infections and
- Acne-prone skin[25]
- Wound care

Considered cooling in Ayurvedic medicine and is indicated for Pitta skin conditions

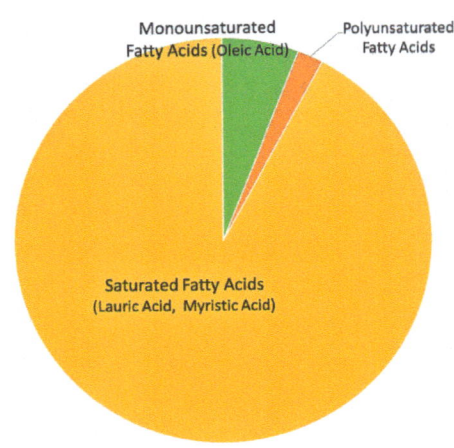

Research

Human Studies

In a randomized, double-blind clinical trial, researchers studied the effects of topical virgin coconut oil (VCO) and mineral oil on SCORAD (SCORing of Atopic Dermatitis) index values, TEWL, and skin capacitance in 105 pediatric patients, ages 1 through 13 years old, with mild to moderate atopic dermatitis AD.

Each patient's parents applied 5 ml of the assigned oil twice daily for several seconds to all body surfaces, excluding the diaper area/inguinal area and the scalp. All parents bathed the patients once daily with warm water for 5–10 minutes and applied the assigned oil immediately after bathing and at night.

In this study, VCO improved all outcomes significantly better than mineral oil. VCO exhibited emollient properties, decreased severity of atopic dermatitis, improved skin barrier function, relieved itchiness, and reduced TEWL.[26]

Another randomized, double-blind controlled clinical trial involving 34 patients examined the efficacy and safety of virgin coconut oil compared to mineral oil in treating mild to moderate xerosis. The study showed that coconut oil and mineral oil have comparable effects, and both were able to improve skin hydration and increase skin surface lipid levels.[27]

Animal Studies (*In vivo*)

In a study utilizing three (3) groups of young rats, researchers applied different concentrations of virgin coconut oil (VCO) to two groups' wounds over ten days, with the control group receiving no treatment. The VCO-treated wounds healed much faster with an increase in vascularization, proliferation of fibroblasts, and increased collagen turnover.[28]

In Vitro

One study demonstrated that VCO suppressed inflammatory markers and enhanced skin barrier function. The researchers concluded that topical use of VCO could be appropriate for skin disorders with permeability barrier dysfunction, especially in cases demonstrating a decrease in epidermal protein expression, such as atopic dermatitis and eczema.[29]

Should I Use Fractionated Coconut Oil in My Cosmetic Formulations?

When formulating natural therapeutic products, we usually prefer our ingredients result from physical extraction methods rather than chemical extraction methods. Fractionated coconut oil (FCO) is an example of a refined oil that may be an appropriate ingredient in some situations.

To produce FCO, manufacturers heat coconut oil to melt all the fatty acids with fewer than 12 carbon atoms, those shorter than lauric acid (C12:0). Using hydrolysis and steam distillation, they separate the solid (long-chain) fatty acids from the rest of the oil, resulting in an odorless, tasteless, colorless, clear oil that remains a liquid at room temperature. Three forms of liquid coconut oil can be produced this way: FCO for cosmetic use, liquid coconut oil, and medium-chain triglyceride (MCT) oil.

Cosmetic use FCO, liquid coconut oil, and MCT oil are similar products, but they also have distinct differences. MCT oil, for instance, can include medium-chain fatty acids from palm kernel oil in addition to coconut fatty acids, and liquid coconut oil is created as a refined cooking oil. Cosmetic grade FCO is less refined than liquid coconut oil and should only include fatty acids from coconut.

FCO contains some of the unsaponifiable fraction and other short-chain fatty acids found in virgin coconut oil, but its major components are caprylic acid (C8:0) and capric acid (C10:0). Although lauric acid (C12:0) is the primary active fatty acid that gives coconut oil its therapeutic qualities, caprylic (C8:0) and capric (C10:0) acid have also demonstrated properties one might desire in a therapeutic formulation.

Capric and caprylic acids' therapeutic qualities (mostly *in vitro* research):
- Skin penetration enhancers in lipophilic solvents[30]
- Antimicrobial activity (specific pathogens)[31,32,33] – internally & topically
- Inhibit biofilm formation[34] or eradicate biofilms[35]

Fractionated coconut oil (CAS #73398-61-5) is an emollient and skin conditioner, like virgin coconut oil, but it is less greasy and absorbs more quickly. FCO also resists oxidation with a shelf-life of 2-3 years. Considering FCO's physical qualities and the clinical evidence supporting the antimicrobial benefits of the primary components, FCO can also be an appropriate topical carrier choice.

Pros:	Cons:
<ul><li>Long shelf-life (2-3 years)</li><li>Liquid at room temperature</li><li>Fragrance-free</li><li>Non-greasy, easily absorbed</li><li>Emollient, moisturizing</li><li>Suitable for those with sensitive skin</li><li>Antimicrobial activity</li></ul>	<ul><li>Refined, manufactured</li><li>Simple chemical composition</li><li>Fewer target therapeutic applications</li><li>More expensive than virgin coconut oil</li></ul>

Cupuaçu

Theobroma grandiflorum

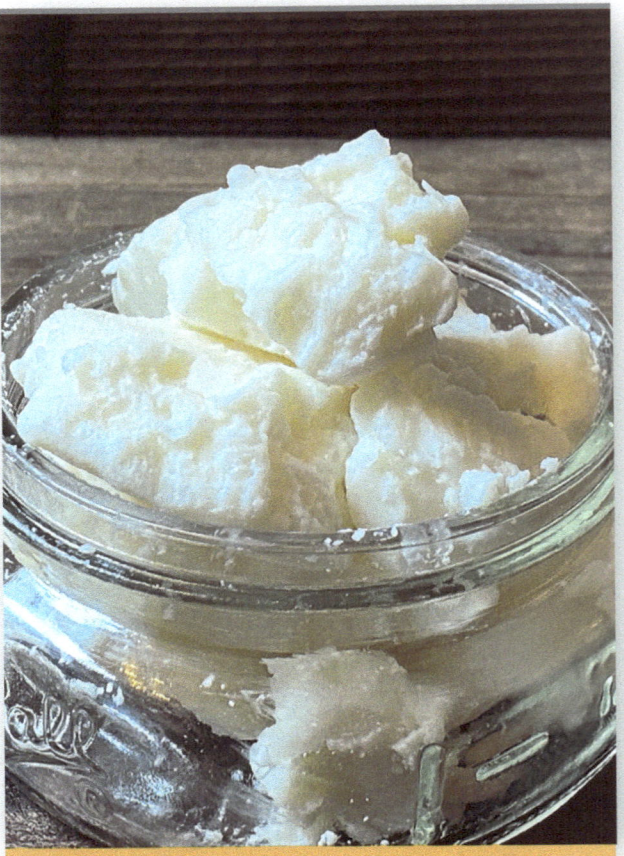

Common name: Cupuaçu (pronounced coo-poo-AH-soo), cupuassu, cupu assu, copoasu, cupuaú
Scientific name: *Theobroma grandiflorum* (Willdenow ex Sprengel) Schumann
Synonym: *Bubroma grandiflorum* Willd. Ex Spreng.
Botanical family: Malvaceae (previously in the Sterculiaceae family)
Conservation status: Least concern[36]

Description: The genus *Theobroma* comprises about 20 species, several of which produce edible seeds, most notably cacao and cupuaçu. The cupuaçu tree is a tropical rainforest native to the Brazilian Amazon, reaching 20 m tall in the wild and 6 to 8 m when cultivated. The tree is widely cultivated in Brazil, Costa Rica, Colombia, Ecuador, and other South American countries.

Young cupuaçu tree large leaves are pink with rusty hairs, becoming dark green upon maturity. The tree produces flowers either singly or in groups of five. The fruit of the cupuaçu tree is the largest of the *Theobroma* genus. It has the characteristics of a drupe and a berry; each berry weighs between 500 – 4500 g and contains five vertical rows of 9-62 seeds surrounded by a white-yellowish pulp that exudes a pleasant aroma. The cupuaçu tree can produce fruit for more than eighty years.

The name cupuaçu is derived from Tupi, the extinct language of the largest pre-colonial native Brazilian tribe, where *kupu* means "similar to cocoa" and *uasu* means "large" or "great."[37]

Ethnobotany: The fruit is utilized as food and medicine by indigenous tribes of the rainforest.[38] The Tikuna tribe used the beans inside the fruit seed pods to treat abdominal pain. Traditional shamans would offer cupuaçu seeds to laboring women to ease labor pain.[39] The flesh of this brown fruit is sour, cream-colored, very fragrant, and has been used to make butter, desserts, ice cream, jellies, liquors, candy, and juices.[40] In skincare, the fatty butter from the cupuaçu

EXTRACTION INFORMATION

Country of origin: Brazil
Part of plant: Seed
Oil content: 40-60%
Extraction method: Cold pressing

MANUFACTURING INFORMATION

CAS number: 394236-97-6
EC number: n/a
INCI name: Theobroma Grandiflorum Seed Butter
CosIng (functions): Skin conditioning

SHELF LIFE

2 years

tree is considered a plant-based alternative to lanolin and can attract and hold more water (440% of its weight) than either shea butter (289% of its weight) or lanolin (250% of its weight).[41]

The seeds are processed not only for the butter but also to produce a chocolate-like product called "cupulate."

Native peoples in Brazil are fighting a Japanese effort to patent their extraction and cupuaçu chocolate-making process, which effectively interferes with the Brazilian people's right to benefit from this historic industry.[42]

NUTRIENT PROFILE

Rich in oleic acid and stearic acid with an unusually high amount of arachidic acid (9- 12%).

Cupuaçu Butter[43, 44, 45]	
Saturated fatty acids	
Palmitic acid (C16:0)	5.8 - 12.0%
Stearic acid (C18:0)	**22 - 35%**
Arachidic acid (C20:0)	9.49 - 12%
Behenic acid (C22:0)	1.2 - 1.72%
Monounsaturated fatty acids	
Oleic acid (C18:1 n-9)	**38 - 47%**
Polyunsaturated fatty acids	
Linoleic acid (C18:2 n-6)	2.37 - 9.0%
Alpha-linolenic acid (C18:3 n-3)	0.13 - 1.0%
Unsaponifiable fraction	
Sterols 2480 mg/kg	Beta-sitosterol (1960 mg/kg), stigmasterol (230 mg/kg), cycloartenol (170 mg/kg), campesterol (90 mg/kg)
Tocopherols 130 mg/kg	Gamma-tocopherol (122 mg/kg), delta-tocopherol (6 mg/kg)

Formulating with Cupuaçu Butter

Sensory info: Light yellow color; medium to hard solid at room temperature; slow to melt on the skin; very light fruity, nutty aroma.

Therapeutic actions: emollient, helps regulate lipid production in the skin,[46] supports skin elasticity, improves skin hydration,[41] antioxidant, anti-inflammatory, wound healing[48]

Therapeutic applications:
- Regenerative skin care[47]
- Dry, sore, chapped skin conditions
- Chapped lips; rough skin
- Wrinkles
- Mature skin
- Premature aging skin
- Inflammatory skin conditions,
- Sun-damaged skin
- Eczema
- Psoriasis

Note: Acts as an emulsifier in cream formulations

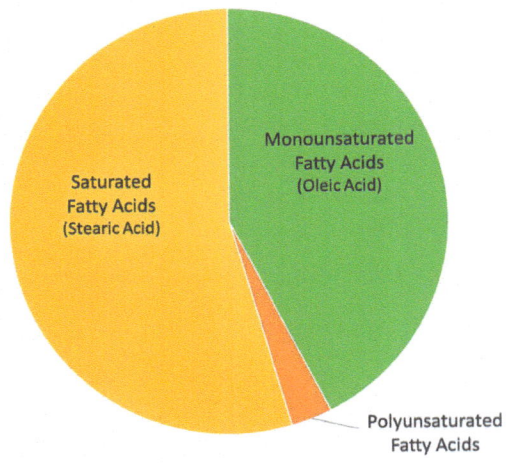

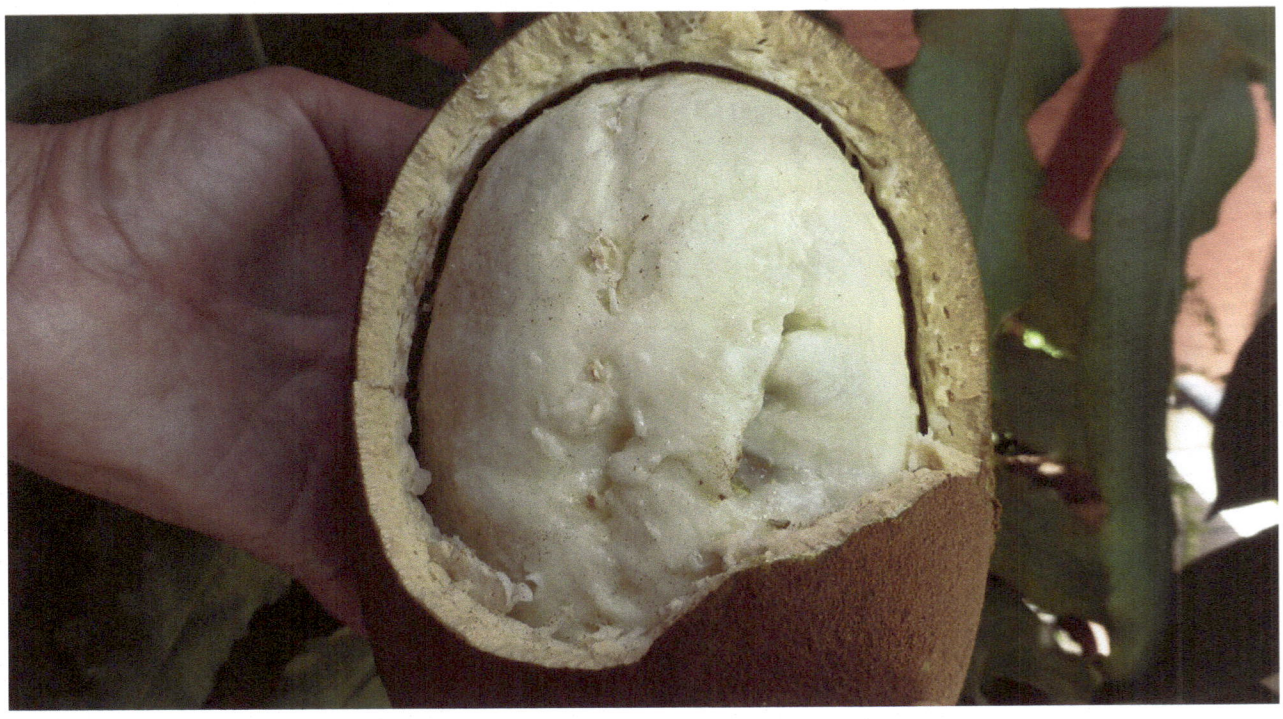

Kokum

Garcinia indica

Common names: Kokam, goa butter tree, kokum butter tree, bindin, biran, katambi, wild mangosteen
Scientific name: *Garcinia indica* (Thouars) Choisy
Botanical family: Clusiaceae syn. Guttiferae
Conservation status: Vulnerable (population decreasing)[49]

Description: The kokum tree is indigenous to the Western Ghats region of India and is one of the most valuable *Garcinia* species growing in the area. It is an evergreen, slender tree that grows 15 - 20 m tall. Its branches droop and provide a dense canopy of dark green leaves. The flowers are solitary or spread in clusters and are a dark pink color. The fruit is brown to brown-gray with yellow and becomes a dark purple-to-red tinged with yellow upon maturation. The round-to-oval fruit contains 3-8 large kidney-shaped flattened seeds embedded in a juicy, sweet-tasting, white pulp. The fat contained within the seeds is also referred to as Garcinia butter.[50,51]

Ethnobotany: Ayurvedic medicine has a long history of using kokum to treat different health-related problems like sores, dermatitis, diarrhea, dysentery, ear infections, and support healthy digestion.[52] Raw kokum fruits are eaten to remedy gastric issues, including acidity, flatulence, constipation, and indigestion.[53]

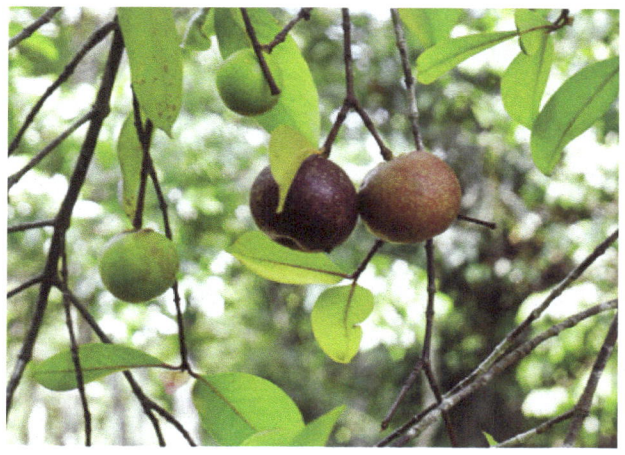

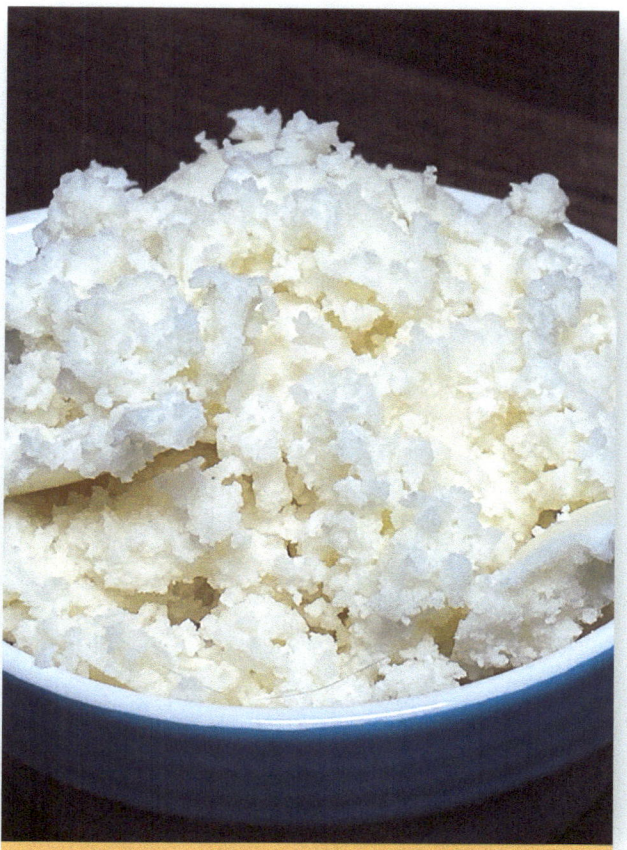

EXTRACTION INFORMATION

Country of origin: India
Part of plant: Seed
Oil content: 23-26%
Extraction method: Aqueous extraction, Expeller pressing, Solvent extraction Note: Often refined

MANUFACTURING INFORMATION

CAS number: n/a*
EC number: n/a*
INCI name: Garcinia Indica Seed Butter
CosIng (functions): Skin conditioning

*Kokum butter is often given CAS and EC numbers to classify it as a "Naturally Occurring Substance" and "Vegetable Oil."

SHELF LIFE

12-24 months

NUTRIENT PROFILE

Kokum Butter[51, 52, 54]	
SATURATED FATTY ACIDS	
Palmitic acid (C16:0)	2.5 - 6%
Stearic acid (C18:0)	**49 - 60%**
MONOUNSATURATED FATTY ACIDS	
Oleic acid (C18:1 n-9)	**30 - 42%**
Gondoic acid (C20:1 n-9)	2.25%
POLYUNSATURATED FATTY ACIDS	
Linoleic acid (C18:2 n-6)	0 - 5.25%
UNSAPONIFIABLE FRACTION 1 - 2%	
Sterols	1.02%
Tocopherols	200.1 mg/kg

Formulating with Kokum Butter

Sensory info: Greyish-white to white. Very light aroma. Solid at room temperature.

Therapeutic actions: emollient, demulcent, astringent, reduces inflammation, moisturizing, antioxidant, protects skin and hair from elements (wind, cold, heat)

Therapeutic applications:
- Psoriasis
- Atopic dermatitis
- Itchy conditions
- Wound healing
- Chapped or cracked skin
- Hair care

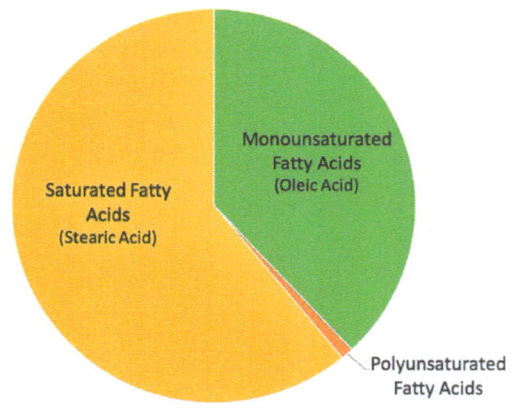

Note: Kokum butter may be used for suppositories.

Kombo

Pycnanthus angolensis

Common name: Kombo butter, African nutmeg, false nutmeg, wild nutmeg
Scientific name: *Pycnanthus angolensis* (Welw.) Warb.
Synonyms: *Pycnanthus kombo* (Baill.) Warb.
Botanical family: Myristicaceae
Conservation status: Least concern[55]

Description: *Pycnanthus angolensis* belongs to the Myristicaceae family, and while true nutmeg (*Myristica fragrans*) is also in the same family, the two plants are quite different. *P. angolensis* is an evergreen tree that grows in forests throughout tropical Africa, reaching 25-35 m in height. When the grey, fissured bark is slashed, it exudes a sticky honey-colored sap that turns red. The rust-colored flowers cluster together at the ends of the branches, and the fruits are oblong spherical drupes. The seeds are wrapped in bright crimson arils and somewhat resemble nutmeg seeds, hence its name, African nutmeg.[56] The seeds yield 45-70% of a yellow to reddish-brown solid fat (butter) called "kombo butter" or "Angola tallow."[57]

Pycnanthus comes from the Greek language. The literal meaning is "dense flowers," referring to the numerous flowers crowded together.

Ethnobotany: An extract from the bark of the kombo tree has been used in Nigerian folk medicine to treat complaints such as toothache, headache, sore throat, ulcers, and wounds.[58] Researchers have studied kombo butter's potential in treating arthritis and joint inflammation.[59]

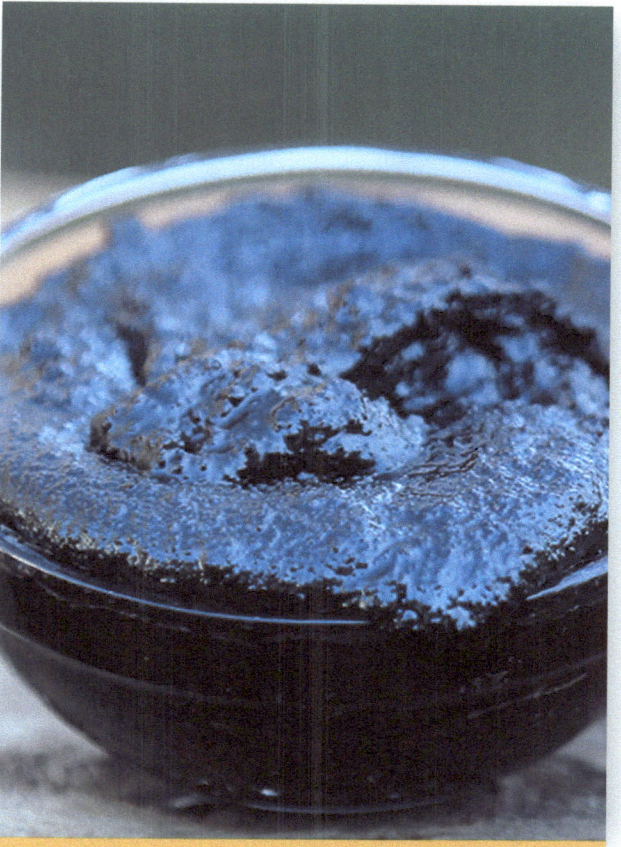

EXTRACTION INFORMATION

Country of origin: West Africa
Part of plant: Kernel
Oil yield: 41-74%
Extraction method: Cold pressing, Expeller pressing

MANUFACTURING INFORMATION

CAS number: n/a
EC number: n/a
INCI name: Pycnanthus Angolensis (African Nutmeg) Nut Oil
CosIng (functions): Skin conditioning - emollient

SHELF LIFE

2 years

NUTRIENT PROFILE

Kombo Butter[60, 61]	
SATURATED FATTY ACIDS	
Myristic acid (C14:0)	55 - 73%
Lauric acid (C12:0)	5.6%
Palmitic acid (C16:0)	2.2 - 7%
Stearic acid (C18:0)	< 3.0%
MONOUNSATURATED FATTY ACIDS	
Myristoleic acid (C14:1)	10 - 19.4%
Palmitoleic acid (C16:1 n-7)	0.3 - 2.8%
Oleic acid (C18:1 n-9)	5 - 13%
POLYUNSATURATED FATTY ACIDS	
Linoleic acid (C18:2 n-6)	< 2.0 %
UNSAPONIFIABLE FRACTION 1.2 - 1.3%[62]	

Myristoleic acid is a precursor of cetyl myristoleate, an ester, which has been found to help treat arthritis and joint pain.[60, 63] Kombo butter contains kombic acid, a highly unsaturated resin acid considered an antioxidant component of the butter.[64]

Formulating with Kombo Butter

Sensory info: Rich deep red-brown color, very medicinal smelling, pungent/bitter, semi-solid at room temperature

Therapeutic actions: anti-inflammatory,[60, 65] antioxidant, lubricates joints

Therapeutic applications:
- Joint pain
- Pain due to inflammation

Notes: This is a potent butter, so using it at 0.5 to 1% in a blend of carrier oils can be sufficient. Its aroma can be overwhelming in higher concentrations. It can also irritate sensitive skin.

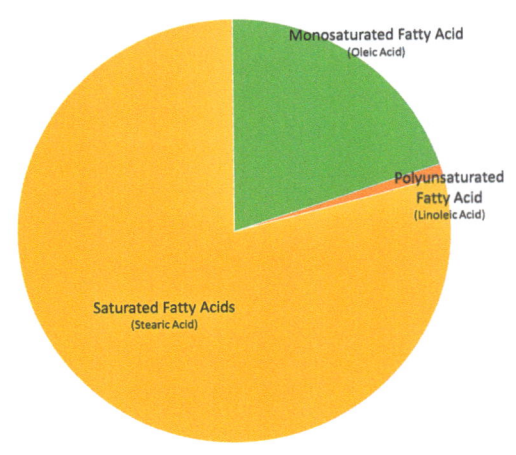

Kpangnan
Pentadesma butyracea

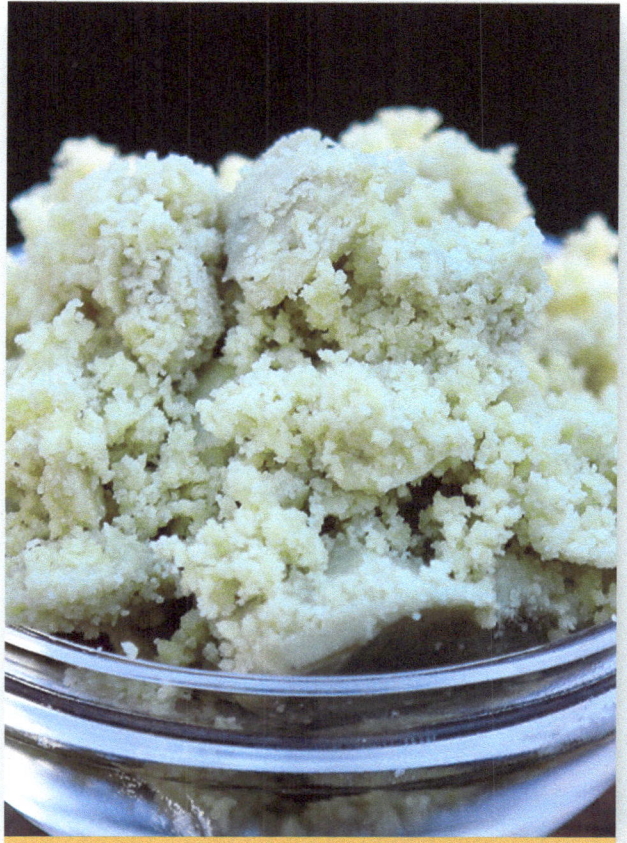

Common name: Kpangnan (PAN-ya), kanya butter, painya butter, tallow tree, African butter tree
Scientific name: *Pentadesma butyracea* Sabine
Botanical family: Clusiaceae
Conservation status: Least concern yet population is decreasing[66]

Description: *Pentadesma butyracea* is native to Africa and is widely distributed from Sierra Leone on the southwest coast to central Africa's Democratic Republic of the Congo. A tropical rainforest tree belonging to the Clusiaceae family, *P. butyracea* grows in wet swamps and riparian forests (located next to rivers) where it can reach a height of 20 - 35 m. The name kpangnan comes from the Republic of Benin, a country in West Africa, where kpangnan grows in riparian forest galleries.[67] Due to overexploitation, *P. butyracea* is becoming increasingly rare in the wild even though the IUCN Red List currently lists it as "least concern with population decreasing."

The trunk of the tree grows straight and has rough brown bark. The glossy, dark green leaves grow in clusters and are oval to elongated with a rounded top and base. The leaves contain resin glands. The tree produces 5-lobed greenish-white to whitish-red flowers with an intense aroma reminiscent of rancid butter. The spherical reddish-green berries (fruit) contain 3 to 10 flattened seeds and yellow flesh.[68]

Ethnobotany: To extract the butter, indigenous women gather the fruits and place them under trees where they are covered and allowed to decay and ferment for up to 10 days. This decaying process prepares the seeds for easier removal and crushing.[69] They then use two different methods to prepare the seeds before extracting the butter from the kernels. In Benin and west-central Nigeria, the Waama, Yom, and Batombu people use a boiling technique, while the Otamari of Benin and Togo use a roasting method. The first step, boiling ground kernels for two hours or roasting them for 48 hours over a wood fire in a large dirt oven, is all that differs. After the boiling or

EXTRACTION INFORMATION

Country of origin: West Africa, Benin Republic, Ghana, Togo
Part of plant: Kernel
Oil content: 40-50%, (35% yield)[75]
Extraction method: Aqueous extraction, Cold pressing

MANUFACTURING INFORMATION

CAS number: 94349-99-2
EC number: 305-217-7
INCI name: Pentadesma Butyracea Seed Butter
CosIng (functions): Skin conditioning – emollient

SHELF LIFE

2 years

roasting step, the kernels dry in the sun for up to three days. The people churn the powdered kernels with warm water to release the creamy butter, which they cool and skim off the water's surface.[70] These forms of heating the seeds do not seem to affect the fatty acid contents of the resulting butters.[71]

Indigenous people produce diverse products from *Pentadesma butyracea*. They use the timber for wood carving and building structures. They use the leaves, bark, and roots for medicinal purposes, including treating parasitic skin diseases, as an antidiuretic, and treating intestinal worms. Traditional medicine has used the butter for chest pain, children's coughs, muscle strains, abscesses,[72] massage, and to care for the skin and hair, as well as for its ability to soften and heal the skin. The butter is also used in the manufacture of soap. The kernels, full of the rich, edible butter, are consumed like kola nuts.[73, 74]

NUTRIENT PROFILE

The fatty acid profile of *Pentadesma* butter is similar to that of shea butter.[87] In the United States, kpangnan butter is sometimes sold as "golden shea butter" or "yellow shea butter."

Kpangnan Butter[70, 71, 74, 78]	
Saturated fatty acids	
Palmitic acid (C16:0)	2.7 - 3.7%
Stearic acid (C18:0)	**38 - 49.8%**
Monounsaturated fatty acids	
Oleic acid (C18:1 n-9)	**45.3 - 58%**
Polyunsaturated fatty acids	
Linoleic acid (C18:2 n-6)	0.5 - 1.4%
Unsaponifiable fraction <2%	
Sterols 1354 - 2205 mg/kg	Stigmasterol (891 - 1358 mg/kg), campesterol (242 - 560 mg/kg), beta-sitosterol (57 - 148 mg/kg), brassicasterol (48 - 110 mg/kg)
Tocopherols 95.3 - 194.7 mg/kg	Beta-tocopherol (8.3 - 107.8 mg/kg), alpha-tocopherol (29.2 - 97.4 mg/kg), delta-tocopherol (9.3 - 31.1 mg/kg), gamma-tocopherol (3.7 - 18.4 mg/kg)

Formulating with Kpangnan Butter

Sensory info: Light yellow with a tint of green. The dry, powdery solid melts on contact with skin. Garden soil-like aroma.

Therapeutic actions: anti-inflammatory (high stigmasterol content), emollient

Therapeutic applications:
- Itchy skin
- Irritated skin
- Dry hair
- Eczema
- Muscle soreness
- Soap-making

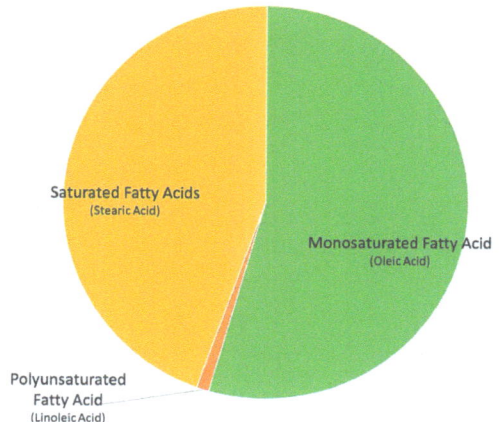

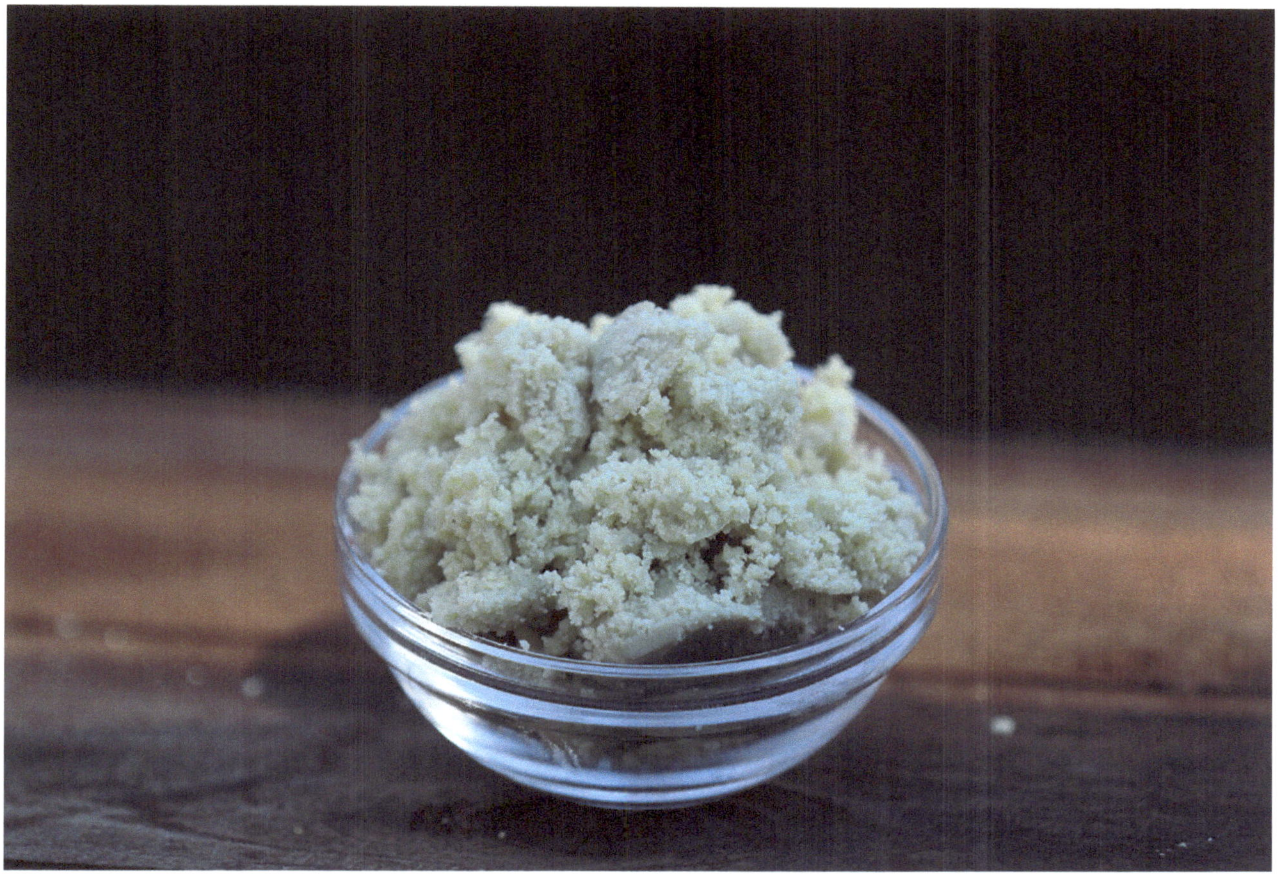

Mango

Mangifera indica

Common name: Mango
Scientific name: *Mangifera indica* L.
Botanical family: Anacardiaceae
Conservation status: Data deficient[79]

Description: The mango tree is native to tropical Asia and has been cultivated in India for over 4000 years. It is now widely cultivated and naturalized in tropical regions worldwide, including Asia, South and Central America, and Africa.

Mango is a large evergreen tree that can reach 10 - 45 m tall. It is a fast-growing, erect tree with a rounded, upright canopy. The tree produces 4000 - 5000 tiny whitish-red or yellowish-green flowers in panicles, although only a small percentage develop into fruit. With over 500 varieties of mango, the fruit, a large drupe, can have a variety of sizes, shapes, aromas, and colors. The soft mango fruit contains a thick yellow pulp with a single seed (kernel) contained within a hard, woody endocarp. Upon ripening, the skin is a yellow to slightly red color. The trees are long-lived, with some still producing fruit at 300 years old.[80, 81]

Ethnobotany: Mango, popular for its desirability as a delicious fruit, is known in India as the "King of Fruits." The chocolate industry sometimes includes mango butter in its chocolates.

Mango has played an important role in Ayurveda and the medicinal traditions of indigenous peoples. The leaves, bark, roots, fruits, and flowers have been used in traditional medicine to prevent and treat a wide range of diseases, and their use differs depending on the country where the tree grows.[82] While each part has been used to treat different conditions, all parts have treated diarrhea, indigestion, liver disorders, asthma, heatstroke, abscesses, and a host of other diseases or ailments.[83]

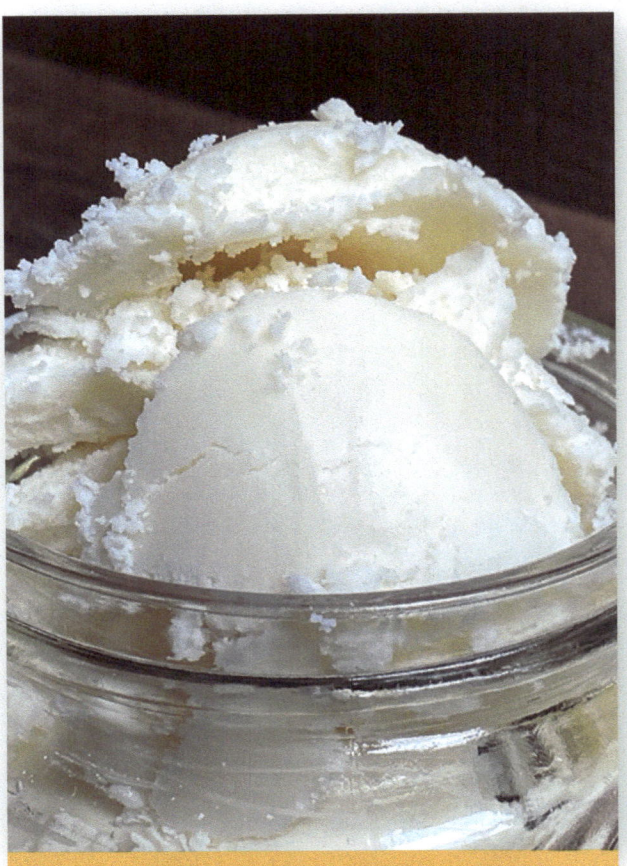

EXTRACTION INFORMATION

Country of origin: India, China, Thailand, Indonesia, Mexico, Pakistan, Brazil
Part of plant: Seed
Oil yield: 12-15%
Extraction method: Cold pressing, Expeller pressing

MANUFACTURING INFORMATION

CAS number: 90063-86-8
EC number: 290-045-4
INCI name: Mangifera Indica Seed Butter
CosIng (functions): Skin conditioning
Additional commercial oil name: Mango Kernel Fat and Mango Oil

SHELF LIFE

2 years

NUTRIENT PROFILE

Mango Butter[84, 85, 86, 87]	
SATURATED FATTY ACIDS	
Palmitic acid (C16:0)	5 - 12.8%
Stearic acid (C18:0)	**31 - 45%**
Arachidic acid (C20:0)	1 - 4%
MONOUNSATURATED FATTY ACIDS	
Oleic acid (C18:1 n-9)	**40 - 58%**
POLYUNSATURATED FATTY ACIDS	
Linoleic acid (C18:2 n-6)	2 - 4%
Alpha-linolenic acid (C18:3 n-3)	n.d. - 2.4%
UNSAPONIFIABLE FRACTION 0.94-2.83%[85]	
Sterols 990 - 1895 mg/kg	Sitosterol (460 - 1195 mg/kg), stigmasterol (190 - 430 mg/kg), campesterol (139 - 160 mg/kg), delta-5-avenasterol (110 mg/kg)
Tocopherols 259 - 266 mg/kg	Alpha-tocopherol (140 - 256 mg/kg), gamma-tocopherol (63 mg/kg), delta-tocopherol (62 mg/kg)

Formulating with Mango Butter

Sensory info: Light grey/yellow color; soft butter texture at room temperature; no aroma to very light, shea-like aroma.

Therapeutic actions: supports skin elasticity and suppleness, prevents and heals dry skin, emollient

Therapeutic applications:

- Dry skin
- Psoriasis
- Dry eczema
- Cracked heels or elbows
- Aging skin
- Itchy skin
- During pregnancy to prevent or reduce stretch marks, sunburn
- Haircare

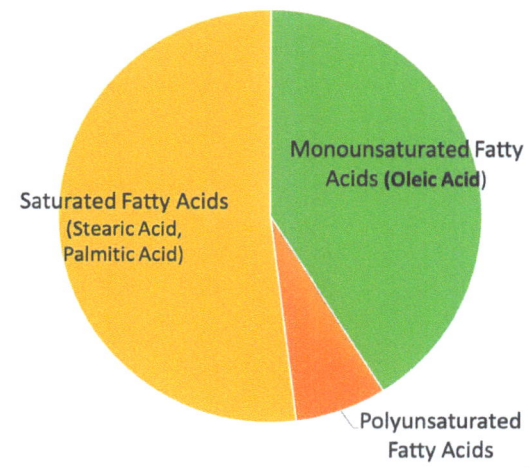

Palm
Elaeis guineensis

Common name: Palm
Scientific name: *Elaeis guineensis* Jacq.
Botanical family: Arecaceae syn. Palmaceae
Conservation status: Least concern[89] (Palm oil has other sustainability issues.)

Description: The African oil palm is an erect, single-stemmed palm tree in the Arecaceae family native to Africa. Although the African oil palm grows as an ornamental in some subtropical regions, it is cultivated for commercial purposes throughout West and Central Africa, Malaysia, and Indonesia.

Elaeis guineensis typically grows 20-30 m tall, with a cylindrical stem up to 75 cm in diameter. The stems of young palms are covered with petiole bases, while older trees (>10-12 years old) are smooth. The root system forms a dense mat in the top 35 cm of the soil, with a small number of roots reaching depths of 1 meter.

Juvenile leaves are lanceolate and entire, gradually becoming pinnate. Mature leaves are spirally arranged, even-pinnate, spiny, and up to 7.5 m long. Fruits are ovoid-oblong drupes 2 - 5 cm long, densely packed in large ovoid bunches of 1000-3000 fruits. The drupes feature a thin exocarp, an oil-producing mesocarp, and a rigid and woody endocarp that contains the embryo and solid endosperm.[90]

Many tiny flowers crowd on short branches and develop into large clusters of fruits. The fruits are black with a red base and, when ripe, contain a single oily seed known as the kernel. Palm kernel oil is pressed from this kernel.[91]

Three different fixed oils come from the African oil palm. Steaming and pressing the fruit produces crude palm oil, which we often call "red palm oil" because of its red-orange color, and palm oil, which is a refined product. Palm kernel oil comes from the seed or kernel. Refined palm oil is a ubiquitous ingredient in multiple industries that produce soaps, cosmetics, pharmaceuticals, candles, biofuels, lubricating greases, process tinplate and coat iron plates, and food

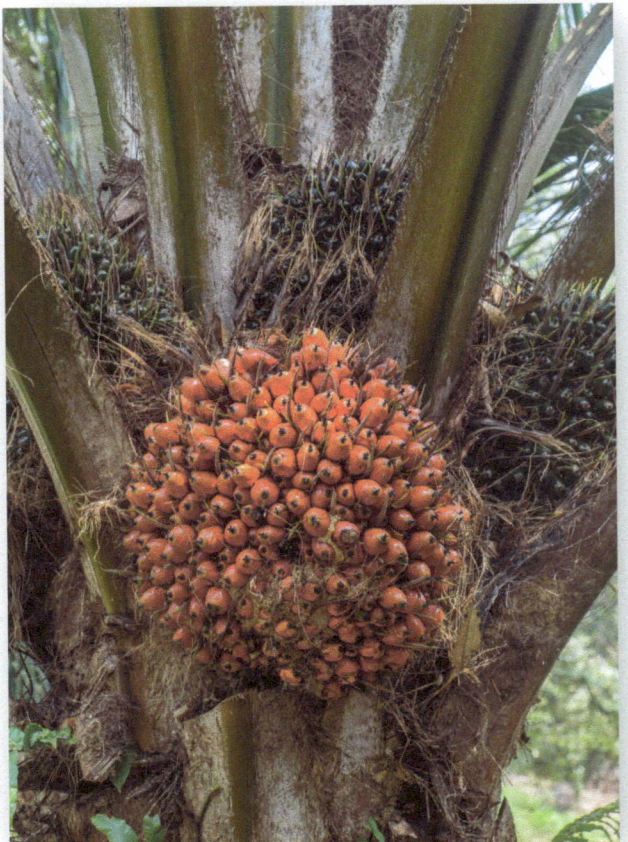

EXTRACTION INFORMATION

Country of origin: Indonesia, Malaysia, South America
Part of plant: Seed /Kernel
Oil content: 50%
Oil yield: 4-10%
Extraction method: Cold pressing

MANUFACTURING INFORMATION

CAS number: 8002-75-3
EC number: 232-316-1
INCI name: Elaeis Guineensis Butter
CosIng (functions): Fragrance, Skin conditioning, Skin conditioning – emollient, Viscosity-controlling

SHELF LIFE

2 years

products (including margarine, ice cream, confections, cookies, and bread). The fruit and kernels produce oils with significantly different nutrient profiles. Crude and refined palm oil are about 90% a combination of palmitic acid and unsaturated acids (oleic and linoleic acid) in contrast to palm kernel oil, which is about 70% lauric acid and myristic acid. Crude or red palm oil is also high in carotenoids (500-2000 mg/kg) and tocopherols (150-1500 mg/kg).[7]

The rapid expansion of the palm oil industry in the late 20th century and the associated destruction of native rainforest to clear the way for new plantations cause serious concern. Significant swaths of Indonesia, Malaysia, and Africa have been deforested using slash-and-burn methods, a practice that fragments natural forests and destroys the habitats of native animals and plants.

Experts consider palm oil one of the most important vegetable oils worldwide. Explosive demand has required palm oil production to increase steadily; production has doubled worldwide every ten years for the past 40 years. The palm industry has caused massive environmental degradation in Indonesia and Malaysia, which produce about 85% of the world's palm oil. Latin America and Africa's expansion of oil palm plantations is expected to exert a problematic impact on local communities in the years to come.[92]

Sustainability Issues: The primary concerns regarding palm oil production include the harmful effects on local water supplies, wildlife populations, biodiversity, climate change, and local communities as large global producers buy land for new monoculture plantations. Efforts to promote sustainable agricultural practices have been slow to take hold, resulting in some environmental groups encouraging consumers to boycott palm oil altogether.[93] Others feel it is more helpful to support palm oil producers working toward responsible management of the palm oil industry.[94]

It is of profound importance to acknowledge that the environmental concerns surrounding palm oil are specific to the industry's harmful practices. It is both possible and practical to cultivate the African oil palm with respect for existing people and environments. The African oil palm is indigenous to West Africa and is an essential traditional crop with an incredible variety of applications. In its native habitat, *E. guineensis* grows wild, or communities sustainably cultivate the trees by integrating them into fields with other crops, unlike the monoculture plantations used for global production.[92]

Ethnobotany: Archeological records dating back to 4000-5000 BC indicate human use of the African oil palm, and the tree was cultivated in West Africa as early as 3600-3200 BC. Palm kernel oil was reportedly recognized for its medicinal value in Ayurvedic medicine as early as 2000 BC.

African palm tree cultivation is closely associated with human settlements and movement. All parts of the African oil palm are used for a range of purposes, including food, drink (the fermented sap produces an effervescent wine), medicine, cosmetics, as a material for building, making clothing, baskets, and fishnets, fuel, and as a component in rituals and religious practices.

The Anaang, an ethnic group in Nigeria, used oil palm to treat cancer, headache, and rheumatism in their traditional medicine. Nigerians used the oil palm as an aphrodisiac, diuretic, liniment, vermifuge, laxative, and antidote to poison. The roots, stem bark, kernel, and oil have been used to treat malaria, diarrhea, asthma, measles, boils, convulsions, and mental disorders. In Ghana, the leaves, bark, fruits, and oil are valued for their wound healing properties. In Togo, the tree is used to treat epilepsy and stomach disorders. Various parts of the oil palm have been used in traditional African medicine to treat gonorrhea, menorrhagia, bronchitis, and skin infections.

Palm kernel oil is one of the most frequently used traditional medicine ingredients. Several African cultures administer palm kernel oil internally (orally and as an enema), as an ointment, and via scarification practices. It has been used to regulate convulsive children's body temperature, treat lumbago, headache, scabies and other skin diseases, malaria, stomach disorders, and as a poison antidote.[95]

NUTRIENT PROFILE

Like coconut oil, palm kernel oil is high in lauric acid. It also has significant proportions of myristic and palmitic acids.

Palm Kernel Oil[7]	
SATURATED FATTY ACIDS	
Caprylic acid (C8:0)	2.4 - 6.2%
Capric acid (C10:0)	2.6 - 5.0%
Lauric acid (C12:0)	45 - 55%
Myristic acid (C14:0)	14 - 18%
Palmitic acid (C16:0)	6.5 - 10.0%
Stearic acid (C18:0)	1.0 - 3.0%
MONOUNSATURATED FATTY ACIDS	
Oleic acid (C18:1 n-9)	12.0 - 19.0%
POLYUNSATURATED FATTY ACIDS	
Linoleic acid (C18:2 n-6)	1.0 - 3.5%
UNSAPONIFIABLE FRACTION 0.94-2.83%	
Sterols 700-1400 mg/kg	Beta-sitosterol (438.2 - 1023.4 mg/kg), stigmasterol (84 - 232.4 mg/kg), campesterol (58.8 - 177.8 mg/kg), delta-5-avenasterol (9.8 - 126 mg/kg), cholesterol (4.2 - 51.8 mg/kg)
Tocopherols n.d. - 260 mg/kg	Gamma-tocopherol (n.d. - 257 mg/kg), beta-tocopherol (n.d. - 248 mg/kg), alpha-tocopherol (n.d. - 44 mg/kg)

Formulating with Palm Kernel Oil

Sensory info: Brown to orange in color; warm, pungent nutty aroma; consider using a smaller amount to keep aroma from overwhelming the product.

Therapeutic actions: emollient, cooling, anti-inflammatory

Therapeutic applications:

- Dry skin
- Itchy skin
- Regenerative skincare

Note: As there are significant ethical and ecological issues regarding palm oil production, confirm that your source follows established responsible sustainability guidelines if you choose to use palm oil.

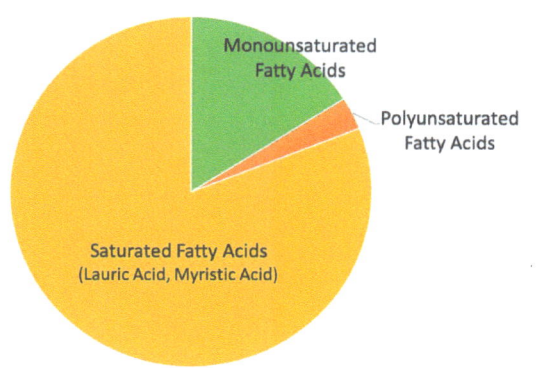

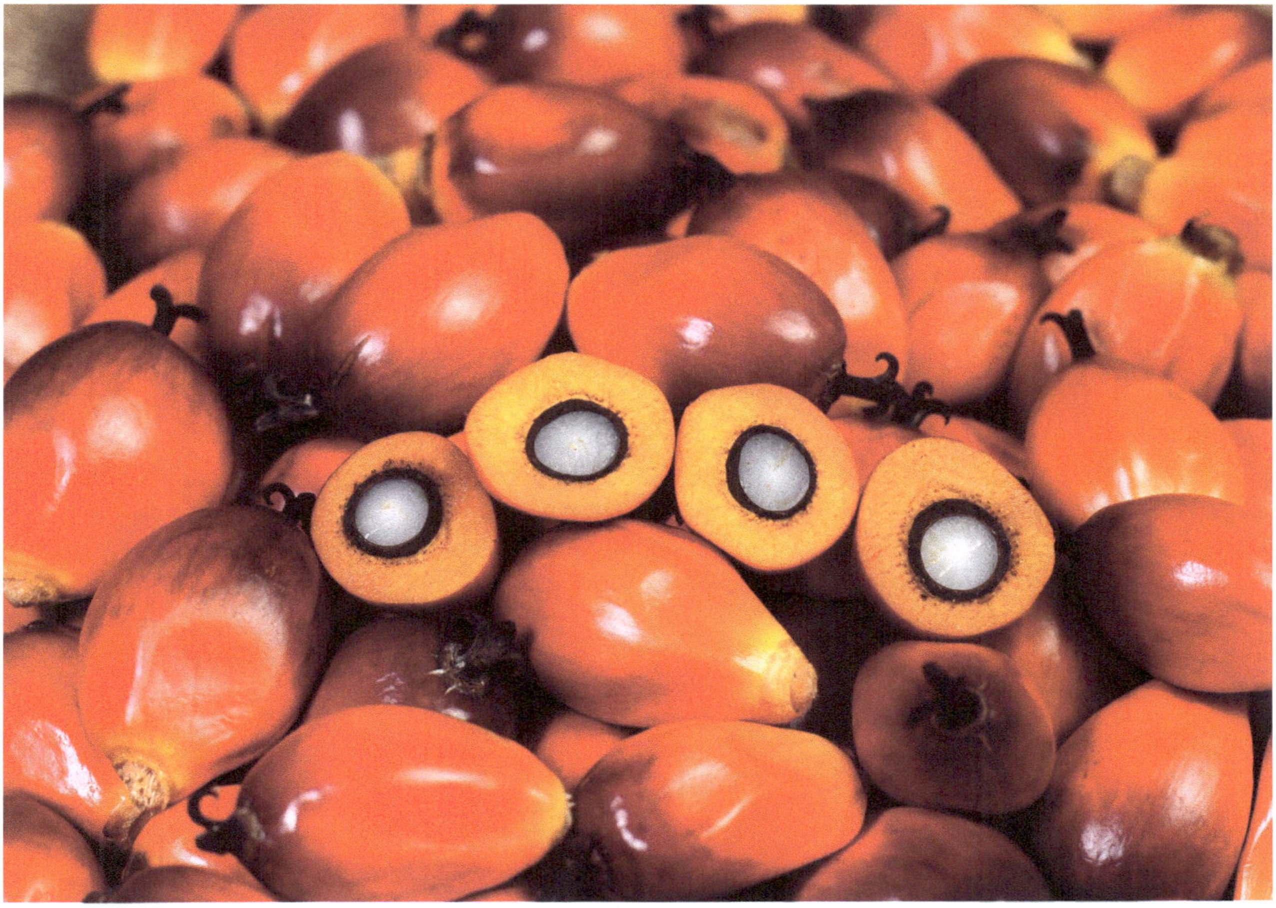

Shea
Vitellaria paradoxa

Common name: Shea, karité
Scientific name: *Vitellaria paradoxa* G. Don
Synonym: *Butyrospermum parkii* C.F. Gaertn.
Botanical family: Sapotaceae
Conservation status: Vulnerable[96]

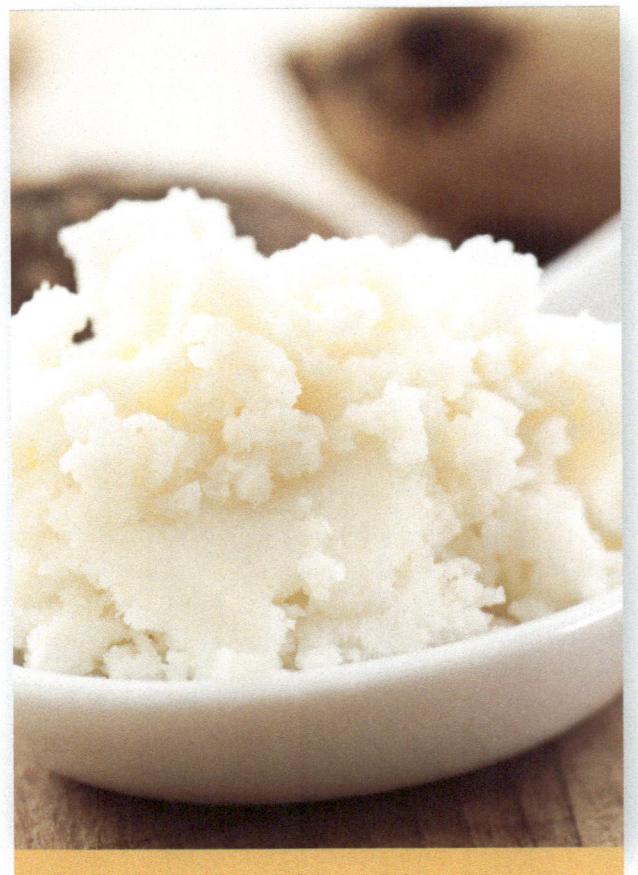

Description: The shea tree is a medium-sized deciduous tree in the Sapotaceae family indigenous to Africa. It grows in a belt that crosses Africa, from Senegal to the Sudan/Ethiopian border. It thrives in dry, sandy, clay soils rich in humus and suffers in swampy sites. The tree's extensive root system enables it to survive the seasonal droughts of savanna climates. The currently accepted botanical name is *Vitellaria paradoxa*, but the cosmetic industry continues to recognize shea's former botanical name, *Butyrospermum parkii*.[97]

Shea trees typically grow up to 25 m tall, with corky bark and a spreading crown. Leaves are oblong and clustered at the ends of branches, while white flowers cluster at the end of shoots. Flat, round fruits contain an edible pulp and up to four shiny brown seeds. The seeds have a fat-rich kernel from which edible shea butter is extracted. The shea tree begins to fruit at 10 - 15 years, with peak production occurring between 20 and 30 years of age.

Women in rural Africa extract shea butter using a laborious process; indeed, shea butter is often referred to as "women's gold." In this process, they first remove the pulp of the shea fruit for food, separating it from the seeds. They boil and then dry the seeds in the sun or a kiln. They then crack open the dried seeds to separate the kernels, which are dried again before being ground and kneaded into a paste. The paste is added to water and boiled until a grey fat rises to the surface. This fat is skimmed off, washed to remove impurities, then molded into various forms for use and distribution. The process is inefficient and labor-intensive, and some communities prefer mechanization over traditional practices.[98]

EXTRACTION INFORMATION

Country of origin: West Africa (Cote d'Ivoire, Ghana, Nigeria, Cameroon, Chad) Indonesia, East Africa (Uganda, Sudan)
Part of plant: Seed
Oil content: 42%
Extraction method: Cold pressing, Aqueous extraction

MANUFACTURING INFORMATION

CAS number: 91080-23-8
EC number: 293-515-7
INCI name: Butyrospermum Parkii Seed Butter
CosIng (functions): Skin conditioning - emollient, Viscosity controlling

SHELF LIFE

Up to 2 years, if stored correctly.

Ethnobotany: *Vitellaria paradoxa* has a stunning diversity of traditional uses; all parts of the tree play valuable roles in spiritual practices, food, medicine, building materials, and environmental management. The tree is sacred to many African ethnic groups and is used in religious ceremonies. Latex extracted from the tree bark is mixed with palm oil to make an adhesive. The sticky black residue that remains after clarifying the butter fills cracks in hut walls. It is also an effective fire starter for cooking and community fires. Poor quality butter applied to the exterior walls of mud huts, doors, windows, and traditional beehives acts as a waterproofing agent. Rancid butter can be repurposed in soap-making. The wood ash is used in dyes. *V. paradoxa* also plays a significant role in traditional apiculture, and beehives are often placed in the tree's branches to provide the bees with abundant nectar and pollen.[99] *V. paradoxa* is planted for ecological conservation purposes, and the termite-resistant wood is used as a building material, fuelwood, and for making charcoal.

Shea butter is commonly used in cooking, pastries, and confectionaries, as well as making cosmetics, soaps, and candles. Despite their mild laxative properties, mature fresh fruits are considered an important food source and are commonly eaten in the savanna as they ripen during periods of land preparation and planting. The flowers of the shea tree are made into fritters, and a reddish latex extruded from deep cuts in the bark is used as chewing gum.

Shea butter is applied topically to relieve rheumatism or joint pain and heal wounds, swellings, dermatitis, bruises, and other skin ailments. Shea butter applied to the nostrils has been used to relieve nasal congestion and rhinitis. Shea leaves have been taken internally to treat stomachache and added to steam baths to ease headaches. Ground roots and bark have been used to treat diarrhea, jaundice, and stomachache. Decocted bark teas have been used to ward off dysentery, facilitate childbirth, stimulate lactation, and, as an eyewash, serve as an antidote to spitting-cobra venom.[98]

NUTRIENT PROFILE

V. paradoxa grows in West Africa, whereas *V. paradoxa nilotica* grows in East Africa. West African shea butter tends to be higher in stearic acid than East African, which is higher in oleic acid.[100]

Shea butter[101, 102, 103]	
SATURATED FATTY ACIDS	
Palmitic acid (C16:0)	2 - 10%
Stearic acid (C18:0)	**25 - 50%**
Arachidic acid (C20:0)	< 3.5%
MONOUNSATURATED FATTY ACIDS	
Oleic acid (C18:1 n-9)	**32 - 62%**
POLYUNSATURATED FATTY ACIDS	
Linoleic acid (C18:2 n-6)	1 - 11%
UNSAPONIFIABLE FRACTION 8%	
Sterols 3974 mg/kg	Sitosterol (2735.9 mg/kg), stigmasterol (902.6 mg/kg), campesterol 266.3 mg/kg), delta-5-avenasterol (68.6 mg/kg)
Tocopherols 44 - 786 mg/kg	Alpha-tocopherol (23 – 414 mg/kg), gamma-tocopherol (0 – 222 mg/kg), delta-tocopherol (0 – 129 mg/kg), beta-tocopherol (0 – 120 mg/kg)

Formulating with Shea Butter

Sensory info: Rich to light ivory or yellow color; very light nutty aroma; soft texture at room temperature

Therapeutic actions: emollient, antioxidant,[104] anti-inflammatory, moisturizing, anti-irritant, UV-protective, good penetrative properties, prevents dryness, improves elasticity of the skin, protects skin from elements (wind, cold, heat)

Therapeutic applications:

- Eczema
- Dermatitis
- Psoriasis
- Dry skin
- Cracked skin
- Irritated skin
- Chapped lips
- Nasal decongestant - place small amount directly into the nose
- Preventing or reducing premature skin aging

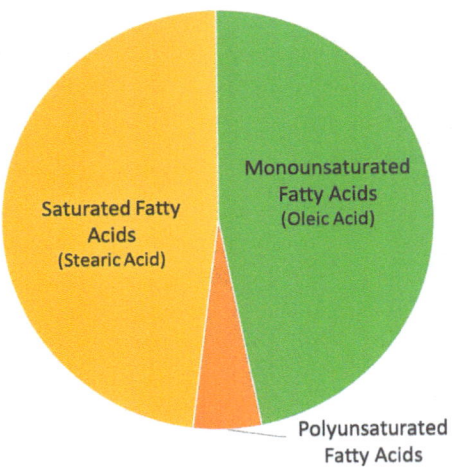

Formulation notes:
- Shea is sensitive to heat. When combining with melted oil or waxes, remove melted blend from heat and let cool slightly before adding shea.
- If you are going to be formulating using cocoa butter and shea, please remember to put melted mixture directly into refrigerator or freezer for at least 15-20 minutes, until mostly solid. The rapid cooling will help prevent crystallization (graininess) and bloom in your final product.

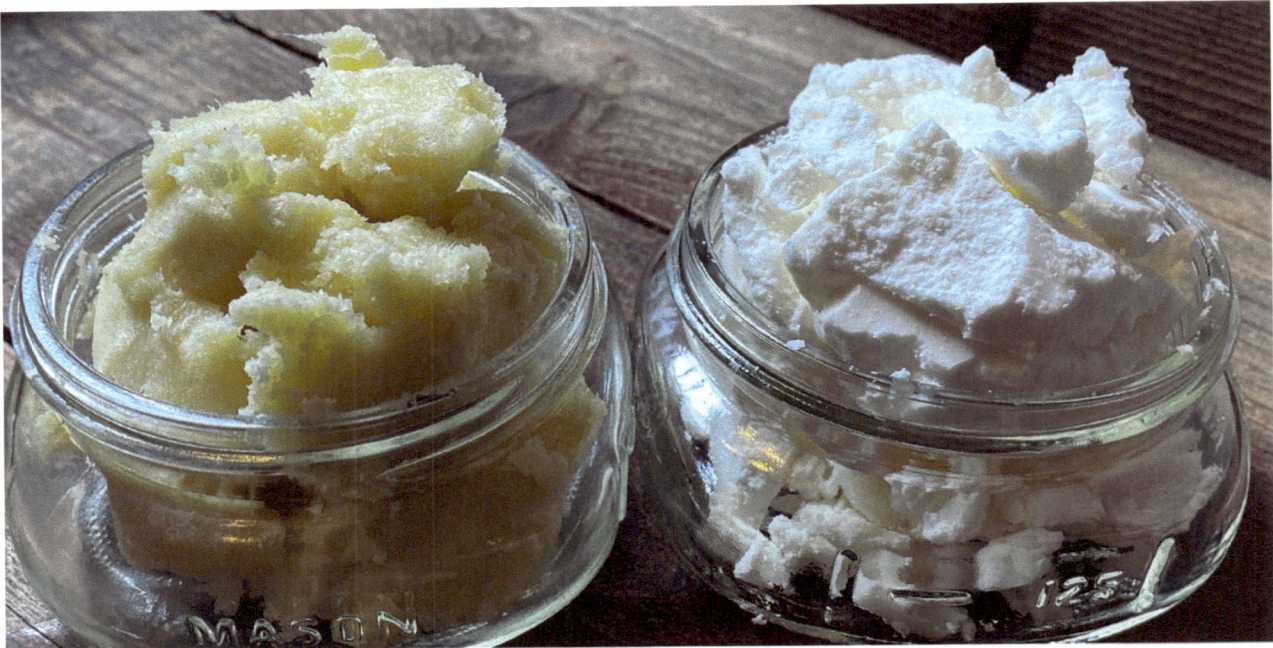

Image: Unrefined (left) and refined (right) shea butter

Appendices

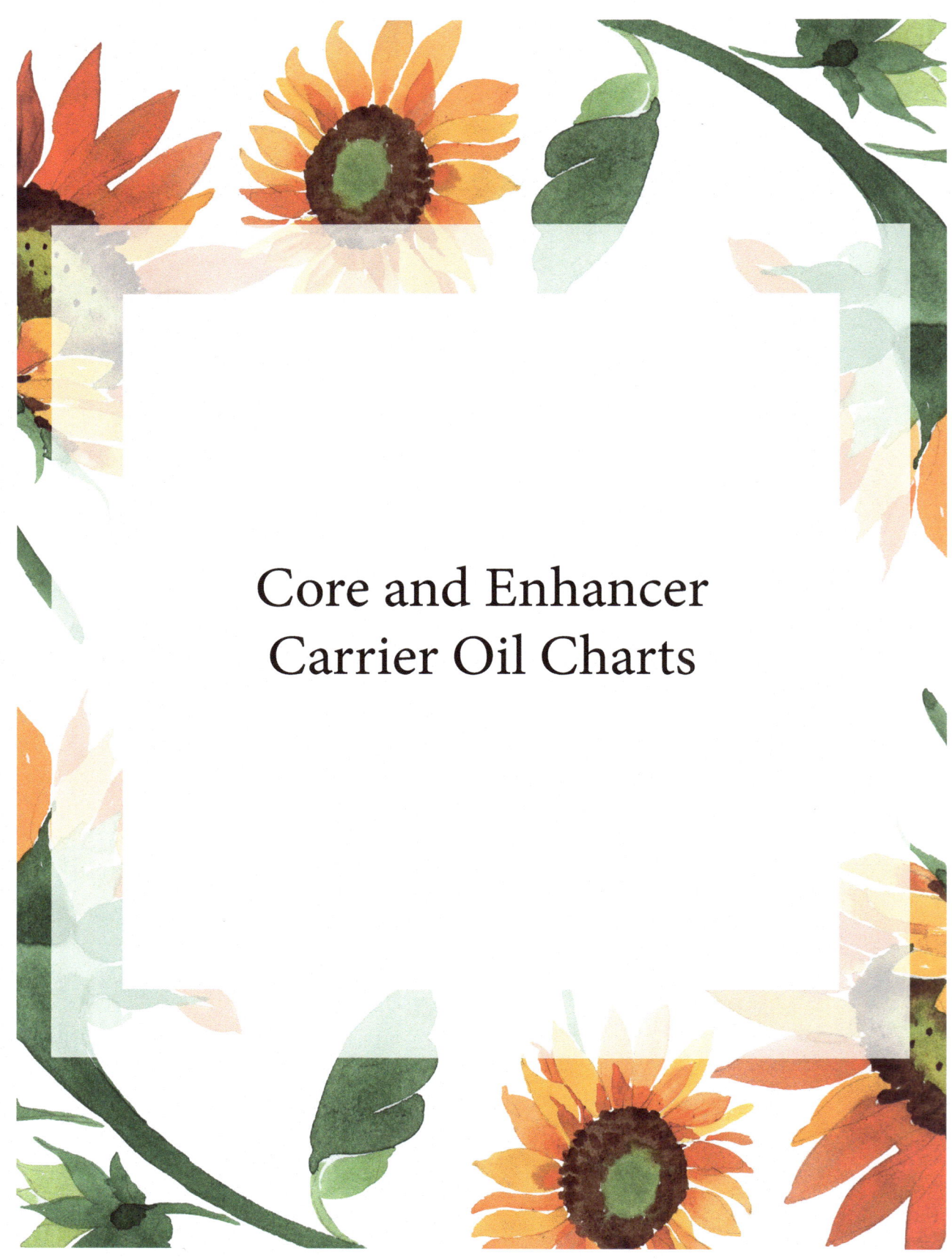

Core and Enhancer Carrier Oil Charts

Core Carrier Oils Chart

Fixed Oil	Nutrient Profile	Therapeutic Actions
Sweet almond oil *Prunus amygdalis* **Absorption rate:** Wet, absorbs slowly **Dilution:** Can be used 100% or in a blend of other oils.	**Monounsaturated/ Polyunsaturated oil** Rich in oleic acid (60-86%) with linoleic acid (15 - 30%)	• A good emollient, it protects and nourishes the skin. • Helps relieve skin itching, soreness, dryness, and inflammation e.g., eczema. • Suitable for all skin types, particularly dry skin.
Apricot kernel oil *Prunus armeniaca* **Absorption rate:** Wet, absorbs more slowly **Dilution:** Can be used 100% or in a blend of other oils.	**Monounsaturated/ Polyunsaturated oil** Rich in oleic acid (62-72%), with linoleic acid (20 - 25%)	• All skin types: mature, dry, sensitive, or inflamed skin. • Protects the skin from free radicals, reduces inflammation, supports wound healing, and promotes skin barrier homeostasis. • Useful for relieving inflammation, itchiness, and dry skin • Massage combination: 50/50 apricot kernel + sunflower oil.
Argan oil *Argania spinosa* **Absorption rate:** Wet, absorbs slowly **Dilution:** Can be used 25-100%	**Monounsaturated/ Polyunsaturated oil** Rich in oleic acid (41-55%), and linoleic acid (28 - 38%)	• Beneficial for mature, aging, or damaged skin. • Improves skin elasticity and skin hydration in post-menopausal women. • Daily dermal application of argan oil may reduce TEWL and restore a damaged skin barrier. • It may be useful in gels or creams to prevent wrinkles or for around the eyes as a nourishing oil or cream. • Indicated for problematic skin and acne. • Argan oil combined with rosehip seed oil may support healthy scar formation and prevent stretch marks.
Baobab oil *Adansonia digitata* **Absorption:** Wet, slow to absorb **Dilution:** Can be used 100% or in a blend of other oils.	**Monounsaturated/ Polyunsaturated/ Saturated oil** Rich in oleic acid (30 - 44%) and linoleic acid (27 - 37%) with palmitic acid (18 - 30%)	• Improves the skin's elasticity, • Relieves inflamed skin condition, e.g., dry eczema and psoriasis • Cell regenerative • May alleviate pain from burns • May improve the appearance of stretch marks and scars • Can improve texture and shine to hair

Core Carrier Oils Chart

Fixed Oil	Nutrient Profile	Therapeutic Actions
Camelina oil *Camelina sativa* **Absorption rate:** Medium **Dilution:** Can be used 100% or in a blend of other oils.	**Polyunsaturated oil** Rich in linoleic acid (16 - 23%) and alpha-linolenic acid (31 - 53%)	• Improve skin elasticity and suppleness • Recommended for mature skin • Anti-inflammatory properties helpful for acne, eczema, and psoriasis. • Address EFA deficiency • Enhance skin's barrier function • Protect skin from UV-induced skin damage • 0.2-2% for shampoo and conditioners and 10% for hair masks. • Indicated for Vata
Jojoba oil *Simmondsia chinensis* **Absorption rate:** Dry, readily absorbs into skin **Dilution:** Can be used 100 percent or in a blend of other oils	**Liquid Wax** 97% wax esters of monounsaturated, straight-chain fatty acids and alcohols with high-molecular weights	• Used for acne to dissolve clogged pores. • Antibacterial and anti-inflammatory properties make it helpful for eczema, psoriasis, and inflamed skin. • Supports wound healing. • Great oil for the hair, relieving dry scalp and dandruff. Recommend a conditioning blend of 50% jojoba and 50% sesame oils. • Great for the nails and cuticles. • Recommended for regenerative skin care and preventative aging care. • Improves and reduces stretch marks; popular for tattoo aftercare. • Indicated for oily, combination, or acne skin types, although all skin types will benefit. • Vata, Pitta, and Kapha Doshas will all benefit from jojoba. • Adding jojoba to other oils can enhance their oxidative stability.
Marula oil *Sclerocarya birrea* **Absorption rate:** Wet, medium to slow **Dilution:** Can be used 100 percent or in a blend of other oils.	**Monounsaturated oil** Rich in oleic acid (70 - 78%)	• Nourishes and protects the skin • Soothing to sunburns and chapped/irritated skin. • Beneficial for inflamed skin conditions such as dry eczema, dermatitis, and psoriasis. • Traditionally used to prevent stretch marks. • Suitable for all Doshas, particularly Vata. • Indicated for dry and cracking skin and dry, damaged, and fragile hair. • Used for herbal infusions of fragrant flowers.

Core Carrier Oils Chart

Fixed Oil	Nutrient Profile	Therapeutic Actions
Olive oil *Olea europaea* **Absorption rate:** Wet, absorbs more slowly **Dilution:** Can be used at 100% percent or in a blend of other oils.	**Monounsaturated oil** Rich in oleic acid (55 - 83%)	• Wound healing, dry skin, eczema, aging skin, hair care and can be used as a skin cleanser. • Maintains skin and muscle suppleness, heals abrasions, and soothes the burning and drying effects of sun and water. • Excellent antioxidant activity. • Serves as a penetration enhancer, making it a helpful carrier for essential oils.
Safflower oil *Carthamus tinctorius* **Absorption rate:** Oleic acid-rich: Slow to absorb Linoleic acid-rich: Absorbs readily **Dilution:** Can be used 100% percent or in a blend of other oils.	**#1: Polyunsaturated oil** Rich in linoleic acid (67 - 83%) with monounsaturated fatty acid: oleic acid (8 - 21%) **#2: Monounsaturated oil** Rich in oleic acid (70 - 84%)	• Suitable for all skin types, emollient and soothing to the skin. • Great for massage and skincare lotions. • Linoleic acid-rich safflower oil is recommended for inflamed, irritated skin as well as for atopic dermatitis and eczema due to its anti-inflammatory and skin-soothing properties. • Oleic acid-rich safflower oil strengthens hair.
Sesame seed oil *Sesamum indicum* **Absorption rate:** Medium **Dilution:** Can be used 100% percent or in a blend of other oils.	**Monounsaturated/ Polyunsaturated oil** Rich in oleic acid (35 - 42%) and linoleic acid (41 - 48%)	• Skin restructuring and emollient properties while also reinforcing the integrity of the skin. • Free radical scavenging. • Used extensively in Ayurvedic medicine and is indicated specifically to pacify Vata due to its warming properties. • Particularly good in dry and/or cold climates because it is heavy and penetrates the skin, going deep into the tissue. • Very nourishing to the skin and helps prevent the skin from getting excessively dry. • Nourishes the scalp and restores the natural oil balance and luster of hair. • Adding sesame oil to other oils can enhance their oxidative stability.

Core Carrier Oils Chart		
Fixed Oil	**Nutrient Profile**	**Therapeutic Actions**
Sunflower oil *Helianthus annuus* **Absorption rate:** **Oleic acid-rich:** Slow to absorb **Linoleic acid-rich:** Absorbs readily **Dilution:** Can be used 100% percent or in a blend of other oils.	**#1: Polyunsaturated oil** Rich in linoleic acid (67 - 83%) with oleic acid (8-21%) **#2: Monounsaturated oil** Rich in oleic acid (70 - 84%)	• Suitable for all skin types, emollient and soothing to the skin. • Oleic-rich sunflower oil is great for herbal oil infusions. • Linoleic acid-rich sunflower oil is recommended for inflamed, irritated skin as well as for atopic dermatitis and eczema due to its anti-inflammatory and skin-soothing properties. Regenerative skincare. • Massage combination: 50/50 apricot kernel + sunflower oil

Enhancer Carrier Oils Chart

Fixed Oil	Nutrient Profile	Therapeutic Actions
Avocado oil *Persea americana* **Absorption rate:** Dry, readily absorbs into skin **Dilution:** Can be used 5 - 25% in a blend of other carrier oils.	**Monounsaturated oil** Rich in oleic acid (47 - 67%), with palmitic acid (12 - 28%) **Other:** Carotenoids (1.9 - 48.7 mg/kg)	• Moisturizing, emollient, skin-penetrating, antibacterial, antiwrinkle, antioxidant, revitalizing, cell-regenerating, hydrating • Increase collagen synthesis and reduce itching • Suitable for all skin types, especially post-menopausal, dry, dehydrated, fragile, or mature skin, or skin experiencing premature aging • Helpful for dry eczema or psoriasis
Black cumin oil *Nigella sativa* **Absorption rate:** Slow-to-average, slight oily feeling on skin **Dilution:** Recommended up to 10% for cosmetic/topical use	**Polyunsaturated oil** Rich in linoleic acid (56 - 64%) with oleic acid (20 - 24%)	• Soothing, emollient, and skin-nourishing • Anti-inflammatory and potent antioxidant activity address eczema, psoriasis, acne, injured skin, dry skin, aging skin, and in after-sun care products • Inflammation and pain in joints, such as in arthritis • Antimicrobial for acne and fungal skin infections • Improves scalp and hair health, reducing scalp inflammation and irritation, damage from UV radiation and pollution, and hair loss, while moisturizing hair strands • May be effective in treating vitiligo
Borage seed oil *Borago officinalis* **Absorption rate:** Dry, readily absorbs into the skin **Dilution:** Can be used 10 - 20% percent in a blend of other oils.	**Polyunsaturated oil** Rich in linoleic acid (34 - 38%) and gamma-linolenic acid (21 - 25%)	• Recommended for premature aging, dry and devitalized skin, psoriasis, sensitive skin, and eczema • Anti-inflammatory • Reduces TEWL • Suitable for facial serums or specialty oils • May be beneficial in the treatment of atopic dermatitis • Suitable for infants and children

Enhancer Carrier Oils Chart

Fixed Oil	Nutrient Profile	Therapeutic Actions
Castor oil *Ricinus communis* **Absorption:** Wet, slow to absorb **Dilution:** Can be used 100 percent or, more commonly, at a 10 - 15% dilution in a blend of other oils.	**Monounsaturated oil** Rich in ricinoleic acid (75 -94%)	• Excellent emollient • Adds a shine to lip balms • May be useful for brown patches (age spots), liver spots, or blemishes • Ricinoleic acid has demonstrated antinociceptive, analgesic, and anti-inflammatory activity • May be suitable for muscular aches and pains or to address general tension in the body • Castor packs may ease the passing of difficult bowel movements.
Evening primrose oil *Oenothera biennis* **Absorption:** Dry, readily absorbs into the skin **Dilution:** Can be used 5 - 15% in a blend of other carrier oils.	**Polyunsaturated oil** Rich in linoleic acid (65 - 80%) and gamma-linolenic acid (9 - 27%)	• Strengthens the epidermal barrier, normalizes TEWL, regenerates skin, and improves smoothness after both topical and oral applications • Suitable for premature aging, dry and devitalized skin, psoriasis, eczema, and regenerative skincare • Indicated for atopic dermatitis due to its anti-inflammatory activity • It is also useful where there is a loss of elasticity. • Suitable for facial serums or specialty oils • Suitable for Vata and Pitta skin types
Hemp seed oil *Cannabis sativa* **Absorption:** Dry, readily absorbs into the skin **Dilution:** 3 - 10% of the formulation	**Polyunsaturated oil** Rich in essential fatty acids, linoleic acid (50 - 70%) and alpha-linolenic acid (15 - 25%) **Other:** Carotenoids (31 - 78 mg/kg), polyphenols (21 - 160 mg GAE/g)	• Omega 3:omega 6 ratio is 1:3. • Indicated for nutrient-deficient, dry, flaky skin • May lighten UV-hyperpigmented skin • Anti-inflammatory and skin regenerative • Appropriate for dermatitis, eczema, psoriasis, acne, rosacea, arthritis, and wound care • Anti-aging formulations to reduce fine lines and wrinkles. • Address EFA deficiency • Moisturizing and emollient

Enhancer Carrier Oils Chart

Fixed Oil	Nutrient Profile	Therapeutic Actions
Meadowfoam seed oil *Limnanthes alba* **Absorption:** Dry, readily absorbs into the skin **Dilution:** up to 100%	Monounsaturated/ Polyunsaturated oil (Long-chain fatty acids) Rich in gondoic acid (58 - 65%), erucic acid (10 - 20%), and 5,13-docosadienoic acid (10 - 21%)	• Beneficial for all skin types • Highly moisturizing • Combine meadowfoam with other carrier oils to increase their overall oxidative stability and shelf life • MSO's antioxidant capacity may also counteract free radicals in the skin, helping repair photodamage and slow the effects of skin aging • An appropriate substitute for argan oil
Neem oil *Azadirachta indica* **Absorption:** Wet, Slow to absorb **Dilution:** Can be used 100% but recommended at 10 - 25% due to powerful aroma.	Monounsaturated/ Polyunsaturated oil Rich in oleic acid (18 - 52%) and linoleic acid (13 - 69%) **Active constituent:** azadirachtin	• Antibacterial, antifungal, and anti-inflammatory activity • Indicated for acne, eczema, yeast infections, foot fungus, scabies, and seborrheic dermatitis • Appropriate for treating dandruff or dry, itchy scalps and restoring dry, damaged hair • Effective treatment for lice and as a mosquito repellent • May effectively address various parasitic infestations, such as chiggers, ticks, fleas, scabies, and swimmer's itch • Safe for children and mammalian pets • In Ayurveda, neem oil balances Kapha and Pitta Dosha.
Pomegranate seed oil *Punica granatum* **Absorption:** Dry, readily absorbs into the skin **Dilution:** Use at a 5-15% percent with other carrier oils	Polyunsaturated oil Rich in puricic aid (57 - 79%) **Other:** Squalene (828-1449 mg/kg)	• Excellent anti-inflammatory carrier oil • Indicated for dermal inflammations such as acne, sunburn, psoriasis, and rosacea • Supports cellular regeneration (specifically in the epidermis) • Combats free radicals (antioxidant activity) • Improves skin elasticity, revitalizes premature aging or sun-damaged skin • Beneficial emollient for dry, irritated skin

Enhancer Carrier Oils Chart

Fixed Oil	Nutrient Profile	Therapeutic Actions
Pumpkin seed oil *Cucurbita maxima* **Absorption:** Dry, readily absorbs into the skin **Dilution:** Use at a 2-10% percent with other carrier oils (caution: using too much can stain the skin orange)	**Polyunsaturated oil / Monounsaturated oil** Rich in linoleic acid (53 - 65%) and oleic acid (27 - 38%) **Other:** Carotenoids (5 - 6 mg/kg), Squalene (5913-6325 mg/kg)	• Anti-inflammatory activity and wound healing support • Indicated for acne-prone or inflamed skin, damaged skin, and overly dry skin • Useful for acne blemishes and to reduce the appearance of scarring • Appropriate for burn care
Raspberry seed oil *Rubus idaeus* **Absorption:** Dry, readily absorbs into the skin **Dilution:** Can be used 1 - 5% in a blend of other carrier oils. Increase concentration as desired.	**Polyunsaturated oil** Rich in linoleic acid (49 - 55%) and alpha-linolenic acid (24 - 33%)	• Positively benefit the skin by improving hydration, reducing TEWL, and softening the skin • Antioxidant and anti-inflammatory activity • Indicated for inflamed skin conditions, tissue regeneration (scars, skin burns, etc.), premature aging, dry skin, acne, oily skin • Strengthens the lipid layer of the epidermis and improves sebaceous gland function • Preventative aging (antioxidant) • Suitable for facial serums or specialty oils • Photoprotective - protective role against UV radiation
Rosehip seed oil *Rosa rubiginosa, R. canina* **Absorption:** Dry, readily absorbs into the skin **Dilution:** Use at a 5 - 25% percent with other carrier oils.	**Polyunsaturated oil** Rich in linoleic acid (40 - 55%) and alpha-linolenic acid (20 - 35%) with oleic acid (12 - 22%) **Other:** All-trans-retinoic acid (0.375 mg/L oil)	• Inflamed skin conditions • Preventative premature skin aging (antioxidant) and photoaging • Suitable for facial serums and specialty oils • Skin disorders: eczema, trophic ulcers of the skin, cheilitis (inflammation of the lips, dry, chapped lips) • Best tissue regenerators for scars, skin burns • Exceptional effect in reducing the hyperpigmentation of scars and reducing their appearance • Prevents TEWL

Enhancer Carrier Oils Chart

Fixed Oil	Nutrient Profile	Therapeutic Actions
Sacha inchi oil *Plukenetia volubilis* **Absorption:** Dry, readily absorbs into the skin **Dilution:** May be used up to 100%	**Polyunsaturated oil** Rich in linoleic acid (21 - 53%) and alpha-linolenic acid (10 - 55%) with oleic acid (9 - 23%)	• Antioxidant capacity to the high percentage of PUFAs • Excellent choice for inflamed or UV-exposed skin • Beneficial for all skin types, but it is particularly effective for dry, mature skin, promoting an even skin tone while calming itch and irritation • A preferred ingredient in anti-aging products • Excellent for hair health - Discourages hair loss and can minimize hair breakage • Appropriate for bacterial skin infections and acne
Sea buckthorn seed oil *Hippophaë rhamnoides* **Absorption:** Dry, readily absorbs into the skin **Dilution:** Can be used 1 - 5%	**Polyunsaturated oil** Rich in essential fatty acids linoleic acid (35 - 37%) and alpha-linolenic (29 - 38%) **Other:** Carotenoids (151-545 mg/kg)	• Promotes the recovery of skin conditions, e.g., eczema, burns, poorly healing wounds, skin damaged by the sun, and after radiation treatment • Anti-aging, enhancing microcirculation, antioxidant, epidermal regeneration, reduces inflammation, natural UV protection • Strengthens the protective lipid barrier of the stratum corneum and prevents TEWL • Improves functioning of sebaceous glands in acne-prone, oily, or problematic skin types - unblocking pores and reducing formation or number of blackheads • Dry, irritated, rough, flaking, or itchy skin • Bedsores, slow-healing wounds • Inflammatory skin conditions • Regenerative skincare • Burns / Sunburn

Enhancer Carrier Oils Chart

Fixed Oil	Nutrient Profile	Therapeutic Actions
Sea buckthorn pulp oil *Hippophaë rhamnoides* **Absorption:** Dry, readily absorbs into the skin **Dilution:** Can be used 1 - 2.5%	**Monounsaturated/ Saturated oil** Rich in palmitoleic acid (32 - 42%) and palmitic acid (28 - 40%) **Other:** Carotenoids (692 - 3420 mg/kg)	• Strengthens the protective lipid barrier of the stratum corneum prevents TEWL • Improves functioning of sebaceous glands in acne-prone, oily, or problematic skin types - unblocking pores and reducing formation or number of blackheads • Dry, irritated, rough, flaking, or itchy skin • Bedsores, slowly or difficult healing of wounds • Preventative aging skin • Inflammatory skin conditions • Regenerative skincare • Burns / Sunburn • Mucous membrane inflammation or damage • Oral hygiene
Tamanu oil *Plukenetia volubilis* **Absorption:** Dry – readily absorbs into the skin. Leaves a slightly tacky feeling on the skin when applied at 100%. **Dilution:** Dilutions of 10 - 25% combined with other carriers are recommended. Can be used at 100%.	**Monounsaturated/ Polyunsaturated/ Saturated oil** Rich in oleic acid (28 - 31%), linoleic acid (24 - 31%), and stearic acid (14 - 29%)	• Wound healing, relieves pain and supports skin health • Improves the appearance of scar tissue • Promotes the formation of new tissue and accelerates healing and growth of healthy skin • Antibacterial, antioxidant • Antimicrobial activity: may be effective in treating Tinea infections (ringworm) and shingles • Highly effective anti-inflammatory oil • Antioxidant and anti-UV properties at a 1% dilution • Indicated for cuts, scrapes, burns, insect bites or stings, abrasions, acne, acne scars, psoriasis, diabetic sores, anal fissures, sunburn, dry or scaly skin, blisters, eczema, herpes sores, and to reduce foot or body odor • May also be indicated for sciatica, neuralgia, and rheumatism • Addresses Kapha and Pitta imbalances

Carrier Oils/Butters, Sustainability, and Zero Waste

As natural product formulators, we care about the quality and provenance of our ingredients. Some of these valuable plants flourish under domestication and sustainable farming practices, while other components are wildcrafted and collected in specific parts of the world. When we understand the socio-economic and environmental factors that affect the production of our precious ingredients, we can engage pro-actively with the retailers and producers to ensure our ingredients' sustainable futures.

Multiple factors affect the sustainability of plant populations. Climate change, habitat destruction, disease, and other threats are often the result of human activities. However, the link between our actions and the effect on the ingredient is not always obvious. We also often find ourselves caught in a Catch-22 situation where our increasing utilization of a specific plant leads to its overuse and possible population decrease or even extinction. Yet it is also that demand for the plant that might encourage the industry, or even an individual, to develop a better management plan that ultimately leads to an adequately high, sustainable yield.

A few carrier oils are considered zero-waste, as they are by-products of a different industry. The fruit jam and juice industries have no use for the fruit seeds, so many of our precious seed oils are by-products of jam or juice production. Strawberry seed, raspberry seed, blueberry seed, blackberry seed, cranberry seed, apple seed, pomegranate seed, tomato seed, cucumber seed, and apricot kernel oils can all be produced as zero-waste ingredients.

At this time, the demand for apricot kernel oil, for example, has increased beyond the demand for jam and juice. Some of the oil must now come from growing apricots specifically to produce the oil from their seeds. While apricots are currently sustainable, the oil sector of the industry is no longer completely zero-waste.

Another challenge that faces us is when various industries compete for shares of the produced oil. Meadowfoam seed, sunflower, and jojoba are examples of oils that play critical roles in a laundry list of industries, including the natural cosmetic industry. The cosmetic industry must compete for its share of a finite resource while simultaneously demanding the highest quality oils for its products.

One of the most challenging sustainability issues is preventing certain plants from becoming extinct. We must balance our demand with the supply or find new, sustainable production methods to meet the increasing demand.

Other sustainability issues, for instance, those surrounding palm fruit and kernel oils, are less direct. The concern with palm oil is not that we will run out of palm trees. In this case, to meet the increasing demand for palm oil, farmers have cleared thousands of acres of forest to increase the land available to their palm plantations. This deforestation, which includes habitat destruction for other threatened plant and animal species, as well as strong-arm tactics and land-grabs, has led to significant environmental damage and socio-economic concerns. Concerned individuals have formed several different non-governmental organizations, who have worked with the palm oil industry to develop, implement, and certify worldwide standards for sustainable palm oil production.

As with organic certification, some ingredients, like palm oil, can now carry organizational certifications, demonstrating their production now has a minimal negative impact on the environment and local people. These certifications do not always reflect a perfect system, but they require companies to innovate and meet specific standards. Looking for and recognizing these labels is one way we can contribute to developing sustainable and ethical production of the plants we value so highly.

Our participation and careful consideration of all socio-economic and environmental factors are also necessary to ensure our future access to these precious plants and their extracts. We can also look for our favorite retailers' mission and vision statements to see if they discuss such topics as organics, fair trade, sustainability, socio-economic equity, and zero waste. Look at the type of packaging they use when they ship your products to you. Are their actions in line with their words? We can talk with them when we have concerns or questions, and we should let them know that we care too.

A Few of the Organizations/Certifications to Consider for Ethical Ingredient Selection:

- Roundtable on Sustainable Palm Oil (RSPO)
- High Carbon Stock Approach
- Certified Sustainable Palm Oil (CSPO)
- World Wildlife Fund Palm Oil Buyers Scorecard https://palmoilscorecard.panda.org/#/scores
- Palm Oil Innovation Group (POIG)
- Certified Organic
- International Sustainability and Carbon Certification (ISCC)
- Roundtable on Sustainable Biomaterials (RSB)
- Rainforest Alliance
- B Corporation
- For Life
- Fair for Life
- Fair Trade

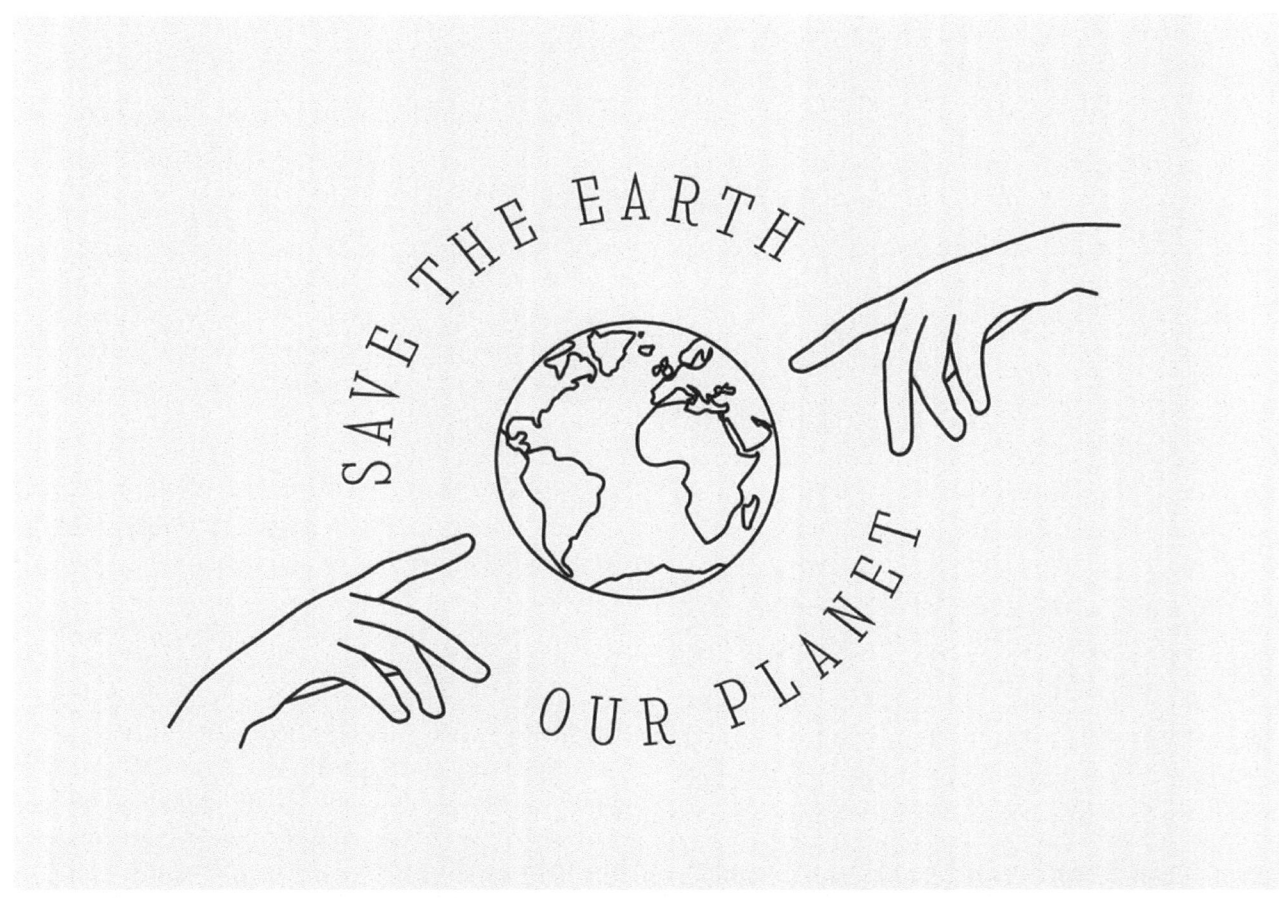

Limited Glossary of Terms

Antioxidant Prevents oxidation. Antioxidants chemically react with free radicals, so the antioxidant molecules are oxidized instead of other desirable molecules, such as fatty acids or molecules in living cells. Antioxidants prevent fats from going rancid. (see Preservative, Rancid)

Carrier oil Any fixed oil used to care for the skin and hair or as a carrier for other substances, usually therapeutic compounds from herbal oils, essential oils, or other plant extracts.

Essential oil Essential oils are plant extracts that contain only volatile, aromatic molecules. Essential oils are not fats or oils, but they are lipophilic. They will dissolve in organic solvents, especially carrier oils. Steam or hydro- distillation is the extraction process for essential oils. The exception is the citrus oils, which are often expressed. (see Fixed oil, Vegetable oil)

Fixed oil A fixed oil is primarily comprised of triglycerides, fatty acids, and wax esters. These constituents are "fixed" and do not evaporate. Cold pressing, expeller pressing, and SFE CO_2 extraction are the primary means of extracting fixed oils for cosmetic use. This term is often preferable to "vegetable oil" since the oils are usually extracted from seeds and fruits, not the vegetative parts of the plant. (see Vegetable oil, Essential oil)

Hydrate Hydration provides the skin with moisture. This is important in situations of dehydration or dehydrated skin. Dehydrated skin is often a product of general physical dehydration, so drinking enough water is a first defense against dehydrated skin. Hydrating skincare products and thin and will absorb quickly. (see Moisturize)

Lipid A substance that is generally insoluble in water but is soluble in organic solvents. Lipids serve both structural and energy functions in plants and animals. They may be liquid or solid at room temperature. In carrier oils, lipids comprise both the saponifiable and unsaponifiable fractions. Examples of lipids are waxes, triglycerides, and phospholipids (phosphoglycerides and sphingolipids,) hydrocarbons, terpene alcohols, sterols, tocopherols, pigments, and other phenolic compounds. (see Fixed oil, Vegetable oil)

Moisturize Moisturization maintains skin moisture. A product that prevents TEWL will moisturize the skin. Moisturizing products are thicker and more likely to stay on the skin surface or absorb more slowly. (see Hydrate)

Preservative Antimicrobial. Prevents deterioration due to bacterial, viral, or fungal growth. Preservatives prevent fats from rotting or decomposing. (see Antioxidant)

Rancid Rancidity is the result of oxidation, a chemical reaction. Rancid oils often smell unpleasant, have a color change (fade or turn brown), and feel sticky. (see Antioxidant)

SFE CO_2 extraction Supercritical Fluid Extraction by carbon dioxide uses supercritical carbon dioxide, which has the properties of both a gas and a liquid, to extract specific compounds from a plant. Carrier oil and essential oil-type CO_2 extracts exist, sometimes from the same plants. Sometimes an extract may be described as a "Total CO_2," which may contain both the fixed and volatile components. Be sure to select the correct type for your intended purpose.

For example:
Sandalwood nut (seed) CO_2 – fixed oil
Sandalwood CO_2 extract – volatile extract (like an essential oil)

TEWL Transepidermal water loss is when water is lost from the skin through evaporation.

Vegetable oil A vegetable oil is primarily comprised of triglycerides, fatty acids, and wax esters. Cold pressing, expeller pressing, and SFE CO_2 extraction are the primary means of extracting fixed oils for cosmetic use. (see Fixed oil, Essential oil)

Carrier Oil Charts and Information

Shelf Lives of Fixed Oils and Butters

6-9 months	6-12 months	12-24 months	2-4 years	4-5 years
Avocado (unrefined) Borage seed*	Apricot kernel Avocado (refined) Evening Primrose Hemp seed* Raspberry seed* Rosehip seed* Pumpkin seed Safflower (LA) Sea Buckthorn pulp Sunflower (LA)	Sweet Almond Argan Black Cumin seed Camelina Castor Coconut Marula Neem Olive Pomegranate seed* Sacha inchi Safflower (OA) Sea buckthorn seed Sesame seed Sunflower (OA) Most butters	Baobab Fractionated Coconut (FCO)	Jojoba Meadowfoam seed Tamanu Cocoa butter Kombo butter

* Store in a refrigerator.

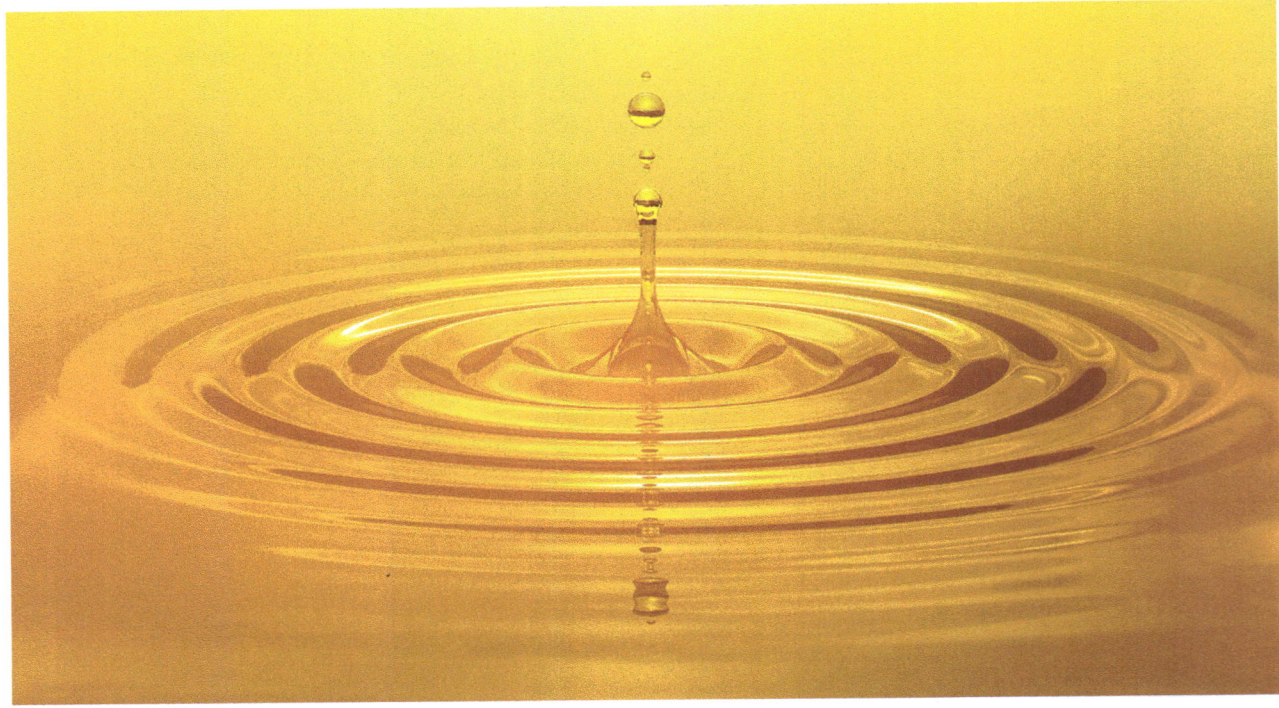

Fixed Oils with >20% Essential Fatty Acids (Linoleic Acid and Alpha-Linolenic Acid)

Fixed Oil	% Linoleic Acid	% Alpha-linolenic acid
Sweet almond oil	20	
Apricot kernel oil	29	
Argan oil	34	2
Baobab oil	25	5
Black cumin seed oil	65	
Borage seed oil	39	
Camelina oil	16	38
Evening primrose oil	74	
Hemp seed oil	56	20
Pumpkin seed oil	51	
Rosehip seed oil	54	19
Sacha inchi oil	34	50
Sea buckthorn seed oil	39	29
Sesame seed oil	45	
Tamanu oil	20	

Omega-3 Fatty Acids (PUFA)
(A carbon-carbon double bond is positioned 3 carbons from the methyl end of the chain)

Alpha-linolenic acid (ALA) (C18:3 n-3)
Eicosapentaenoic acid (EPA) (C20:5 n-3)
Docosahexaenoic acid (DHA) (C22:6 n-3)

Omega-6 Fatty Acids (PUFA)
(A carbon-carbon double bond is positioned 6 carbons from the methyl end of the chain)

Linoleic acid (LA) (C18:2 n-6)
Gamma-linolenic acid (GLA) C18:3 n-6)
Eicosadienoic acid (C20:2 n-6)
Arachidonic acid (AA) (C20:4 n-6)
Docosadienoic acid (C22:2 n-6)
Tetracosatetraenoic acid (C24:4 n-6)
Tetracosapentaenoic acid (C24:5 n-6)

Omega-9 Fatty Acids (MUFA)
(A carbon-carbon double bond is positioned 9 carbons from the methyl end of the chain)

Oleic acid (C18:1 n-9)
Ricinoleic acid (C18:1 n-9)
Gondoic acid (C20:1 n-9)
Erucic acid (C22:1 n-9)
Nervonic acid (C24:1 n-9)

Oleic Acid (Omega-9) Content >50%

Oil	%
Sweet almond oil	60 - 86%
Apricot kernel oil	62 - 71%
Avocado oil	47 - 68%
Kpangnan butter	45 - 58%
Marula oil	70 - 78%
Neem oil	18 - 52%
Olive oil	55 - 83%
High-oleic safflower oil	70 - 84%
High-oleic sunflower oil	80 - 90%

Linoleic Acid (Omega-6) Content >50%

Oil	%
Black cumin seed oil	56 - 64%
Evening primrose oil	65 - 80%
Hemp seed oil	50 - 70%
Neem oil	13 - 69%
Pumpkin seed oil	59 - 65%
Raspberry seed oil	49 - 55%
Rosehip seed oil	41 - 59%
Sacha inchi	21 - 53%
High-linoleic safflower oil	68 - 83%
High-linoleic sunflower oil	48 - 74%

Alpha-Linolenic Acid (Omega-3) Content >25%

Oil	%
Camelina oil	31 - 54%
Hemp seed oil	15 - 25%
Raspberry seed oil	24 - 33%
Rosehip seed oil	20 - 35%
Sacha inchi oil	10 - 55%
Sea buckthorn seed oil	29 - 38%

Gamma-Linolenic Acid (Omega-6) Content >10%

Oil	%
Borage seed oil	21 - 25%
Evening primrose oil	9 - 27%

Oils with Notable Omega-6:Omega-3 ratio

Camelina oil	1:2
Hemp oil	3:1
Rosehip seed oil	1:1
Sacha inchi oil	1:1
Sea buckthorn seed oil	1:1

Sources of Less Common Fatty Acids and Influential Compounds

Carrier Oil	Influential Compounds
Babassu oil	Lauric acid, myristic acid
Black cumin seed oil	Thymoquinone
Castor oil	Ricinoleic acid
Cocoa butter	Stearic acid
Coconut oil	Caprylic acid, capric acid, lauric acid, myristic acid, stearic acid
Cupuaçu butter	Stearic acid
Jojoba oil	Gondoic acid, erucic acid, nervonic acid, wax esters
Kokum butter	Stearic acid
Kpangnan butter	Stearic acid
Kombo butter	Myristic acid, myristoleic acid, kombic acid
Mango butter	Stearic acid
Meadowfoam seed oil	Gondoic acid, erucic acid, docosadienoic acid
Neem oil	Azadirachtin
Olive oil	Polyphenols
Palm kernel oil	Lauric acid, myristic acid
Pomegranate seed oil	Punicic acid
Rosehip seed oil	All-trans-retinoic acid
Sea buckthorn pulp oil	Palmitic acid, palmitoleic acid
Sesame oil	Sesamin, Sesamolin
Shea butter	Stearic acid
Tamanu oil	Calophyllolide

Oils High in Medium Chain (C8-C12) Fatty Acids

Babassu oil
Coconut oil
Palm kernel oil

Oils High in Very Long Chain (C20 and C22) Fatty Acids

Jojoba oil
Meadowfoam seed oil

Significant Sources of Carotenoids

Hemp seed oil
Neem oil
Olive oil
Palm fruit oil
Pumpkin seed oil
Rosehip seed oil
Sea buckthorn fruit oil
Sunflower oil
Tamanu oil

Tocopherol Content >1700 mg/kg

Carrier Oil	Tocopherol Content	Predominant Tocopherol
Black cumin seed oil	1718-1745 mg/kg	(Gamma tocopherol)
Pomegranate seed oil	680-4950 mg/kg	(Gamma-tocopherol)
Pumpkin seed oil	2069-4264 mg/kg	(Gamma-tocopherol)
Raspberry seed oil	2952-3019 mg/kg	(Gamma-tocopherol)
Sacha inchi oil	700-3300 mg/kg	(Gamma-tocopherol)
Sea buckthorn seed oil	1700-4026 mg/kg	(Alpha-tocopherol)
Sea buckthorn pulp oil	716-1700 mg/kg	(Alpha-tocopherol)

Carrier Oils High in Squalene

Carrier Oil	Squalene mg/kg
Argan oil	3030 - 3210 mg/kg
Avocado oil	190 - 1327 mg/kg
Olive oil	800 - 12000 mg/kg
Pomegranate seed oil	828 - 1449 mg/kg
Pumpkin seed	5913 - 6325 mg/kg

Sterol Content > 3000 mg/kg

Carrier Oil	Sterol Content
Apricot kernel oil	2157 - 9736 mg/kg
Avocado oil	2906 - 5955 mg/kg
Borage seed oil	1820 - 4900 mg/kg
Cocoa butter	4960 – 6441 mg/kg
Evening primrose oil	6024 - 10390 mg/kg
Jojoba oil	3977 mg/kg
Pomegranate seed oil	4864 - 5938 mg/kg
Pumpkin seed oil	1895-8052 mg/kg
Raspberry seed oil	5384 mg/kg
Rosehip seed oil	4835 - 5837 mg/kg
Safflower oil	2100 - 4600 mg/kg
Sea buckthorn pulp oil	6684 - 8627 mg/kg
Sesame seed oil	5400 mg/kg
Shea butter	3974 mg/kg
Sunflower oil	2400 - 5000 mg/kg

Oils That Can Extend the Shelf Life of Other Oils
Jojoba oil
Meadowfoam seed oil

Top Recommended Base Oils for Herbal Infusion
Sweet almond oil
Olive oil
Sunflower oil (oleic-acid rich)

For floral infusions – vanilla, neroli, etc.
Coconut oil
Jojoba oil
Marula oil

Carrier Oils for Wound Healing or Skin Regeneration
Babassu oil
Baobab seed oil
Black cumin seed oil
Hemp seed oil
Neem oil
Tamanu oil

Suitable for Ayurvedic Doshas
*specialized indications

Kapha	Pitta	Vata
	Babassu	
		Camelina
	Coconut	
	Evening Primrose	Evening Primrose
Jojoba	Jojoba	Jojoba
Marula	Marula	Marula
Neem	Neem	
Sesame	Sesame	Sesame
Tamanu	Tamanu	

Oil-Bearing Plant Botanical Families

Anacadiaceae
Marula
Mango

Arecaceae syn. Palmaceae
Babassu
Coconut
Palm

Asteraceae syn. Compositae
Safflower
Sunflower

Boraginaceae
Borage

Brassicaceae
Camelina

Calophyllaceae syn. Clusiaceae
Tamanu
Kokum
Kpangnan

Cannabaceae
Hemp

Cucurbitaceae
Pumpkin

Elaeagnaceae
Sea Buckthorn

Euphorbiaceae
Castor
Sacha inchi

Lauraceae
Avocado

Limnanthaceae
Meadowfoam

Lythraceae
Pomegranate

Malvaceae
Baobab
Cocoa
Cupuaçu

Meliaceae
Neem

Myristiaceae
Kombo

Oleaceae
Olive

Onagraceae
Evening primrose

Pedaliaceae
Sesame

Ranunculaceae
Black cumin (Nigella)

Rosaceae
Sweet almond
Apricot
Raspberry
Rose

Sapotaceae
Argan
Shea

Simmondsiaceae
Jojoba

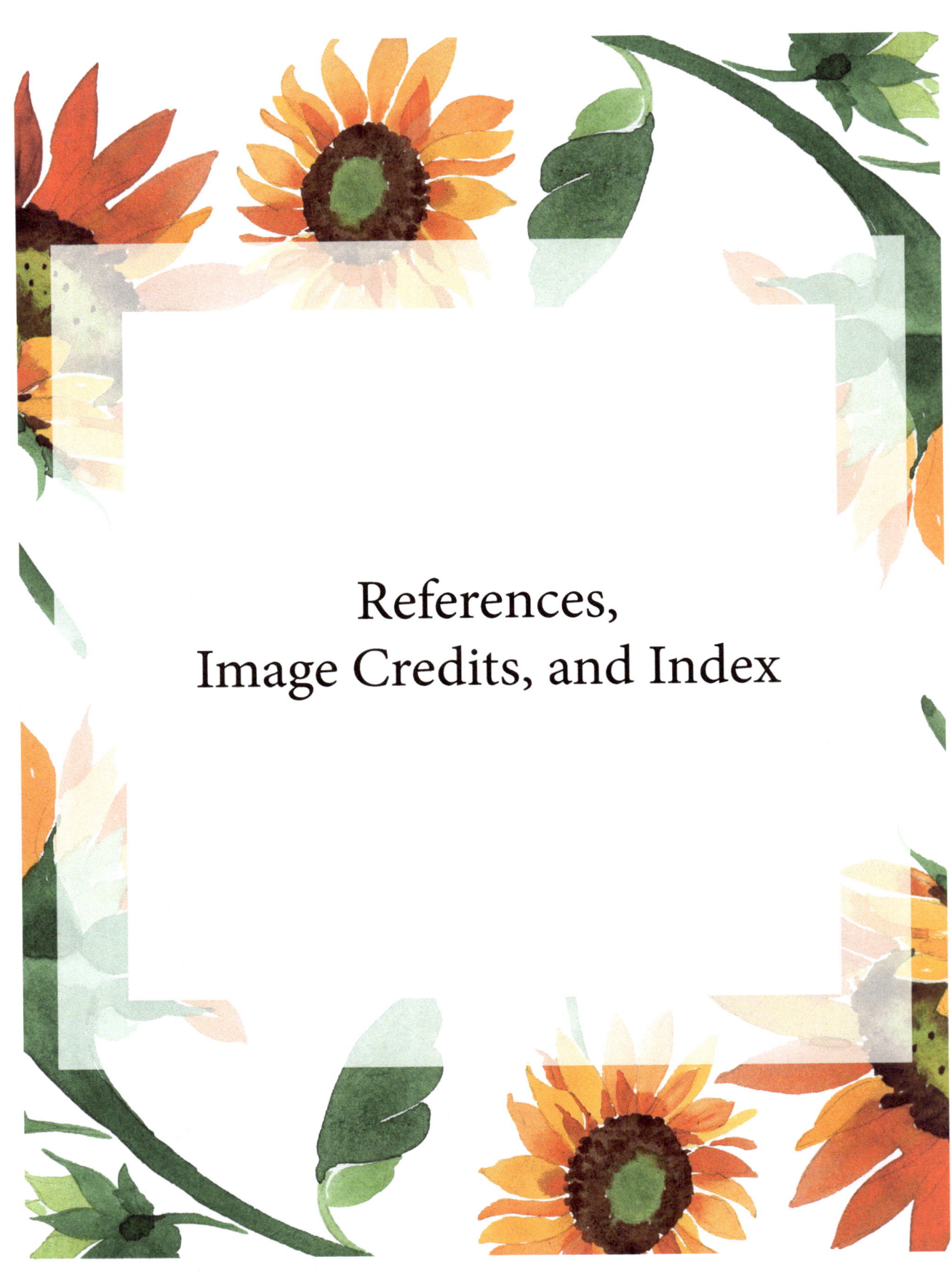

References, Image Credits, and Index

References
Part One: About Carrier Oils

1. Kusmirek, J. (2002). *Liquid sunshine.* Foramicus.

2. Codex Alimentarius Commission. (1999). Codex Standard for Named Vegetable Oils. Codex-Stan 210-1999. Food and Agriculture Organization of the United Nations. Retrieved from https://www.fao.org/3/y2774e/y2774e04.htm# TopOfPage

3. Schaufler, R. (2013, December 12). Processing Edible Oils. PennState Extension. https://extension.psu.edu/processing-edible-oils

4. Ergonul, P.G., & Nergiz, C. (2015). The effect of different filter aid materials and winterization periods on the oxidative stability of sunflower and corn oils. *CyTA - Journal of Food, 13*(2), 174-180. DOI: 10.1080/19476337.2014.931889

5. Helmenstine, A.M. (2020, August 27). *Saponification definition and reaction.* ThoughtCo. https://www.thoughtco.com/definition-of-saponification-605959

6. Stuchlík, M., & Žák, S. (2002). Vegetable lipids as components of functional foods. *Biomedical Papers, 146*(2), 3-10. DOI:10.5507/bp.2002.001

7. Miller, S. (2014, January 21). Essential fatty acids are the holy grail of skin health. Naked Chemist. Retrieved April 9, 2021, from https://thenakedchemist.com/essential-fatty-acids/

8. Fatty Acid Nomenclature. (n.d.). Lumen Nutrition. https://courses.lumenlearning.com/pierce-nutritionmaster/chapter/fatty-acid-naming-food-sources/

9. Dijkstra, A.J. (2021). Trivial names of fatty acids. AOCS. Lipid Library. https://lipidlibrary.aocs.org/resource-material/trivial-names-of-fatty-acids-part-1

10. Moss, G.P. (1976). Nomenclature of lipids: Recommendations Lip-1 and Lip-2. IUPAC-IUB Commission on Biochemical Nomenclature. https://iupac.qmul.ac.uk/lipid/lip1n2.html

11. Yoon, B.K., Jackman, J. A., Valle-Gonzalez, E.R., & Cho, N.-J. (2018). Antibacterial free fatty acids and monoglycerides: Biological activities experimental testing and therapeutic applications. *International Journal of Molecular Sciences, 19*(4), 1114. https://doi.org/10.3390/ijms19041114

12. Huang, W.-C., Tsai, T.-H., Chuang, L.-T., Li, Y.-Y., Zouboulis, C.C., & Tsai, P.-J. (2014). Anti-bacterial and anti-inflammatory properties of capric acid against Propionibacterium acnes: A comparative study with lauric acid. *Journal of Dermatological Science, 73*(3), 232-240. doi: 10.1016/j.jdermsci.2013.10.010

13. Nakatsuji, T., Kao, M., Fang, J-Y., Zouboulis, C., Zhang, L., Gallo, R., & Huang, C-M. (2009). Antimicrobial property of lauric acid against Propionibacterium acnes: Its therapeutic potential for inflammatory acne vulgaris. *Journal of Investigative Dermatology, 129*(10), 2480-2488. doi:10.1038/jid.2009.93

14. Pornpattananangkul, D., Fu, V., Thamphiwatana, S., Zhang, L., Chen, M., Vecchio, J., Gao, W., Huang, C. M., & Zhang, L. (2013). In vivo treatment of Propionibacterium acnes infection with liposomal lauric acids. *Advanced Healthcare Materials, 2*(10), 1322–1328. https://doi.org/10.1002/adhm.201300002

15. Alonso-Castro, A.J., Serrano-Vega, R., Gutierrez, S.P., Isiordia-Espinoza, M.A., & Solorio-Alvarado, C.R. (2021). Myristic acid reduces skin inflammation and nociception. *Journal of Food Biochemistry, 46*(1), e14013. https://doi.org/10.1111/jfbc.14013

16. Mariod, A.A., Matthäus, B., Idris, Y.M.A., & Abdelwahab, S.I. (2010). Fatty acids, tocopherols, phenolics and the antimicrobial effect of Sclerocarya birrea kernels with different harvesting dates. *Journal of the American Oil Chemists' Society, 87*(4), 377–384. https://doi.org/10.1007/s11746-009-1510-4

17. National Cattlemen's Beef Association. (n.d.). Stearic acid. [Technical Summary]. *Human Nutrition Research.* Retrieved April 7, 2021, from https://www.beefresearch.org/resources/human-nutrition/white-papers/stearic-acid

18. Bindu, N., & Kumar, V. (2014). Cocoa butter and its alternatives: A review. *Journal of Bioresource Engineering and Technology*, 1, 7-17. Retrieved February 5, 2022, from http://jakraya.com/journal/pdf/2-jbetArticle_1.pdf

19. Maranz, S., Wiesman, Z., Bisgaard, J. & Bianchi, G. (2004). Germplasm resources of Vitallaria paradoxa based on variations in fat composition across the species distribution range. *Agroforestry Systems*, 60, 71-76. https://doi.org/10.1023/B:AGFO.0000009406.19593.90

20. Marsinach, M.S. & Cuenca, A.P. (2019). The impact of sea buckthorn oil fatty acids on human health. *Lipids in Health and Disease, 18*(1), 145. DOI: 10.1186/s12944-019-1065-9

21. Davidson, K.G., Bersten, A.D., Barr, H.A., Dowling, K.D., Nicolas, T.E., & Doyle, R. (2000). Lung function, permeability and surfactant composition in oleic acid-induced acute lung injury in rats. *American Journal of Physiology. Lung Cellular and Molecular Physiology, 279*(6), L1091-L1102. doi: 10.1152/ajplung.2000.279.6.L1091

22. Mack Correa, M.C., Mao, G., Saad, P., Flach, C.R., Mendelsohn, R., & Walters, R.M. (2014). Molecular interactions of plant oil components with stratum corneum lipids correlate with clinical measures of skin barrier function. *Experimental Dermatology, 23*(1), 39–44. https://doi.org/10.1111/exd.12296

23. Elias, P.M., Brown, B.E., & Ziboh, V.A. (1980). The permeability barrier in essential fatty acid deficiency: Evidence for a direct role for linoleic acid in barrier function. *Journal of Investigative Dermatology, 74*(4), 230–233. doi:10.1111/1523-1747.ep12541775

24. Moreira, T.S.A., de Sousa, V.P., & Pierre, M.B.R. (2010). A novel transdermal delivery system for the anti-inflammatory lumiracoxib: Influence of oleic acid on in vitro percutaneous absorption and in vivo potential cutaneous irritation. *AAPS PharmSciTech, 11*(2), 621–629. doi: 10.1208/s12249-010-9420-1

25. Lin, T. K., Zhong, L., & Santiago, J. L. (2017). Anti-inflammatory and skin barrier repair effects of topical application of some plant oils. International *Journal of Molecular Sciences, 19*(1), 70. https://doi.org/10.3390/ijms19010070

26. de Oliveira, M.L.M., Sousa Nunes-Pinheiro, D.C., Tomé, A.R., Freitas Mota, E., Lima-Verde, I.A., de Melo Pinheiro, F.G., Campello, C.C., & de Morais, S.M. (2010). In vivo topical anti-inflammatory and wound healing activities of the fixed oil of Caryocar coriaceum Wittm. seeds. *Journal of Ethnopharmacology, 129*(2), 214-219. https://doi.org/10.1016/j.jep.2010.03.014

27. Cardoso, C.R., Favoreto, Jr., S., Oliveira, L.L., Vancim, J.O., Barban, G.B., Ferraz, D.B., & Silva, J.S. (2011). Oleic acid modulation of the immune response in wound healing: A new approach for skin repair.

Immunobiology, 216(3), 409–415. DOI: 10.1016/j.imbio.2010.06.007

28. Cardoso, C.R., Souza, M.A., Ferro, E.A., Favoreto, S., Jr, & Pena, J.D. (2004). Influence of topical administration of n-3 and n-6 essential and n-9 nonessential fatty acids on the healing of cutaneous wounds. *Wound Repair and Regeneration, 12*(2), 235–243. https://doi.org/10.1111/j.1067-1927.2004.012216.x

29. Orsavova, J., Misurcova, L., Ambrozova, J. V., Vicha, R., & Mlcek, J. (2015). Fatty acids composition of vegetable oils and its contribution to dietary energy intake and dependence of cardiovascular mortality on dietary intake of fatty acids. *International Journal of Molecular Sciences, 16*(6), 12871–12890. doi:10.3390/ijms160612871

30. Wertz, P. & Downing D T. (1990) Metabolism of linoleic acid in porcine epidermis. *Journal of Lipid Research, 31*(10), 1839-1844.

31. Timoszuk, M., Bielawska, K., & Skrzydlewska, E. (2018). Evening primrose (Oenothera biennis) biological activity dependent on chemical composition. *Antioxidants, 7*(8), 108. https://doi.org/10.3390/antiox7080108

32. Zheng, C.J., Yoo, J.S., Lee, T.G., Cho, H.Y., Kim, Y.H., & Kim, W.G. (2005). Fatty acid synthesis is a target for antibacterial activity of unsaturated fatty acids. *FEBS letters, 579*(23), 5157–5162. https://doi.org/10.1016/j.febslet.2005.08.028

33. Zielińska, A. & Nowak, I. (2014). Fatty acids in vegetable oils and their importance in cosmetic industry. *Chemik*, 68, 103-110.

34. Silva, J.R., Burger, B., Kuhl, C.M.C., Candreva, T., dos Anjos, M.B.P., & Rodrigues, H.G. (2018). Wound healing and omega-6 fatty acids: From inflammation to repair. *Mediators of Inflammation*, 2018, Article ID 2503950. https://doi.org/10.1155/2018/2503950

35. Ando, H., Ryu, A., Hashimoto, A., Oka, M., & Ichihashi, M. (1998). Linoleic acid and alpha-linolenic acid lightens ultraviolet-induced hyperpigmentation of the skin. *Archives of Dermatological Research, 290*(7), 375–381. https://doi.org/10.1007/s004030050320

36. Timoszuk, M., Bielawska, K., & Skrzydlewska, E. (2018). Evening primrose (Oenothera biennis) biological activity dependent on chemical composition. *Antioxidants, 7*(8), 108. https://doi.org/10.3390/antiox7080108

37. Ziboh, V.A., Miller, C.C., & Cho, Y. (2000). Metabolism of polyunsaturated fatty acids by skin epidermal enzymes: Generation of anti-inflammatory and antiproliferative metabolites. *American Journal of Clinical Nutrition*, 71(suppl): 361S–6S. DOI:10.1093/ajcn/71.1.361s

38. Ren, J., & Chung, S.H. (2007). Anti-inflammatory effect of alpha-linolenic acid and its mode of action through the inhibition of nitric oxide production and inducible nitric oxide synthase gene expression via NF-kappaB and mitogen-activated protein kinase pathways. *Journal of Agricultural and Food Chemistry, 55*(13), 5073–5080. https://doi.org/10.1021/jf0702693

39. Eskin, N.A.M. (2008). Borage and evening primrose oil. *European Journal of Lipid Science and Technology, 110*(7), 651-654. https://doi.org/10.1002/ejlt.200700259

40. Fabrikov, D., Guil-Guerro, J.L., Gonzalez-Fernandez, M.J. Rodriquez-Garcia, I., Gomez-Mercado, F., Urrestarazu, M., Lao, M.T., Rincon-Cervera, M.A., Alvaro, J.E, & Lyashenko, S. (2019). Borage oil: Tocopherols, sterols and squalene in farmed and endemic-wild Borago species. *Journal of Food Composition and Analysis*, 83. 103299. https://doi.org/10.1016/j.jfca.2019.103299

41. Storey, A., McArdle, F., Friedmann, P. S., Jackson, M. J., & Rhodes, L. E. (2005). Eicosapentaenoic acid and docosahexaenoic acid reduce UVB- and TNF-alpha-induced IL-8 secretion in keratinocytes and UVB-induced IL-8 in fibroblasts. *The Journal of Investigative Dermatology, 124*(1), 248–255. https://doi.org/10.1111/j.0022-202X.2004.23543.x

42. Cert, A., Moreda, W., & Pérez-Camino, M.C. (2000). Chromatographic analysis of minor constituents in vegetable oils. *Journal of Chromatography A, 881*(1-2), 131–148. https://doi.org/10.1016/s0021-9673(00)00389-7

43. Ayegnon, B.P., Adjanohoun, G., & Kayode, A.P.P. (2019). Technological application of the butter of Pentadesma butyracea: A comparative evaluation of its cosmetic behavior with Vitellaria paradoxa butter. *Journal of Cereals and Oil Seeds, 10*(2), 43-53. DOI:10.5897/JCO2019.0199

44. Grajzer, M., Szmalcel, K., Kuźmiński, Ł., Witkowski, M., Kulma, A., & Prescha, A. (2020). Characteristics and antioxidant potential of cold-pressed oils-Possible strategies to improve oil stability. *Foods, 9*(11), 1630. https://doi.org/10.3390/foods9111630

45. Koskovac, M., Cupara, S., Kipic, M., Barjaktarevic, A., Milovanovic, O., Kojicic, K., & Markovic, M. (2017). Sea buckthorn oil—A valuable source for cosmeceuticals. *Cosmetics, 4*(4), 40. https://doi.org/10.3390/cosmetics4040040

46. Sajfrtová, M., Licková, I., Wimmerová, M., Sovová, H., & Wimmer, Z. (2010). b-Sitosterol: supercritical carbon dioxide extraction from sea buckthorn (Hippophae rhamnoides L.) seeds. *International Journal of Molecular Sciences, 11*(4), 1842–1850. doi:10.3390/ijms11041842

47. Huang, Z.R., Lin, Y.K., & Fang, J.Y. (2009). Biological and pharmacological activities of squalene and related compounds: potential uses in cosmetic dermatology. *Molecules, 14*(1), 540–554. https://doi.org/10.3390/molecules14010540

48. Balic, A., & Mokos, M. (2019). Do we utilize our knowledge of the skin protective effects of carotenoids enough? *Antioxidants*, 8, 259. doi:10.3390/antiox8080259

49. Aluyor, E.O., Ozigagu, C.E., Oboh, O.I. and Aluyor, P. (2009). Chromatographic analysis of carrier oils: A review. *Scientific Research and Essay, 4*(4), 191-197.

50. Zielińska, A., & Nowak, I. (2017). Abundance of active ingredients in sea-buckthorn oil. *Lipids in Health and Disease, 16*(1), 95. doi:10.1186/s12944-017-0469-7

51. Azadmard-Damirchi, S., Emami, S., Hesari, J., Peighambardoust, S.H., & Nemati, M. (2011). Nuts composition and their health benefits. International *Journal of Nutrition and Food Engineering, 5*(9), 544-548.

52. Sajfrtová, M., Licková, I., Wimmerová, M., Sovová, H., & Wimmer, Z. (2010). b-Sitosterol: supercritical carbon dioxide extraction from sea buckthorn (Hippophae rhamnoides L.) seeds. *International Journal of Molecular Sciences, 11*(4), 1842–1850. doi:10.3390/ijms11041842

53. Dweck, A. (2003). *The role of natural ingredients in anti-aging of the skin*. Australian Society of Cosmetic Chemists Annual Congress, Hamilton Island.

54. Dulf, F.V., Unguresan, M.L., Vodnar, D.C., & Socaciu, C. (2010). Free and esterified sterol distribution in four Romanian vegetable oil. *Notulae Botanicae Horti Agrobotanici Cluj-Napoca, 38*(2), 91-97. https://doi.org/10.15835/nbha3824753

55. Kamal-Eldin, A. (2005). Minor Components of Fats and Oils. In F. Shahidi (Ed.), *Bailey's industrial oil and fat products.* (6th ed.). John Wiley

& Sons, Ltd. https://doi.org/10.1002/047167849X.bio012

56. Yang, R., Xue, L., Zhang, L., Wang, X., Qi, X., Jiang, J., Yu, L, Wang, X., Zhang, W., Zhang, Q., & Li, P. (2019). Phytosterol contents of edible oils and their contributions to estimated phytosterol intake in the Chinese diet. *Foods, 8*(8), 334. doi:10.3390/foods8080334

57. Azadmard-Damirchi, S., Emami, S., Hesari, J., Peighambardoust, S.H., & Nemati, M. (2011). Nuts composition and their health benefits. International *Journal of Nutrition and Food Engineering, 5*(9), 544-548.

58. Gupta, M.B., Nath, R., Srivastava, N., Shanker, K., Kishor, K., & Bhargava, K.P. (1980). Anti-inflammatory and antipyretic activities of beta-sitosterol. *Planta Medica, 39*(2), 157–163. https://doi.org/10.1055/s-2008-1074919

59. Bouic, P.J.D., & Lamprecht J.H. (1999). Plant sterols and sterolins: A review of their immune-modulating properties. *Alternative Medicine Review, 4*(3), 170-177.

60. Vermaak, I., Kamatou, G.P.P., Komane-Mofokeng, B., Viljoen, A.M., & Beckett, K. (2011). African seed oils of commercial importance – Cosmetic applications. *South African Journal of Botany, 77*(4), 920-933. http://dx.doi.org/10.1016/j.sajb.2011.07.003

61. Vazquez, L., Torres. C.F., Senorans, F.J., Reglero, G. (2007). Recovery of squalene from vegetable oil sources using countercurrent supercritical carbon dioxide extraction. *The Journal of Supercritical Fluids, 40*(1), 59-66.

62. Grompone, M. (2005). Sunflower and high-oleic sunflower oils. In F. Shahidi (Ed.), *Bailey's industrial oil and Fat products*. (6th ed.). John Wiley and Sons, Inc. https://doi.org/10.1002/047167849X.bio017.pub2

63. Schmidt, S. & Pokorny, J. (2005). Potential applications of oilseeds as sources of antioxidants for food lipids – A review. *Czech Journal of Food Sciences, 23*(3), 93-102. DOI:10.17221/3377-CJFS

64. Azadmard-Damirchi, S., Emami, S., Hesari, J., Peighambardoust, S.H., & Nemati, M. (2011). Nuts composition and their health benefits. International *Journal of Nutrition and Food Engineering, 5*(9), 544-648.

65. Tavakkol, A., Nabi, Z., Soliman, N., & Polefka, T.G. (2004). Delivery of vitamin E to the skin by a novel liquid skin cleanser: comparison of topical versus oral supplementation. *Journal of Cosmetic Science, 55*(2), 177-87.

66. National Institutes of Health. (2021, March 6). Vitamin A: Fact sheet for health professionals. National Institutes of Health Office of Dietary Supplements. http://ods.od.nih.gov/factsheets/VitaminA-HealthProfessional/

67. Varani, J., Warner, R.L., Gharaee-Kermani, M., Phan, S., Kang, S., Chung, J.H., Wang, Z.Q., Datta, S., Fisher, G.J., & Voorhees, J.J. (2000). Vitamin A antagonizes decreased cell growth and elevated collagen-degrading matrix metalloproteinases and stimulates collagen accumulation in naturally aged human skin. *Journal of Investigative Dermatology, 114*(3), 480–486. doi:10.1046/j.1523-1747.2000.00902.x

68. Wisse, B. (2020, January 26) Hypervitaminosis A. National Library of Medicine. Medline Plus. Retrieved April 7, 2021, from https://medlineplus.gov/ency/article/000350.htm

69. Golan, R. (1995). *Optimal wellness*. Ballantine Books.

70. Gloria, N.F., Soares, N., Brand, C., Oliveira, F.L., Borojevic, R., & Teodoro, A.J. (2014). Lycopene and beta-carotene induce cell-cycle arrest and apoptosis in human breast cancer cell lines. *Anticancer Research, 34*(3), 1377-86.

71. Pizzorno, J.E. & Murray, T. (1999). *Textbook of natural medicine*. Churchill Livingstone.

72. El Meshad, A.N., & Tadros, M.I. (2011). Transdermal delivery of an anti-cancer drug via w/o emulsions based on alkyl polyglycosides and lecithin: Design, characterization, and in vivo evaluation of the possible irritation potential in rats. *AAPS PharmSciTech, 12*(1), 1–9. doi: 10.1208/s12249-010-9557-y

References
Part Two: Lipids and the Skin

1. Drakou, K., Tsianni, A., Vrani, F., Kefala, V., & Rallis, E. (2021). Revealing the correlation between altered skin lipids composition and skin disorders. *Cosmetics, 8*(3), 88. http://dx.doi.org/10.3390/cosmetics8030088

2. Sanford, J.A., & Gallo, R.L. (2013). Functions of the skin microbiota in health and disease. *Seminars in Immunology, 25*(5), 370–377. https://doi.org/10.1016/j.smim.2013.09.005

3. Grice, E.A., Kong, H.H., Conlan, S., Deming, C.B., Davis, J., Young, A.C., NISC Comparative Sequencing Program, Bouffard, G.G., Blakesley, R.W., Murray, P.R., Green, E.D., Turner, M.L., & Segre, J.A. (2009). Topographical and temporal diversity of the human skin microbiome. *Science, 324*(5931), p. 1190. https://doi.org/10.1126/science.1171700

4. Christensen, G.J., & Brüggemann, H. (2014). Bacterial skin commensals and their role as host guardians. *Beneficial Microbes, 5*(2), 201–215. https://doi.org/10.3920/BM2012.0062

5. Ellis, S.R., Nguyen, M., Vaughn, A.R., Notay, M., Burney, W.A., Sandhu, S., & Sivamani, R.K. (2019). The skin and gut microbiome and its role in common dermatologic conditions. *Microorganisms, 7*(11), 550. https://doi.org/10.3390/microorganisms7110550

6. Baviera, G., Leoni, M.C., Capra, L., Cipriani, F., Longo, G., Maiello, N., Ricci, G., Galli, E. (2014). Microbiota in healthy skin and in atopic eczema. *BioMed Research International*, 2014. Article ID 436921, 6 pages. https://doi.org/10.1155/2014/436921

7. Kong, H.H., Oh, J., Deming, C., Conlan, S., Grice, E.A., Beatson, M.A., Nomicos, E., Polley, E.C., Komarow, H.D., NISC Comparative Sequence Program, Murray, P.R., Turner, M.L., & Segre, J.A. (2012). Temporal shifts in the skin microbiome associated with disease flares and treatment in children with atopic dermatitis. *Genome Research, 22*(5), 850–859. https://doi.org/10.1101/gr.131029.111

8. Xu, H., & Li, H. (2019). Acne, the skin microbiome, and antibiotic treatment. *American Journal of Clinical Dermatology, 20*(3), 335–344. https://doi.org/10.1007/s40257-018-00417-3

9. Zaidi, A.K., Spaunhurst, K., Sprockett, D., Thomason, Y., Mann, M.W., Fu, P., Ammons, C., Gerstenblith, M., Tuttle, M.S., & Popkin, D.L. (2018). Characterization of the facial microbiome in twins discordant for rosacea. *Experimental Dermatology, 27*(3), 295–298. https://doi.org/10.1111/exd.13491

10. Benhadou, F., Mintoff, D., Schnebert, B., & Thio, H. B. (2018). Psoriasis and microbiota: A systematic review. *Diseases, 6*(2), 47. https://doi.org/10.3390/diseases6020047

11. Misic, A.M., Gardner, S.E., & Grice, E.A. (2014). The wound microbiome: Modern approaches to examining the role of microorganisms

in impaired chronic wound healing. *Advances in Wound Care, 3*(7), 502–510. https://doi.org/10.1089/wound.2012.0397

12. Elias, A.E., McBain, A.J., & O'Neill, C.A. (2021). The role of the skin microbiota in the modulation of cutaneous inflammation - Lessons from the gut. *Experimental Dermatology, 30*(10), 1509–1516. https://doi.org/10.1111/exd.14420

13. Nakatsuji, T., Chen, T.H., Butcher, A.M., Trzoss, L.L., Nam, S.J., Shirakawa, K.T., Zhou, W., Oh, J., Otto, M., Fenical, W., & Gallo, R.L. (2018). A commensal strain of Staphylococcus epidermidis protects against skin neoplasia. *Science Advances, 4*(2), eaao4502. https://doi.org/10.1126/sciadv.aao4502

14. Zakany, N., Olah, A., Markovics, A., Takacs, E. Aranyasz, A., Nicolussi, S., Piscitelli, F., Allara, M., Por, A., Kovacs, I., Zouboulis, C.C., Gertsch, J. Di Marzo, V., Biro, T., & Szabo, T. (2018). Endocannabinoid tone regulates human sebocyte biology. *Dermatology, 138*(8), 1699-1706. DOI: 10.1016/j.jid.2018.02.022

15. Pappas A. (2009). Epidermal surface lipids. *Dermato-endocrinology, 1*(2), 72–76. https://doi.org/10.4161/derm.1.2.7811

16. Drake, D. R., Brogden, K. A., Dawson, D. V., & Wertz, P. W. (2008). Thematic review series: Skin lipids. Antimicrobial lipids at the skin surface. *Journal of Lipid Research, 49*(1), 4–11. https://doi.org/10.1194/jlr.R700016-JLR200

17. Kuo, S.-H., Shen, C.-J., Shen, C.-F., & Cheng, C.-M. (2020). Role of pH value in clinically relevant diagnosis. *Diagnostics, 10*(2), 107. https://doi.org/10.3390/diagnostics10020107

18. Ali, S.M., & Yosipovitch, G. (2013). Skin pH: From basic science to basic skin care. *Acta Dermato-Venereologica, 93*(3), 261-267. DOI: 10.2340/00015555-1531

19. Rippke, F., Schreiner, V., & Schwanitz, H. J. (2002). The acidic milieu of the horny layer: New findings on the physiology and pathophysiology of skin pH. *American Journal of Clinical Dermatology, 3*(4), 261–272. https://doi.org/10.2165/00128071-200203040-00004

20. Kusmirek, J. (2002). *Liquid sunshine*. Foramicus.

21. Belkaid, Y., & Tamoutounour, S. (2016). The influence of skin microorganisms on cutaneous immunity. *Nature Reviews Immunology, 16*(6), p. 353. https://doi.org/10.1038/nri.2016.48

22. Drakou, K., Tsianni, A., Vrani, F., Kefala, V., & Rallis, E. (2021). Revealing the correlation between altered skin lipids composition and skin disorders. *Cosmetics, 8*(3), 88. http://dx.doi.org/10.3390/cosmetics8030088

23. Wertz P. W. (2018). Lipids and the permeability and antimicrobial barriers of the skin. *Journal of Lipids*, 2018, Article ID 5954034. https://doi.org/10.1155/2018/5954034

24. Bensouilah, J. & Buck, P. (2006). *Aromadermatology*. Radcliffe Publishing Company.

25. Wertz, P. (2000). Lipids and barrier function of the skin. *Acta Dermato-Venereologica*, 2000(Supplement 208), 7-11. DOI: 10.1080/000155500750042790

26. Nguyen, A. V., & Soulika, A. M. (2019). The dynamics of the skin's immune system. *International Journal of Molecular Sciences, 20*(8), 1811. https://doi.org/10.3390/ijms20081811

27. Angelo, G. (2012, February). *Essential fatty acids and skin health*. Linus Pauling Institute. Retrieved on April 2, 2022, from https://lpi.oregonstate.edu/mic/health-disease/skin-health/essential-fatty-acids

28. Fowler, J. (2012). Understanding the role of natural moisturizing factor in skin hydration. *Practical Dermatology, July 2012*, 36-40. https://practicaldermatology.com/articles/2012-jul/understanding-the-role-of-natural-moisturizing-factor-in-skin-hydration

29. Spada, F., Barnes, T.M., & Greive, K.A. (2018). Skin hydration is significantly increased by a cream formulated to mimic the skin's own natural moisturizing systems. *Clinical, Cosmetic and Investigational Dermatology*, 11, 491–497. https://doi.org/10.2147/CCID.S177697

30. Khnykin, D., Miner, J.H., & Jahnsen, F. (2011). Role of fatty acid transporters in epidermis: Implications for health and disease. *Dermato-Endocrinology, 3*(2): 53–61. DOI: 10.4161/derm.3.2.14816

31. Vaughn, A.R., Clark, A.K., Sivamani, R.K., & Shi, V.Y. (2018). Natural oils for skin-barrier repair: Ancient compounds now backed by modern science. *American Journal of Clinical Dermatology, 19*(1), 103–117. https://doi.org/10.1007/s40257-017-0301-1

32. Truchetet, E., Brändle, I., & Grosshans, E. (1988). Hautveränderungen, Pathophysiologie und Therapie bei Mangel an essentiellen Fettsäuren [Skin changes, pathophysiology and therapy in deficiency of essential fatty acids]. *Zeitschrift für Hautkrankheiten, 63*(4), 290–301.

33. Choe, S.J., Kim, D., Kim, E.J., Ahn, J.-S., Choi, E.-J., Son, E.D., Lee, T.R., & Choi, E.H. (2018). Psychological stress deteriorates skin barrier function by activating 11b-hydroxysteroid dehydrogenase 1 and the HPA axis. *Scientific Reports*, 8, 6334. https://doi.org/10.1038/s41598-018-24653-z

34. Ahmad, A., & Ahsan, H. (2020). Lipid-based formulations in cosmeceuticals and biopharmaceuticals. *Biomedical Dermatology*, 4, 12. https://doi.org/10.1186/s41702-020-00062-9

35. Purnamawati, S., Indrastuti, N., Danarti, R., & Saefudin, T. (2017). The role of moisturizers in addressing various kinds of dermatitis: A review. *Clinical Medicine & Research, 15*(3-4), 75-87. DOI:10.3121/cmr.2017.1363

36. Angelo, G. (2012, February). *Essential fatty acids and skin health*. Linus Pauling Institute. Retrieved on April 2, 2022, from https://lpi.oregonstate.edu/mic/health-disease/skin-health/essential-fatty-acids

References
Part Three: The Core Carrier Oils

1. BTSA. (n.d.). *The oxidation process in fats and oils*. https://www.btsa.com/en/process-oxidation-fats/

2. Koon, R. (2009, August 4). *Understanding rancidity of nutritional lipids*. Natural Products Insider. https://www.naturalproductsinsider.com/regulatory/understanding-rancidity-nutritional-lipids

3. Missouri Botanical Garden (n.d.). *Prunus dulcis*. Retrieved October 16, 2020, from http://www.missouribotanicalgarden.org/PlantFinder/PlantFinderDetails.aspx?kempercode=d453

4. Ahmad, Z. (2010). The uses and properties of almond oil. *Complementary Therapies in Clinical Practice, 16*(1), 10–12. https://doi.org/10.1016/j.ctcp.2009.06.015

5. Codex Alimentarius Commission. (1999). *Codex Standard for Named Vegetable Oils.* Codex-Stan 210-1999. Food and Agriculture Organization of the United Nations. Retrieved from https://www.fao.org/3/y2774e/y2774e04.htm# TopOfPage

6. Qi, Z., Xiao, J., Ye, L., Chuyun, W., Chang, Z., Shugang, L., & Fenghong, H. (2019). The effect of the subcritical fluid extraction on the quality of almond oils: Compared to conventional mechanical pressing method. *Food, Science, and Nutrition, 7*(7), 2231-2241. DOI:10.1002/fsn3.1023

7. Roncero, J.M., Álvarez-Ortí, M., Pardo-Giménez, A., Rabadán, A., & Pardo, J. E. (2020). Review about non-lipid components and minor fat-soluble bioactive compounds of almond kernel. *Foods, 9*(11), 1646. https://doi.org/10.3390/foods9111646

8. Roussos, P.A., Denaxa, N.-K., Tsafouros, A., Efstathios, N., & Intidhar, B. (2016). Apricot (Prunus armeniaca L.). *Nutritional Composition of Fruit Cultivars,* (M. S. J. Simmonds & V. R. Preedy, Eds.), 19-48. https://doi.org/10.1016/B978-0-12-408117-8.00002-7

9. Plants for a Future. (n.d.). *Prunus armeniaca.* Retrieved October 23, 2020, from https://pfaf.org/user/Plant.aspx?LatinName=Prunus+armeniaca

10. Stryjecka, M., Kiełtyka-Dadasiewicz, A., Michalak, M., Rachoń, L., & Głowacka, A. (2019). Chemical composition and antioxidant properties of oils from the seeds of five apricot (Prunus armeniaca L.) cultivars. *Journal of Oleo Science, 68*(8), 729–738. https://doi.org/10.5650/jos.ess19121

11. Rudzińska, M., Górnaś, P., Raczyk, M., & Soliven, A. (2017). Sterols and squalene in apricot (Prunus armeniaca L.) kernel oils: The variety as a key factor. *Natural Product Research, 31*(1), 84–88. https://doi.org/10.1080/14786419.2015.1135146

12. Hrichi, S., Rigano, F., Chaabane-Banaoues, R., Oulad El Majdoub, Y., Mangraviti, D., Di Marco, D., Babba, H., Dugo, P., Mondello, L., Mighri, Z., & Cacciola, F. (2020). Identification of fatty acid, lipid and polyphenol compounds from Prunus armeniaca L. kernel extracts. *Foods, 9*(7), 896. https://doi.org/10.3390/foods9070896

13. Tian, H.L. & Zhan, P. (2011). Chemical composition and antioxidant activities of ansu apricot oil growing wild in north Xinjiang, China. *Natural Product Research, 25*(12), 1208-1211. DOI: 10.1080/14786419.2010.541882

14. Paniagua-Pérez, R., Flores-Mondragón, G., Reyes-Legorreta, C., Herrera-López, B., Cervantes-Hernández, I., Madrigal-Santillán, O., Morales-González, J. A., Álvarez-González, I., & Madrigal-Bujaidar, E. (2016). Evaluation of the anti-inflammatory capacity of beta-sitosterol in rodent assays. *African Journal of Traditional, Complementary, and Alternative Medicines, 14*(1), 123–130. https://doi.org/10.21010/ajtcam.v14i1.13

15. Gupta, M. B., Nath, R., Srivastava, N., Shanker, K., Kishor, K., & Bhargava, K. P. (1980). Anti-inflammatory and antipyretic activities of beta-sitosterol. *Planta Medica, 39*(2), 157–163. https://doi.org/10.1055/s-2008-1074919

16. Missouri Botanical Garden. (n.d.). *Argania spinosa.* Retrieved October 26, 2020, from https://www.missouribotanicalgarden.org/PlantFinder/PlantFinderDetails.aspx?taxonid=286835&isprofile=0&

17. Villareal, M. O., Kume, S., Bourhim, T., Bakhtaoui, F. Z., Kashiwagi, K., Han, J., Gadhi, C., & Isoda, H. (2013). Activation of MITF by argan oil leads to the inhibition of the tyrosinase and dopachrome tautomerase expressions in B16 murine melanoma cells. *Evidence-based Complementary and Alternative Medicine,* 2013. https://doi.org/10.1155/2013/340107

18. Hanana, M., Mezghenni, H., Ben Ayed, R., Ben Dhiab, A., Jarradi, S., Jamoussi, B., & Hamrouni, L. (2018). Nutraceutical potentialities of Tunisian argan oil based on its physicochemical properties and fatty acid content as assessed through Bayesian network analyses. *Lipids in Health and Disease, 17*(1), 138. https://doi.org/10.1186/s12944-018-0782-9

19. Poljšak, N., Kreft, S., & Kočevar Glavač, N. (2020). Vegetable butters and oils in skin wound healing: Scientific evidence for new opportunities in dermatology. *Phytotherapy Research, 34*(2), 254–269. https://doi.org/10.1002/ptr.6524

20. Charrouf, Z. & Guillaume, D. (2008). Argan oil: Occurrence, composition and impact on human health. *European Journal of Lipid Science and Technology,* 110, 632–636. https://onlinelibrary.wiley.com/doi/pdf/10.1002/ejlt.200700220

21. Boucetta, K. Q., Charrouf, Z., Derouiche, A., Rahali, Y., & Bensouda, Y. (2014). Skin hydration in postmenopausal women: Argan oil benefit with oral and/or topical use. *Przeglad menopauzalny [Menopause review], 13*(5), 280–288. https://doi.org/10.5114/pm.2014.46470

22. Charrouf, Z. & Guillaume, D. (2008). Argan oil: Occurrence, composition and impact on human health. *European Journal of Lipid Science and Technology,* 110, 632–636. Retrieved from https://onlinelibrary.wiley.com/doi/pdf/10.1002/ejlt.200700220

23. Hanana, M., Mezghenni, H., Ben Ayed, R., Ben Dhiab, A., Jarradi, S., Jamoussi, B., & Hamrouni, L. (2018). Nutraceutical potentialities of Tunisian argan oil based on its physicochemical properties and fatty acid content as assessed through Bayesian network analyses. *Lipids in Health and Disease, 17*(1), 138. https://doi.org/10.1186/s12944-018-0782-9

24. Miklavcic, M.B., Taous, F., Valencic, V., Elghali, T., Podgornik, M., Strojnik, L., & Ogrinc, N. (2020). Fatty acid composition of cosmetic argan oil: Provenience and authenticity criteria. *Molecules,* 25, doi: 10.3390/molecules25184080

25. Khallouki, F., Younos, C., Soulimani, R., Oster, T., Charrouf, Z., Spiegelhalder, B., Bartsch, H., & Owen, R.W. (2003). Consumption of argan oil (Morocco) with its unique profile of fatty acids, tocopherols, squalene, sterols and phenolic compounds should confer valuable cancer chemo preventive effects. *European Journal of Cancer Prevention, 12*(1), 67-75. DOI: 10.1097/00008469-200302000-00011

26. Hilali, M., Charrouf, Z., Soulhi, A., Hachimi, L., & Guillaume, D. (2005). Influence of origin and extraction method on argan oil physicochemical characteristics and composition. *Journal of Agricultural and Food Chemistry, 53*(6), 2081–2087. https://doi.org/10.1021/jf040290t

27. Boucetta, K. Q., Charrouf, Z., Aguenaou, H., Derouiche, A., & Bensouda, Y. (2015). The effect of dietary and/or cosmetic argan oil on postmenopausal skin elasticity. *Clinical Interventions in Aging,* 10, 339–349. https://doi.org/10.2147/CIA.S71684

28. Boucetta, K. Q., Charrouf, Z., Derouiche, A., Rahali, Y., & Bensouda, Y. (2014). Skin hydration in postmenopausal women: Argan oil benefit with oral and/or topical use. *Przeglad menopauzalny [Menopause review], 13*(5), 280–288. https://doi.org/10.5114/pm.2014.46470

29. Kusmirek, J. (2002). *Liquid sunshine.* Foramicus.

30. Petruzzello, M. (2021). *baobab.* Encyclopedia Britannica. https://www.britannica.com/plant/baobab-tree-genus

31. Rahul, J., Jain, M.K., Singh, S.P., Kamal, R.K., Anuradha, Naz, A., Gupta, A.K., & Mrityunjay, S.K. (2015). Adansonia digitata L. (baobab): A review of traditional information and taxonomic description. *Asian Pacific Journal of Tropical Biomedicine, 5*(1), 79–84. https://doi.org/10.1016/S2221-1691(15)30174-X

32. Chadare, F.J., Linnemann, A.R., Hounhouigan, J.D., Nout, M.J.R., & Van Boekel, M.A.J.S. (2008). Baobab food products: A review on their composition and nutritional value. *Critical Reviews in Food Science and Nutrition, 49*(3), 254-274. https://doi.org/10.1080/10408390701856330

33. Burnett, C.L., Fiume, M.M., Bergfeld, W.F., Belsito, D.V., Hill, R.A., Klaassen, C.D., Liebler, D., Marks, J.G., Shank, R.C., Slaga, T.J., Snyder, P.W., & Andersen, F.A. (2017). Safety assessment of plant-derived fatty acid oils. *International Journal of Toxicology, 36*(Supp. 3), 51S-129S. https://doi.org/10.1177/1091581817740569

34. Ayaz, M., Rizwani, G.H., Shareef, H., Zia-ul-Haq, M., & Mumtaz, T. (2015). Analytical characterization of Adansonia digitata L. seed oil grown in the Sind region of Pakistan. *International Journal for Pharmaceutical Research Scholars, 3*(4), 285-291. E-ISSN: 2277-7873

35. The Biology of *Camelina sativa* (L.) Crantz (Camelina). (n.d.) Government of Canada. Guidance Document Repository. Retrieved May 18, 2021, from https://inspection.canada.ca/plant-varieties/plants-with-novel-traits/applicants/directive-94-08/biology-documents/camelina-sativa-l-/eng/1330971423348/1330971509470

36. Eynck, C., & Falk, K.C. (2013). Camelina (Camelina sativa). *Biofuel Crops: Production, Physiology and Genetics,* (B.P. Singh, Ed.), 369-391. https://www.cabi.org/isc/FullTextPDF/2013/20133196031.pdf

37. Sampath, A. (2009). *Chemical characterization of camelina seed oil.* [Masters Thesis, Rutgers University]. Retrieved May 27, 2021, from https://rucore.libraries.rutgers.edu/rutgers-lib/25894/PDF/1/play/&lang=en

38. Rode, J. (2008). Study of autochthon Camelina sativa (L.) Crantz in Slovenia. *Journal of Herbs, Spices & Medicinal Plants, 9*(4), 313-318. DOI: 10.1300/J044v09n04_08

39. Ibrahim, F.M., & El Habbasha, S.F. (2015). Chemical composition, medicinal impacts and cultivation of camelina (Camelina sativa): Review. *International Journal of PharmTech Research, 8*(10), 114-122. https://www.researchgate.net/publication/298073329_Chemical_composition_medicinal_impacts_and_cultivation_of_camelina_Camelina_sativa_Review

40. Tsui, V. (2014). Cooking oil: Which one should you be using? *EatNorth.* Retrieved May 31, 2021, from https://eatnorth.com/vincci-tsui/cooking-oil-which-one-should-you-be-using

41. The Biology of *Camelina sativa* (L.) Crantz (Camelina). (n.d.) Government of Canada. Guidance Document Repository. Retrieved May 18, 2021, from https://inspection.canada.ca/plant-varieties/plants-with-novel-traits/applicants/directive-94-08/biology-documents/camelina-sativa-l-/eng/1330971423348/1330971509470

42. Grajzer, M., Szmalcel, K., Kuźmiński, Ł., Witkowski, M., Kulma, A., & Prescha, A. (2020). Characteristics and antioxidant potential of cold-pressed oils: Possible strategies to improve oil stability. *Foods, 9*(11), 1630. https://doi.org/10.3390/foods9111630

43. Angelo, G. (2012). Essential fatty acids and skin health. Linus Pauling Institute, Oregon State University, Micronutrient Information Center. Retrieved from https://lpi.oregonstate.edu/mic/health-disease/skin-health/essential-fatty-acids#delivery

44. Making Cosmetics. (n.d.). *Camelina oil.* Retrieved May 19, 2021, from https://www.makingcosmetics.com/Camelina-Oil_p_180.html?locale=en

45. Ladybird Johnson Wildflower Center. (2015). Simmondsia chinensis. The University of Texas at Austin. Retrieved from https://www.wildflower.org/plants/result.php?id_plant=sich

46. Gentry, H.S. (1958). The natural history of jojoba (Simmondsia chinensis) and its cultural aspects. *Economic Botany, 12*(3), 261–295. https://doi.org/10.1007/BF02859772

47. Orwa, C., Mutua, A., Kindt, R., Jamnadass, R., & Simons, A. (2009). *Simmondsia chinensis. Agroforestry Database: A tree reference and selection guide 4.0.* Retrieved February 1, 2021, from http://apps.worldagroforestry.org/treedb2/AFTPDFS/Simmondsia_chinensis.PDF

48. Gad, H.A., Roberts, A., Hamzi, S.H., Gad, H.A., Touiss, I., Altyar, A.E., Kensara, O.A., & Ashour, M.L. (2021). Jojoba oil: An updated and comprehensive review on chemistry, pharmaceutical uses, and toxicity. *Polymers* (13), 1711. https://doi.org/10.3390/polym 13111711

49. Miwa, T.K. (1971). Jojoba oil wax esters and derived fatty acids and alcohols: Gas chromatographic analyses. *Journal of the American Oil Chemists Society, 48*(6), 259–264. https://doi.org/10.1007/BF02638458

50. Tietel, Z., Kahremany, S., Cohen, G., & Ogen-Shtern, N. (2021). Medicinal properties of jojoba (Simmondsia chinensis). *Israel Journal of Plant Sciences, 68*(1-2), 38-47. http://dx.doi.org/10.1163/22238980-bja10023

51. Tada, A., Jin, Z. L., Sugimoto, N., Sato, K., Yamazaki, T., & Tanamoto, K. (2005). Analysis of the constituents in jojoba wax used as a food additive by LC/MS/MS. *Shokuhin eiseigaku zasshi [Journal of the Food Hygienic Society of Japan], 46*(5), 198–204. https://doi.org/10.3358/shokueishi.46.198

52. Agarwal, S., Arya, D., & Khan, S. (2018). Comparative fatty acid and trace elemental analysis identified the best raw material of jojoba (Simmondsia chinensis) for commercial applications. *Annals of Agricultural Sciences, 63,* 37-45. https://doi.org/10.1016/j.aoas.2018.04.003

53. El-Mallah, M. H., & El-Shami, S. M. (2009). Investigation of liquid wax components of Egyptian jojoba seeds. *Journal of Oleo Science, 58*(11), 543–548. https://doi.org/10.5650/jos.58.543

54. Meier, L., Stange, R., Michalsen, A., & Uehleke, B. (2012). Clay jojoba oil facial mask for lesioned skin and mild acne: Results of a prospective, observational pilot study. *Forschende Komplementarmedizin, 19*(2), 75–79. https://doi.org/10.1159/000338076

55. Umaiyal, M.P., Gayathri, R., Vishnupriya, V., & Geetha, R.V. (2016). Anti microbial activity of jojoba oil against selected microbes: An invitro study. *Journal of Pharmaceutical Sciences & Research, 8*(6), 528-529.

56. Al-Ghamdi, A., Elkholy, T., Abuhelal, S., Al-Abbadi, H., Qahwaji, D., Khalefah, N., Sobhy, H., & Abu-Hilal, M. (2019). Against antibacterial and antifungal activity of jojoba wax liquid (Simmondsia chinensis). *Pharmacognosy Journal, 11*(1), 191-194. DOI: 10.5530/pj.2019.11.31

57. Habashy, R.R., Abdel-Naim, A.B., Khalifa, A.E., & Al-Azizi, M.M. (2005). Anti-inflammatory effects of jojoba liquid wax in experimental models. *Pharmacological Research, 51*(2), 95– 105. https://doi.org/10.1016/j.phrs.2004.04.011

58. Ranzato, E., Martinotti, S., & Burlando, B. (2011). Wound healing properties of jojoba liquid wax: An in vitro study. *Journal of Ethnopharmacology, 134*(2), 443–449. https://doi.org/10.1016/j.jep.2010.12.042

59. Vermaak, I., Kamatou, G.P.P., Komane-Mofokeng, B., Viljoen, A.M., & Beckett, K. (2011). African seed oils of commercial importance: Cosmetic applications. *South African Journal of Botany, 77*(4), 920-933. https://doi.org/10.1016/j.sajb.2011.07.003

60. Mokgolodi, N.C., Ding, Y.F., Setshogo, M.P., Ma, C., & Liu, Y.-J. (2011). The importance of an indigenous tree to southern African communities with specific relevance to its domestication and commercialization: A case of the marula tree. *Forestry Studies in China*, 13, 36–44. https://doi.org/10.1007/s11632-011-0110-1

61. Mariod, A.A., Matthaus, B., Idris, Y.M.A., & Abdelwahab, S.I. (2009). Fatty acids, tocopherols, phenolics and the antimicrobial effect of Sclerocarya birrea kernels with different harvesting dates. *Journal of the American Oil Chemists' Society*, 87(4), 377-384. https://doi.org/10.1007/s11746-009-1510-4

62. Magos Brehm, J., Draper Munt, D. & Kell, S.P. (2016). *Olea europaea*. The IUCN Red List of Threatened Species. Retrieved October 29, 2020, from https://www.iucnredlist.org/species/181959/7774051

63. Missouri Botanical Garden (n.d.). *Olea europaea*. Retrieved October 26, 2020, from https://www.missouribotanicalgarden.org/PlantFinder/PlantFinderDetails.aspx?taxonid=283004&isprofile=0&

64. Crisosto, C. H., Ferguson, L., & Nanos, G. (2011). Olive (Olea europaea L.). P*ostharvest biology and technology of tropical and subtropical fruits*, (M. Yahia, Ed.), 63–87e. https://doi.org/10.1533/9780857092618.63

65. Rupp, R. (2016). The bitter truth about olives. *National Geographic: The Plate*. Retrieved April 5, 2021, from https://www.nationalgeographic.com/culture/article/olives--the-bitter-truth

66. Hashmi, M. A., Khan, A., Hanif, M., Farooq, U., & Perveen, S. (2015). Traditional uses, phytochemistry, and pharmacology of Olea europaea (Olive). *Evidence-Based Complementary and Alternative Medicine*. https://doi.org/10.1155/2015/541591

67. Tripoli, E., Giammanco, M., Tabacchi, G., DiMajo, D., Giammanco, S., & La Guardia, M. (2005) The phenolic compounds of olive oil: Structure, biological activity and beneficial effects on human health. *Nutrition Research Reviews*, 18(1), 98-112. https://doi.org/10.1079/NRR200495

68. Dabbou, S., Issaoui, M., Servili, M., Taticchi, A., Sifi, S., Montedoro, G.F. & Hammami, M. (2009). Characterisation of virgin olive oils from European olive cultivars introduced in Tunisia. *European Journal of Lipid Science and Technology*, 111(4), 392-401. https://doi.org/10.1002/ejlt.200800032

69. Issaoui, M., Flamini, G., Brahmi, F., Dabbou, S., Ben Hassine, K., Taamali, A., Chehab, H., Ellouz, M., Zarrouk, M, & Hammami, M. (2010). Effect of the growing area conditions on differentiation between Chemlali and Chétoui olive oils. *Food Chemistry*, 119(2010), 220-225. https://doi.org/10.1016/j.foodchem.2009.06.012

70. Codex Alimentarius Commission. (1999). Codex standard for olive oils and olive pomace oils. Codex-Stan 210-1989-2021. Food and Agriculture Organization of the United Nations. https://www.fao.org/3/y2774e/y2774e04.htm#bm4.2

71. Lopez, S., Bermudez, B., Montserrat-de la Paz, S., Jaramillo, S., Varela, L. M., Ortega-Gomez, A., Abia, R., & Muriana, F. J. (2014) Membrane composition and dynamics: A target of bioactive virgin olive oil constituents. *Biochimica et Biophysica Acta*, 1838(6), 1638–1656. https://doi.org/10.1016/j.bbamem.2014.01.007

72. Čižinauskas, V., Elie, N., Brunelle, A., & Briedis, V. (2017). Skin penetration enhancement by natural oils for dihydroquercetin delivery. *Molecules*, 22(9), 1536. https://doi.org/10.3390/molecules22091536

73. Ferns, K. (2019). *Carthamus tinctorius*. Useful Tropical Plants. http://tropical.theferns.info/viewtropical.php?id=Carthamus+tinctorius

74. Delshad, E., Yousefi, M., Sasannezhad, P., Rakhshandeh, H., & Ayati, Z. (2018). Medical uses of Carthamus tinctorius l. (Safflower): A comprehensive review from traditional medicine to modern medicine. *Electronic Physician*, 10(4), 6672–6681. https://doi.org/10.19082/6672

75. Liu, L., Guan, L.L., Wu, W., & Wang, L. (2016). A review of fatty acids and genetic characterization of safflower (Carthamus tinctorius L.) seed oil. *Organic Chemistry Current Research*, 5(1), 160. Doi: 10.4172/2161-0401.1000160

76. Katkade, M.B., Syed, H.M., Andhale, R.R., & Sontakke, M.D. (2018). Fatty acid profile and quality assessment of safflower (Carthamus tinctorius) oil at region. *Journal of Pharmacognosy and Phytochemistry*, 7(2), 3581-3585. Retrieved from https://www.phytojournal.com/archives/2018/vol7issue2/PartAX/7-2-364-260.pdf

77. Golkar, P. (2014). Breeding improvements in safflower (Carthamus tinctorius L.): A review. *Australian Journal of Crop Science*, 8(7), 1079-1085. Retrieved from http://www.cropj.com/golkar_8_7_2014_1079_1085.pdf

78. Elias, P.M., Brown, B.E., & Ziboh, V.A. (1980). Permeability barrier in essential fatty acid deficiency: Evidence for a direct role for linoleic acid in barrier function. *The Journal of Investigative Dermatology*, 74(4), 230-233. doi: 10.1111/1523-1747.ep12541775

79. Mack Correa, M.C., Mao, G., Saad, P., Flach, C.R., Mendelsohn, R., & Walters, R.M. (2014). Molecular interactions of plant oil components with stratum corneum lipids correlate with clinical measures of skin barrier function. *Experimental Dermatology*, 23(1), 39-44. https://doi.org/10.1111/exd.12296

80. The Editors of Encyclopedia Britannica. (2020). Sesame. *Encyclopedia Britannica*. https://www.britannica.com/plant/sesame-plant

81. American Botanical Council (n.d.). Sesame oil. *HerbalGram*. Retrieved October 25, 2020, from http://cms.herbalgram.org/healthyingredients/SesameOil.html

82. Gharby, S., Harhar, H., Bouzoubaa, Z., Asdadi, A., El Yadini, A., & Charrouf, Z. (2017). Chemical characterization and oxidative stability of seeds and oil of sesame grown in Morocco. *Journal of the Saudi Society of Agricultural Sciences*, 16, 105-111. http://dx.doi.org/10.1016/j.jssas.2015.03.004

83. Aued-Pimentel, S., Takemoto, E., Antoniassi, R., & Gastaldo Badolato, E.S. (2006). Composition of tocopherols in sesame seed oil: An indicative of adulteration. *Grasas y Aceites (Fats and Oils)*, 57(2), 205–210. https://doi.org/10.3989/gya.2006.v57.i2.38

84. The Editors of Encyclopedia Britannica. (2020). Sunflower. *Encyclopedia Britannica*. https://www.britannica.com/plant/sunflower-plant

85. Adeleke, B. S. & Babalola, O.O. (2020). Oilseed crop sunflower (Helianthus annus) as a source of food: Nutritional and health benefits. *Food Science and Nutrition*, 8(9), 4666-4684. https://doi.org/10.1002/fsn3.1783

86. National Sunflower Association. (n.d.). Sunflower seed/kernel. Retrieved from https://www.sunflowernsa.com/seed/

87. National Sunflower Association. (2010). Sunflower oil fact sheet. *National Sunflower Association*. Retrieved from https://www.sunflowernsa.com/uploads/35/sunflower-oil-fact-sheet_062510.pdf

88. Aparicio, R., García González, D.L., & Aparicio-Ruiz, R. (2018).

Vegetable oils. *Food integrity handbook on food authenticity issues and related analytical techniques* (J.F. Morin & M. Lees, Eds.), 359-382. https://doi.org/10.32741/fihb

89. Akkaya, M.R. (2018). Fatty acid compositions of sunflowers (Helianthus annuus L.) grown in east Mediterranean region. *Rivista Italiana Delle Sostanze Grasse [Italian Magazine of Fatty Substances], 45*(4), 239-247. Retrieved from https://www.researchgate.net/publication/328143287_Fatty_acid_compositions_of_sunflowers_Helianthus_annuus_L_grown_in_east_Mediterranea_region

90. Elias, P.M., Brown, B.E., & Ziboh, V.A. (1980). Permeability barrier in essential fatty acid deficiency: Evidence for a direct role for linoleic acid in barrier function. *The Journal of Investigative Dermatology, 74*(4), 230-233. DOI: 10.1111/1523-1747.ep12541775

91. Marques, S.R., Peixoto, C.A., Messias, J.B., De Albuquerque, A.R., & Da Silva, Jr., V.A. (2004). The effects of topical application of sunflower-seed oil on open wound healing in lambs. *Acta Cirurgica Brasileira [Brazilian Surgical Record], 19*(3), 196-209. Retrieved from https://www.scielo.br/pdf/acb/v19n3/20406.pdf

92. Mack Correa, M.C., Mao, G., Saad, P., Flach, C.R., Mendelsohn, R., & Walters, R.M. (2014). Molecular interactions of plant oil components with stratum corneum lipids correlate with clinical measures of skin barrier function. *Experimental Dermatology, 23*(1), 39–44. https://doi.org/10.1111/exd.12296

References
Part Four: The Enhancer Carrier Oils

1. Dąbrowska, M., Maciejczyk, E., & Kalemba, D. (2019). Rose hip seed oil: Methods of extraction and chemical composition. *European Journal of Lipid Science and Technology, 121*(8), 1800440. https://doi.org/10.1002/ejlt.201800440

2. del Valle, J.M., Bello, S., Thiel, J., Allen, A., & Chordia, L. (2000). Comparison of conventional and supercritical CO2-extracted rosehip oil. *Brazilian Journal of Chemical Engineering, 17*(3), 335-348. https://doi.org/10.1590/S0104-66322000000300010_

3. Pereira, C.G., & Meireles, M.A.A. (2010). Supercritical fluid extraction of bioactive compounds: Fundamentals, applications and economic perspectives. *Food Bioprocess Technology, 3*, 340-372. DOI 10.1007/s11947-009-0263-2

4. Wegier, A., Lorea Hernández, F., Contreras, A., Tobón, W. & Mastretta-Yanes, A. (2017). *Persea americana* (errata version published in 2018). The IUCN Red List of Threatened Species 2017: e.T96986556A129765464. Retrieved November 13, 2020, from https://dx.doi.org/10.2305/IUCN.UK.2017-3.RLTS.T96986556A96986588.en

5. Missouri Botanical Garden. (n.d.). *Persea americana*. Retrieved October 17, 2020, from http://www.missouribotanicalgarden.org/PlantFinder/PlantFinderDetails.aspx?taxonid=281661

6. Bauman, H., & Moyer, T. (2017). Food as medicine: Avocado (Persea americana, Lauraceae). *HerbalEGram, 14*(6). Retrieved March 3, 2022, from http://cms.herbalgram.org/heg/volume14/06June/FoodasMedicine_Avocado.html

7. Woolf, A., Wong, M., Eyres, L., McGhie, T., Lund, C., Olsson, S., Wang, Y., Bulley, C., Wang, M., Friel, E., & Requejo-Jackman, C. (2009). Avocado oil. In Moreau, R.A. & Kamal-Eldin, A. (Eds.), *Gourmet and health-promoting specialty oils* (pp. 73-125). AOCS Press. https://doi.org/10.1016/B978-1-893997-97-4.50008-5

8. Kusmirek, J. (2002). *Liquid sunshine*. Foramicus.

9. Flores, M., Saravia, C., Vergara, C.E., Avila, F., Valdés, H., & Ortiz-Viedma, J. (2019). Avocado oil: Characteristics, properties, and applications. *Molecules, 24*(11), 2172. https://doi.org/10.3390/molecules24112172

10. Flores, M.A., Perez-Camino, M.D.C., & Troca, J. (2014). Preliminary studies on composition, quality and oxidative stability of commercial avocado oil produced in Chile. *Journal of Food Science and Engineering, 4*, 21-26.

11. de Oliveira A.P., Franco, E. de S., Barreto, R.R., Cordeiro, D.P., de Melo, R.G., de Aquino, C.M., E Silva, A.A.R., de Medeiros, P.L., da Silva, T.G., Góes, A.J., & Maia, M.B. (2013). Effect of semisolid formulation of Persea americana Mill (avocado) oil on wound healing in rats. *Evidence-Based Complementary and Alternative Medicine*, 2013 (472382), 8 pages. DOI: 10.1155/2013/472382

12. Fernandes, G.D, Gomez-Coca, R.B., Perez-Camino, M.C., Moreda, W., & Barrera-Arellano, D. (2018). Chemical characterization of commercial and single-variety avocado oils. *Grasas Aceites, 69*(2), 256. DOI: https://doi.org/10.3989/gya.0110181

13. Nayak, B.S., Raju, S.S., & Chalapathi Rao, A.V. (2008). Wound healing activity of Persea americana (avocado) fruit: A preclinical study on rats. *Journal of Wound Care, 17*(3), 123–126. https://doi.org/10.12968/jowc.2008.17.3.28670

14. Gunstone, F. (2005) Vegetable oils. In F. Shahidi (Ed.), *Bailey's Industrial Oils and Fat Products* (6th ed.). John Wiley & Sons, Inc.

15. Dweck, A. (2003). *The role of natural ingredients in anti-aging of the skin*. Australian Society of Cosmetic Chemists Annual Congress, Hamilton Island.

16. Finau, K.A. (2011). Literature review on avocado oil for SROS technological purposes. *Scientific Research Organization of Samoa*

17. Ahmad, A., Husain, A., Mujeeb, M., Khan, S. A., Najmi, A.K., Siddique, N.A., Damanhouri, Z.A., & Anwar, F. (2013). A review on therapeutic potential of Nigella sativa: A miracle herb. *Asian Pacific Journal of Tropical Biomedicine, 3*(5), 337–352. https://doi.org/10.1016/S2221-1691(13)60075-1

18. Dajani, E.Z., Shahwan, T.G., & Dajani, N.E. (2018). Overview of the human investigations of Nigella sativa (black seeds): A complementary drug with historical and clinical significance. *General Internal Medicine and Clinical Innovations, 4*(1), 1-16. DOI: 10.15761/GIMCI.1000171

19. Ali, S.A., Parveen, N., & Ali, A.S. (2018). Links between the Prophet Muhammad (PBUH) recommended foods and disease management: A review in the light of modern superfoods. *International Journal of Health Sciences, 12*(2), 61-69.

20. Ashfaq, S., Khan, N.T., & Ali, G.H. (2021). Nigella sativa (Kalonji), its essential oils and their therapeutic potential. *Biomedical Journal of Scientific and Technical Research, 33*(1), 25448-25454. DOI: 10.26717/BJSTR.2021.33.005335

21. Petruzzello, M. (2018, February 6). *Black cumin*. Encyclopedia Britannica. https://www.britannica.com/plant/black-cumin

22. Gharbi, S., Harhar, H., Guillaume, D., Roudani, A., Boulbaroud, S., Ibrahimi, M., Ahmad, M., Sultana, S., Ben Hadda, T., Chafchaouni-Massaoui, I., & Charrouf, Z., (2015). Chemical investigation of Nigella

sativa L. seed oil produced in Morocco. *Journal of the Saudi Society of Agricultural Sciences*, 14, 172-177. http://dx.doi.org/10.1016/j.jssas.2013.12.001

23. Hassanien, M.M.M, Abdel-Razek, A.G., Ruzinska, M., Siger, A., Ratusz, K., & Przybylski, R. (2014). Phytochemical contents and oxidative stability of oils from non-traditional sources. *European Journal of Lipid Science and Technology*, 116, 1563-1571. DOI: 10.1002/ejlt.201300475

24. Argon, Z.U. & Gokyer, A. (2016). Determination of physicochemical properties of Nigella sativa seed oil from Balikesir Region, Turkey. *Chemical and Process Engineering Research*, 41, 43-46. Retrieved June 9, 2021, from https://core.ac.uk/download/pdf/234689229.pdf

25. European Chemicals Agency. (2021, March 12). *Substance infocard: Nigella sativa*. European Chemicals Agency Substance Information. Retrieved June 4, 2021, from https://echa.europa.eu/substance-information/-/substanceinfo/100.081.872

26. Mohammed, N.K., Manap, M.Y.A., Tan, C.P., Muhialdin, B.J., Alhelli, A.M., & Hussin, A.S.M. (2016). The effects of different extraction methods on antioxidant properties, chemical composition, and thermal behavior of black seed (Nigella sativa L.) oil. *Evidence-Based Complementary and Alternative Medicine*, 2016, (6273817), 1-10. http://dx.doi.org/10.1155/2016/6273817

27. Bordoni, L, Fedeli, D., Nasuti, C., Maggi, F., Papa, F., Wabitsch, M., De Caterina, R., & Gabbianelli, R. (2019). Antioxidant and anti-inflammatory properties of Nigella sativa oil in human pre-adipocytes. *Antioxidants*, 8(2), 51. https://doi.org/10.3390/antiox8020051

28. Tuna, H.I., Babadag, B., Ozkaraman, A., & Alparslan, G.B. (2018). Investigation of the effect of black cumin oil on pain in osteoarthritis geriatric individuals. *Complementary Therapies in Clinical Practice*, 31, 290-294. https://doi.org/10.1016/j.ctcp.2018.03.013

29. Abdul-Ameer, N. & Al-Harchan, H. (2010). Treatment of acne vulgaris with Nigella sativa oil lotion. *The Iraqi Postgraduate Medical Journal*, 9(2), 140-144. Retrieved June 9, 2021, from https://www.iasj.net/iasj/download/d6a1de27a39f5ad5

30. Halawani, E. (2009). Antibacterial activity of thymoquinone and thymohydroquinone of Nigella sativa L. and their interaction with some antibiotics. *Advances in Biological Research*, 3(5-6), 148-152.

31. Dera, A.A., Ahmad, I., Rajagopalan, P., Al Shahrani, M., Saif, A., Alshahrani, M.Y., Alraey, Y., Almari, A.M., Alasmari, S., Makkawi, M., Alkhathami, A.G., Zaman, G., Hakami, A., Alhefzi, R., & Alfhili, M.A. (2021). Synergistic efficacies of thymoquinone and standard antibiotics against multi-drug resistant isolates. *Saudi Medical Journal*, 42(2), 196-204. DOI: 10.15537/smj.2021.2.25706

32. Amin, S., Mir, S.R., Kohli, K., Ali, B., & Ali, M. (2010). A study of the chemical composition of black cumin oil and its effect on penetration enhancement from transdermal formulations. *Natural Product Research*, 24(12), 1151-1157. DOI: 10.1080/14786410902940909

33. Ghorbanibirgani, A., Khalili, A., & Rokhafrooz, D. (2014). Comparing Nigella sativa oil and fish oil in treatment of vitiligo. *Iran Red Crescent Medical Journal*, 16(6), E4515. DOI: 10.5812/ircmj.4515

34. Bilz, M. (2013). *Borago officinalis*. The IUCN Red List of Threatened Species 2013: e.T202942A2758153. Retrieved March 9. 2022, from https://www.iucnredlist.org/species/202942/2758153

35. Asadi-Samani, M., Bahmani, M., & Rafieian-Kopaei, M. (2014). The chemical composition, botanical characteristic and biological activities of Borago officinalis: A review. *Asian Pacific Journal of Tropical Medicine*, 7, S22–S28. https://doi.org/10.1016/S1995-7645(14)60199-1

36. Lozano-Baena, M.-D., Tasset, I., Muñoz-Serrano, A., Alonso-Moraga, Á., & de Haro-Bailón, A. (2016). Cancer prevention and health benefices of traditionally consumed borago officinalis plants. *Nutrients*, 8(1). https://doi.org/10.3390/nu8010048

37. Missouri Botanical Garden (n.d.). *Borago officinalis*. Retrieved October 20, 2020, from https://www.missouribotanicalgarden.org/PlantFinder/PlantFinderDetails.aspx?kempercode=b765

38. Tasset-Cuevas, I., Fernández-Bedmar, Z., Lozano-Baena, M. D., Campos-Sánchez, J., de Haro-Bailón, A., Muñoz-Serrano, A., & Alonso-Moraga, A. (2013). Protective effect of borage seed oil and gamma linolenic acid on DNA: in vivo and in vitro studies. *PloS One*, 8(2), e56986. https://doi.org/10.1371/journal.pone.0056986

39. Eskin, N.A.M. (2008). Borage and evening primrose oil. *European Journal of Lipid Science and Technology*, 110, 651-654. https://doi.org/10.1002/ejlt.200700259

40. Khattab, H., Abdallah, I., Yousef, F. M., & Huwait, E. A. (2017). Efficiency of borage seeds oil against gamma irradiation-induced hepatotoxicity in male rats: possible antioxidant activity. *African Journal of Traditional, Complementary, and Alternative Medicines*, 14(4), 169–179. https://doi.org/10.21010/ajtcam.v14i4.20

41. Fabrikov, D., Guil-Guerro, J.L., Gonzalez-Fernandez, M.J. Rodriquez-Garcia, I., Gomez-Mercado, F., Urrestarazu, M., Lao, M.T., Rincon-cervera, M.A., Alvaro, J.E, & Lyashenko, S. (2019). Borage oil: Tocopherols, sterols and squalene in farmed and endemic-wild Borago species. *Journal of Food Composition and Analysis*, 83. https://doi.org/10.1016/j.jfca.2019.103299

42. Casas-Cardoso, L., Mantell, C., Obregón, S., Cejudo-Bastante, C., Alonso-Moraga, Á., de la Ossa, E., & de Haro-Bailón, A. (2021). Health-promoting properties of borage seed oil fractionated by supercritical carbon dioxide extraction. *Foods*, 10(10), 2471. https://doi.org/10.3390/foods10102471

43. Velasco, L., & Goffman, F.D. (1999). Chemotaxonomic significance of fatty acids and tocopherols in Boraginaceae. *Phytochemistry*, 52(1999), 423-426. https://doi.org/10.1016/S0031-9422(99)00203-4

44. Kapoor, R., & Huang, Y. S. (2006). Gamma linolenic acid: an antiinflammatory omega-6 fatty acid. *Current Pharmaceutical Biotechnology*, 7(6), 531–534. https://doi.org/10.2174/138920106779116874

45. Kanehara, S., Ohtani, T., Uede, K., & Furukawa, F. (2007). Clinical effects of undershirts coated with borage oil on children with atopic dermatitis: A double-blind, placebo-controlled clinical trial. *The Journal of Dermatology*, 34(12), 811–815. https://doi.org/10.1111/j.1346-8138.2007.00391.x

46. Williamson, E., Driver, S. & Baxter, K. (Eds.). (2009). *Stockley's herbal medicines interactions*. Pharmaceutical Press. p. 381.

47. The Editors of Encyclopaedia Britannica. (2018) Castor-oil plant. In *Encyclopedia Brittanica*. Retrieved December 8, 2020, from https://www.britannica.com/plant/castor-oil-plant.

48. Pursell, J. J. (2016). *The Herbal Apothecary: 100 Medicinal herbs and how to use them*. Timber Press.

49. Patel, V. R., Dumancas, G. G., Kasi Viswanath, L. C., Maples, R., & Subong, B. J. J. (2016). Castor oil: Properties, uses, and optimization of processing parameters in commercial production. *Lipid Insights*, 9, 1–12.

https://doi.org/10.4137/LPI.S40233

50. Marwat, S. K., Rehman, F., Khan, E. A., Baloch, M. S., Sadiq, M., Ullah, I., Javaria, S., & Shaheen, S. (2017). Review—Ricinus cmmunis [sic]—Ethnomedicinal uses and pharmacological activities. *Pakistan Journal of Pharmaceutical Sciences, 30*(5), 1815–1827.

51. Harhar, H., Gharby, S., Pioch, D., Kartah, B. Ibrahimi, M., & Charrouf, Z. (2016). Chemical characterization and oxidative stability of castor oil grown in Morocco. *Moroccan Journal of Chemistry, 4*(2), 279-284. https://doi.org/10.48317/IMIST.PRSM/morjchem-v4i2.4117

52. Yeboah, A., Ying, S., Lu, J., Xie, Y., Amoanimaa-dede, H., Boateng, K.G.A., Chen, M., & Yin, X. (2020). Castor oil (Ricinus communis): A review on the chemical composition and physicochemical properties. *Food Science and Technology*. https://doi.org/10.1590/fst.19620

53. Ananth, D.A., Deviram, G., Mahalakshmi, V., Sivasudha, T., & Tietel, Z. (2019). Phytochemical composition and antioxidant characteristics of traditional cold pressed seed oils in South India. *Biocatalysis and Agricultural Biotechnology,* 17, 416-421. https://doi.org/10.1016/j.bcab.2018.12.018

54. Arslan, G.G., & Eser, I. (2011). An examination of the effect of castor oil packs on constipation in the elderly. *Complementary Therapies in Clinical Practice, 17*(1), 58-62. DOI: 10.1016/j.ctcp.2010.04.004

55. Vieira, C., Evangelista, S., Cirillo, R., Terracciano, R., Lippi, A., Maggi, C.A., & Manzini, S. (2000). Antinociceptive activity of ricinoleic acid, a capsaicin-like compound devoid of pungent properties. *European Journal of Pharmacology, 407*(1-2), 109–116. https://doi.org/10.1016/s0014-2999(00)00727-5

56. Vieira, C., Evangelista, S., Cirillo, R., Lippi, A., Maggi, C.A., & Manzini, S. (2000). Effect of ricinoleic acid in acute and subchronic experimental models of inflammation. *Mediators of Inflammation, 9*(5), 223–228. https://doi.org/10.1080/09629350020025737

57. Missouri Botanical Garden (n.d.) *Oenothera biennis*. Retrieved October 20, 2020, from http://www.missouribotanicalgarden.org/PlantFinder/PlantFinderDetails.aspx?taxonid=283027

58. Immel, D.L. (2001). *Common evening primrose.* United States Department of Agriculture, Natural Resources Conservation Service. Retrieved March 5, 2022, from https://plants.usda.gov/DocumentLibrary/plantguide/pdf/cs_oebi.pdf

59. Mehmood, Z., Khan, M.S., Qais, F.A., & Samreen, A.I. (2019). Herb and modern drug interactions: Efficacy, quality, and safety aspects. In M.S. Ahmad Khan, I. Ahmad, & D. Chattopadhyay (Eds.), *New look to phytomedicine: Advancements in herbal products as novel drug leads* (pp. 503–520). Academic Press. https://doi.org/10.1016/B978-0-12-814619-4.00019-7

60. Christie, W.W. (1999). The analysis of evening primrose oil. *Industrial Crops and Products, 10*(2), 73-83. https://doi.org/10.1016/S0926-6690(99)00013-8

61. Timoszuk, M., Bielawska, K., & Skrzydlewska, E. (2018). Evening primrose (Oenothera biennis) biological activity dependent on chemical composition. *Antioxidants), 7*(8), 108. https://doi.org/10.3390/antiox7080108

62. Hudson, B. J. F. (1984). Evening primrose (Oenothera spp.) oil and seed. *Journal of the American Oil Chemists' Society, 61*(3), 540-543. https://doi.org/10.1007/BF02677026

63. Eskin, N.A.M. (2008). Borage and evening primrose oil. European *Journal of Lipid Science and Technology,* 110, 651-654. https://doi.org/10.1002/ejlt.200700259

64. Da Silva, S.A., Sampaio, G.R., & Da Silva Torres, E.A.F. (2020). Phytosterols content in vegetable oils of Brazil: Coconut, safflower, linseed and evening primrose. *Brazillian Archives of Biology and Technology, 63*(e20190216). 8 pages. http://dx.doi.org/10.1590/1678-4324-2020190216

65. Montserrat-de la Paz, S., Fernandez-Arche, M. A., Angel-Martin, M., Garcia-Gimenez, M. D. (2014). Phytochemical characterization of potential nutraceutial ingredients from evening primrose oil (Oenothera biennis L.). *Phytochemistry Letters,* 8, 158–162. https://doi.org/10.1016/j.phytol.2013.08.008

66. Muggli R. (2005). Systemic evening primrose oil improves the biophysical skin parameters of healthy adults. *International Journal of Cosmetic Science, 27*(4), 243–249. https://doi.org/10.1111/j.1467-2494.2005.00274.x

67. Cannabis sativa (hemp). (2021, November 16). CABI: Invasive Species Compendium. Retrieved from https://www.cabi.org/isc/datasheet/14497

68. Farinon, B., Molinari, R., Costantini, L., & Merendino, N. (2020). The seed of industrial hemp (Cannabis sativa L.): Nutritional quality and potential functionality for human health and nutrition. *Nutrients, 2020*(12), 1935. doi:10.3390/nu12071935

69. CABI. (2022). *Cannabis sativa* (hemp). In: Invasive Species Compendium. Wallingford, UK: CAB International. Retrieved March 6, 2022, from https://www.cabi.org/isc/datasheet/14497#21F90A60-4295-4B8E-81A0-37074C206858

70. Callaway, J.C. (2010, March). Hempseed in a Nutshell. American Oil Chemists Society. AOCS.org. Retrieved from https://www.aocs.org/stay-informed/inform-magazine/featured-articles/hempseed-oil-in-a-nutshell-march-2010

71. Schilling, S., Melzer, R., & McCabe, P.F. (2020). Cannabis sativa. *Current Biology Magazine,* 30, R1-R9. Retrieved from https://www.cell.com/action/showPdf?pii=S0960-9822%2819%2931379-X

72. Montserrat-de la Paz, S., Marin-Aguilar, F., Garcia-Gimenez, M.D., & Fernandez-Arche, M.A. (2014). Hemp (Cannabis sativa L.) seed oil: Analytical and phytochemical characterization of the unsaponifiable fraction. *Journal of Agricultural Food Chemistry, 62*(5), 1105-1110. DOI:10.1021/jf404278q

73. Izzo, L., Pacifico, S., Piccolella, S., Castaldo, L., Narvaez, A., Grosso, M., & Ritieni, A. (2020). Chemical analysis of minor bioactive components of cannabidiolic acid in commercial hemp seed oil. *Molecules, 2020*(25), 3710. DOI: 10.3390/molecules25163710

74. Galasso, I., Russo, R., Mapelli, S., Ponzoni, E., Brambilla, I.M., Battelli G., & Reggiani, R. (2016). Variability in seed traits in a collection of Cannabis sativa L. genotypes. *Frontiers in Plant Science,* 7, Article 688. DOI: 10.3389/fpls.2016.00688

75. Oseyko, M., Sova, N., Lutsenko, M., & Kalyna, V. (2019). Chemical aspects of the composition of industrial hemp seed products. *Ukrainian Food Journal, 8*(3), 544-558. DOI: 10.24263/2304-974X-2019-8-3-11

76. Aladic, K., Jokic, S., Moslavac, T., Tomas, S., Vidovic, S., Vladic, J., & Subaric, D. (2014). Cold pressing and supercritical CO2 extraction of hemp (Cannabis sativa) seed oil. *Chemical and Biochemical Engineering Quarterly, 28*(4), 481-490. DOI: 10.15255/CABEQ.2013.1895

77. Mikulcová, V., Kaspárková, V., Humpolicek, P., & Bunková, L.

(2017). Formulation, characterization and properties of hemp seed oil and its emulsions. *Molecules, 22*(5), 700. 13 pages. doi:10.3390/molecules22050700

78. Ando H, Ryu A, Hashimoto A, Oka M, & Ichihashi M. (1998) Linoleic acid and alpha-linolenic acid lightens ultraviolet- induced hyperpigmentation of the skin. *Archives of Dermatological Research, 290*(7), 375-381. DOI: 10.1007/s004030050320.

79. Natural Plant Products, Inc. (n.d.). Meadowfoam: The little flower that's a big deal. Retrieved August 19, 2021, from https://meadowfoam.com/2019/05/29/a-little-flower-thats-a-big-deal/

80. Agricultural Marketing Resource Center. (2018). Meadowfoam. Retrieved September 21, 2021, from https://www.agmrc.org/commodities-products/grains-oilseeds/meadowfoam

81. Natural Plant Products, Inc. (n.d.). 20 reasons to love meadowfoam seed oil. Retrieved October 19, 2021, from https://meadowfoam.com/wp-content/uploads/2019/04/20_reasons_mso_LTR_03032021.pdf

82. Oelke, E.A., Oplinger, E.S., Hanson, C.V., & Kelling, K.A. (1990). Meadowfoam. In Alternative field crops manual. University of Wisconsin-Extension, & University of Minnesota-Extension (Eds.). Retrieved Ocrtober 19, 2021, from https://farmanswers.org/Library/Record/meadowfoam_alternative_field_crops_manual

83. Morin, N.R. (2020). Limnanthes alba. Retrieved October 28, 2021, from http://beta.floranorthamerica.org/Limnanthes_alba

84. Natural Plant Products, Inc. (n.d.). Meadowfoam Seed Oil. Retrieved August 19, 2021, from https://meadowfoam.com/products/meadowfoam-seed-oil/

85. Ghost Democracy. (n.d.). Meadowfoam seed oil. Retrieved October 28, 2021, from https://www.ghostdemocracy.com/blogs/ingredients/meadowfoam-seed-oil

86. Natures Crops International. (n.d.). Meadowfoam. Retrieved October 28, 2021, from https://www.naturescrops.com/our-products/meadowfoam-seed-oil

87. Zielinska, A., Wójcicki, K., Klensporf-Pawlik, D., Dias-Ferreira, J., Lucarini, M., Durazzo, A., Lucariello, G., Capasso, R., Santini, A., Souto, E., & Nowak, I. (2020). Chemical and physical properties of meadowfoam seed oil and extra virgin olive oil: Focus on vibrational spectroscopy. *Journal of Spectroscopy*, Article ID 9970170. 9 pages. https://doi.org/10.1155/2020/8870170

88. Moser, B., Knothe, G., & Cermak, S. (2010). Biodiesel from meadowfoam (Limnanthes alba L.) seed oil: Oxidative stability and unusual fatty acid composition. *Energy & Environmental Science*, 3, 318-327. DOI: 10.1039/b923740m

89. Jolliff, G.D., Tinsley, I.J., Calhoun, W., & Crane, J.M. (1981). Limnanthes alba: Its research and development as a potential new oilseed crop for the Willamette Valley of Oregon. Agricultural Experiment Station, Oregon State University, Corvallis. *Station Bulletin 648*. https://ir.library.oregonstate.edu/downloads/1544bp58m

90. Isbell, T.A., Abbott, T.P., & Carlson, K.D. (1999). Oxidative stability index of vegetable oils in binary mixtures with meadowfoam oil. *Industrial Crops and Products, 9*(1999), 115-123. https://doi.org/10.1016/S0926-6690(98)00022-3

91. Barstow, M. & Deepu, S. (2018). *Azadirachta indica*. The IUCN Red List of Threatened Species 2018. Retrieved September 11, 2020, from https://dx.doi.org/10.2305/IUCN.UK.2018-1.RLTS.T61793521A61793525.en

92. Nicoletti, M. (2020). *Insect-borne diseases in the 21st century*. Elsevier. https://doi.org/10.1016/B978-0-12-818706-7.00007-3

93. Kumar, V.S., & Navaratnam, V. (2013). Neem (Azadirachta indica): Prehistory to contemporary medicinal uses to humankind. *Asian Pacific Journal of Tropical Biomedicine, 3*(7), 505-514. DOI: 10.1016/S2221-1691(13)60105-7

94. *Neem: Benefits, Ayurveda usage, side effects, research*. (n.d.). Easy Ayurveda. Retrieved June 3, 2021, from https://www.easyayurveda.com/2012/11/28/neem-in-ayurveda-benefits-usage-side-effects-full-reference/

95. Biswas, K., Chattopadhyay, I., Banerjee, R.K., & Bandyopadhyay, U. (2002). Biological activities and medicinal properties of neem (Azadirachta indica). *Current Science, 82*(11), 1336-1345. Retrieved June 1, 2021, from ://citeseerx.ist.psu.edu/viewdoc/download?doi=10.1.1.465.5699&rep=rep1&type=pdf

96. U.S. Environmental Protection Agency. (2012, May 7). *Cold pressed neem oil: PC code 025006*. Environmental Protection Agency. Retrieved June 2, 2021, from https://www3.epa.gov/pesticides/chem_search/reg_actions/registration/decision_PC-025006_07-May-12.pdf

97. Mordue (Luntz), A.J. & Nisbet, A.J. (2000). Azadirachtin from neem tree Azadirachta indica: Its action against insects. *Anais da Sociedade Entomologica do Brasil, 29*(4), 615-632. https://doi.org/10.1590/S0301-80592000000400001

98. Abiy, E., Gebre=Michael, T., Balkew, M., & Medhin, G. (2015). Repellent efficacy of DEET, MyggA, neem (Azedirachta indica) oil and chinaberry (Melia azedarach) oil against Anopheles arabiensis, the principal malaria vector in Ethiopia. *Malaria Journal, 14*(187). DOI: 10.1186/s12936-015-0705-4

99. Ayinde, A.A., Morakinyo, O.M., & Sridhar, M.K.C. (2020). Repellency and larvicidal activities of Azadirachta indica seed oil on Anopheles gambiae in Nigeria. *Heliyon, 6*(2020), e03920. https://doi.org/10.1016/j.heliyon.2020.e03920

100. Biswas, K., Chattopadhyay, I., Banerjee, R.K., & Bandyopadhyay, U. (2002). Biological activities and medicinal properties of neem (Azadirachta indica). *Current Science, 82*(11), 1336-1345. Retrieved June 1, 2021, from http://citeseerx.ist.psu.edu/viewdoc/download?doi=10.1.1.465.5699&rep=rep1&type=pdf

101. Chaudhary, S., Kanwar, R.K., Sehgal, A., Cahill, D.M., Barrow, C.J., Sehgal, R., & Kanwar, J.R. (2017). Progress on Azadirachta indica based biopesticides in replacing synthetic toxic pesticides. *Frontiers in Plant Science, 8*(610), 13 pp. DOI: 10.3389/fpls.2017.00610

102. Ismaili, S.A., Harhar, H., Gharby, S., Bourazmi, H., & Tabyaoui, M. (2016). Chemical composition of two non-conventional oils in Morocco: Melia azadirachta and Silybum marianum (L.). *Journal of Materials and Environmental Science, 7*(6), 2208-2213. https://www.jmaterenvironsci.com/Document/vol7/vol7_N6/236-JMES-2307-Alaoui%20Ismaili.pdf

103. Momchilova, S., Antonova, D., Marekov, I., Kuleva, L., Nikolova-Damyanova, B. & Jham, G. (2007). Fatty acids, triacylglycerols, and sterols in neem oil (Azadirachta indica A. Juss.) as determined by a combination of chromatographic and spectral techniques. *Journal of Liquid Chromatography & Related Technologies*, 30, 11-25. DOI: 10.1080/10826070601034188

104. Warra, A.A. (2012). Medicinal and cosmetic potential of neem (Azadirachta indica) seed oil: A review. *Research and Reviews: Journal of Medicinal Chemistry, 1*(1), 5-8. https://www.rroij.com/open-access/

medicinal-and-cosmetic-potential-of-neem-azadiracta-indica-seed-oil-a-review-5-8.pdf

105. Abdel-Ghaffar, F., Al-Quraishy, S., Al-Rasheid, K.A.S., & Mehlhorn, H. (2012). Efficacy of single treatment of head lice with a neem seed extract: An in vivo and in vitro study on nits and motile stages. *Parasitology Research*, 110, 277-280. https://doi.org/10.1007/s00436-011-2484-3

106. Abdel-Ghaffar, F., & Semmler, M. (2006). Efficacy of neem seed extract shampoo on head lice of naturally infected humans in Egypt. *Parasitology Research*, 100, 329-332. https://doi.org/10.1007/s00436-006-0264-2

107. Elson, L., Randu, K., Feldmeier, H., & Fillinger, U. (2019). Efficacy of a mixture of neem seed oil (Azadirachta indica) and coconut oil (Cocos nucifera) for topical treatment of tungiasis. A randomized controlled, proof-of-principle study. *PloS Neglected Tropical Diseases, 13*(11), e0007822. https://doi. org/10.1371/journal.pntd.0007822

108. Participants of the FFI/IUCN SSC Central Asian regional tree Red Listing workshop, Bishkek, Kyrgyzstan (11-13 July 2006). 2020. *Punica granatum* (amended version of 2007 assessment). The IUCN Red List of Threatened Species 2020: e.T63531A173543609. Retrieved September 6, 2020, from https://dx.doi.org/10.2305/IUCN.UK.2020-2.RLTS.T63531A173543609.en

109. Encyclopedia Britannica. (2020). Pomegranate. In *Brittanica.com encyclopedia*. Retrieved January 14, 2021, from https://www.britannica.com/plant/pomegranate

110. Missouri Botanical Garden. (n.d.). *Punica granatum*. Retrieved October 27, 2020, from http://www.missouribotanicalgarden.org/PlantFinder/PlantFinderDetails.aspx?taxonid=286059

111. Rahimi, H.R., Arastoo, M., & Ostad, S.N. (2012). A comprehensive review of Punica granatum (pomegranate) properties in toxicological, pharmacological, cellular and molecular biology researches. *Iranian Journal of Pharmaceutical Research, 11*(2), 385–400. Retrieved from https://www.ncbi.nlm.nih.gov/pmc/articles/PMC3832175/

112. Lansky, E. P., & Newman, R. A. (2007). Punica granatum (pomegranate) and its potential for prevention and treatment of inflammation and cancer. *Journal of Ethnopharmacology, 109*(2), 177–206. https://doi.org/10.1016/j.jep.2006.09.006

113. Ahangari, B. & Sargolzaei, J. (2011). Supercritical fluid extraction of oils from pomegranate seeds. *Journal of the American Oil Chemists Society*, 94. DOI: 10.1007/s11746-011-1789-9

114. Sharma, P., McClees, S. F., & Afaq, F. (2017). Pomegranate for prevention and treatment of cancer: An update. *Molecules, 22*(1), 177. https://doi.org/10.3390/molecules22010177

115. Choi, D.W., Kim, J.Y., Choi, S.H., Jung, H.S., Kim, H.J., Cho, S.Y., Kang, C.S., & Chang, S.Y. (2006). Identification of steroid hormones in pomegranate (Punica granatum) using HPLC and GC-mass spectrometry. *Food Chemistry, 96*(4), 562-571. https://doi.org/10.1016/j.foodchem.2005.03.010

116. Kho, Y.L., Jung, W., Kwon, D., & Kim, J.H. (2010). Identification of estrone in pomegranate (Punica granatum) extracts by liquid chromatography-tandem mass spectrometry. *Food Science and Biotechnology*, 19, 809–813. https://doi.org/10.1007/s10068-010-0113-z

117. Yoshime, L.T., de Melo, I.L.P., Sattler, J.A.G., Torres, R.P., & Mancini-Filho, J. (2019). Bioactive compounds and the antioxidant capacities of seed oils from pomegranate (Punica granatum L.) and bitter gourd (Momordica charantia L.). *Food Science and Technology (Campinas), 39*(Supp.2), 571-580. DOI: 10.1590/fst.23218

118. de Melo, I.L.P., de Carvalho, E.B., Silva, A.M., Yoshime, L.T., Sattler, J.A.G., Pavan, R.T., & Mancini-Filho, J. (2016). Characterization of constituents, quality and stability of pomegranate seed oil (Punica granatum L.). *Food Science and Technology (Campinas), 36*(1), 132-139. DOI: 10.1590/1678-457X.0069

119. Caligiani, A., Bonzanini, F., Palla, G., Cirlini, M., & Bruni, R. (2010). Characterization of a potential nutraceutical ingredient: Pomegranate (Punica granatum L.) seed oil unsaponifiable fraction. *Plant Foods for Human Nutrition (Dordrecht, Netherlands), 65*(3), 277–283. https://doi.org/10.1007/s11130-010-0173-5

120. Eden Botanicals Certificate of Analysis, Pomegranate CO_2 extract. Retrieved March 5, 2022, from https://www.edenbotanicals.com/product_documents/COA/831_Pomegranate_Seed_CO2_Organic_COA_16.pdf

121. The Herbarie. Analysis of Pomegranate seed CO_2 extract. Retrieved March 5, 2022, from https://www.theherbarie.com/Pomegranate-Seed-CO2-Extract.html

122. Liu, G., Xu, X., Hao, Q., Gao, Y. (2009). Supercritical CO_2 extraction optimization of pomegranate (Punica granatum L.) seed oil using response surface methodology. *LWT- Food Science and Technology, 42*(9), 1491-1495. https://doi.org/10.1016/j.lwt.2009.04.011

123. Wang, R., Ding, Y., Liu, R., Xiang, L., & Du, L. (2010). Pomegranate: Constituents, bioactivities and pharmacokinetics. *Fruit, Vegetable and Cereal Science and Biotechnology*, 4 (Special Issue 2), 77-87, 2010. https://www.researchgate.net/publication/228474896_Pomegranate_Constituents_Bioactivities_and_Pharmacokinetics

124. Aslam, M.N., Lansky, E.P., & Varani, J. (2006). Pomegranate as a cosmeceutical source: Pomegranate fractions promote proliferation and procollagen synthesis and inhibit matrix metalloproteinase-1 production in human skin cells. *Journal of Ethnopharmacology, 103*(3), 311–318. https://doi.org/10.1016/j.jep.2005.07.027

125. Castellanos Morales, G., Sánchez de la Vega, G., Aragón Cuevas, F., Contreras, A. & Lira Saade, R. (2019). *Cucurbita pepo*. The IUCN Red List of Threatened Species 2019: e.T20742885A20755901. Retrieved March 6, 2022, from https://dx.doi.org/10.2305/IUCN.UK.2019-2.RLTS.T20742885A20755901.en.

126. The Editors of Encyclopaedia Britannica. (2019, December 4). Pumpkin. *Encyclopedia Britannica*. https://www.britannica.com/plant/pumpkin

127. Salehi, B., Capanoglu, E., Adrar, N., Catalkaya, G., Shaheen, S., Jaffer, M., Giri, L., Suyal, R., Jugran, A.K., Calina, D., Docea, A.O., Kamiloglu, S., Kregiel, D., Antolak, H., Pawlikowska, E., Sen, S., Acharya, K., Selamoglu, Z., Sharifi-Rad, J., Martorell, M., Rodrigues, C.F., Sharopov, F., Martins, N., & Capasso, R. (2019). Cucurbits plants: A key emphasis to its pharmacological potential. *Molecules, 24*(10), 1854. https://doi.org/10.3390/molecules24101854

128. Vujasinovic, V., Djilas, S., Dimic, E., Romanic, R., & Takaci, A. (2010). Shelf life of cold-pressed pumpkin (Cucurbita pepo L.) seed oil obtained with a screw press. *Journal of the American Oil Chemists' Society, 87*(12), 1497-1505. https://doi.org/10.1007/s11746-010-1630-x

129. Rezig, L., Chouaibi, M., Msaada, K., & Hamdi, S. (2012). Chemical composition and profile characterization of pumpkin (Cucurbita maxima) seed oil. *Industrial Crops and Products, 37*(1), 82-87. https://doi.org/10.1016/j.indcrop.2011.12.004

130. Boujemaa, I., El Bernoussi, S., Harhar, H., & Tabyaoui, M. (2020). The influence of the species on the quality, chemical composition and antioxidant activity of pumpkin seed oil. *Oilseeds and Fats, Crops and Lipids, 27*(40), 7 pages. https://doi.org/10.1051/ocl/2020031

131. Akin, G., Arslan, F.N., Karuk Elmas, S.N., & Yilmaz, I. (2018). Cold-pressed pumpkin seed (Cucurbita pepo L.) oils from the central Anatolia region of Turkey: Characterization of phytosterols, squalene, tocols, phenolic acids, carotenoids and fatty acid bioactive compounds. *Grasas Y Aceites, 69*(1), 12 pages. https://doi.org/10.3989/gya.0668171

132. Brusie, C. (19 December 2016). The health benefits of pumpkin seed oil. *Healthline*. Retrieved April 4, 2021, from https://www.healthline.com/health/pumpkin-seed-oil#TOC_TITLE_HDR_1

133. Frey, M. (29 July 2020). The health benefits of pumpkin seed oil. *Verywell Health*. Retrieved April 4, 2021, from https://www.verywellhealth.com/pumpkin-seed-oil-health-benefits-4686960

134. Ibrahim, A.A., Salih, T.F.M., Ibrahimc, S.J., & Al-Noor, T.H. (2018). Facial acne therapy using pumpkin seed oil with its physiocochemical properties. *Applied Science Reports, 23*(1), 39-47. DOI: 10.15192/PSCP.ASR.2018.23.1.3947

135. Bardaa, S., Turki, M., Ben Khedir, S, Mzid, M., Rebai, T., Ayadi, F. & Sahnoun, Z. (2020). The effect of prickly pear, pumpkin, and linseed oils on biological mediators of acute inflammation and oxidative stress markers. *BioMed Research International, 2020*(5643465), 1-11. https://doi.org/10.1155/2020/5643465

136. Bardaa, S., Chabchoub, N., Jridi, M., Moalla, D., Mseddi, M., Rebai, T., & Sahnoun, Z. (2016). The effect of natural extracts on laser burn wound healing. *Journal of Surgical Research, 201*(2), 464-472. DOI: 10.1016/j.jss.2015.11.052

137. Missouri Botanical Garden (n.d.). *Rubus idaeus*. Retrieved December 16, 2020, from http://www.missouribotanicalgarden.org/PlantFinder/PlantFinderDetails.aspx?taxonid=295999

138. Ferlemi, A.-V., & Lamari, F. N. (2016). Berry leaves: An alternative source of bioactive natural products of nutritional and medicinal value. *Antioxidants, 5*(2). https://doi.org/10.3390/antiox5020017

139. Van Hoed, V., De Clercq, N., Echim, C., Andjelkovic, M., Leber, E., et. al. (2009). Berry seeds: a source of specialty oils with high content of bioactives and nutritional value. *Journal of Food Lipids*, 16, 33-49.

140. Oomah, B.D., Ladet, S., Godfrey, D.V., Liang, J.X., Girard, B. (2000). Characteristics of raspberry (Rubus idaeus L.) seed oil. *Food Chemistry*, 69, 187-193. DOI: 10.1016/S0308-8146(99)00260-5

141. Pieszka, M., Migdal, W., Gasior, R., Rudzinska, M., Bederska-Lojewska, D., Pieszka, M. & Szczurek, P. (2015). Native oils from apple, black currant, raspberry, and strawberry seeds as a source of polyenoic fatty acids, tocochromanols, and phytosterols: A health implication. *Journal of Chemistry*, 2015(Article 659541). 8 pages. https://doi.org/10.1155/2015/659541

142. Rätsep, R., Bleive, U., Neppo, H., Tammik, M.L., Kaldmäe, H., Aluvee, A., Kikas, A., Arus, L., & Pääso, P. (2017). Supercritical CO2 extraction of raspberry seed oil. Retrieved March 7, 2022, from https://www.researchgate.net/publication/319876568_Supercritical_CO2_extraction_of_raspberry_seed_oil. DOI:10.13140/RG.2.2.17873.43364

143. Eden Botanicals. (2019). *Certificate of analysis: Raspberry Seed CO2 -Organic*. Eden Botanicals. Retrieved March 6, 2022, from https://www.edenbotanicals.com/product_documents/COA/833_Raspberry_seed_CO2_ORG_COA_8.pdf

144. Nature's Gift. (2018). *Certificate of anaylsis: Raspberry seed CO2*. Batch GE-161121. Nature's Gift Raspberry Seed Total CO2. Retrieved March 6, 2022, from: https://naturesgift.com/product/raspberry-seed-total-co2/

145. Yang, B., Ahotupa, M., Maatta, P., Kallio, H. (2011). Composition and antioxidantive activities of supercritical CO2-extracted oils from seeds and soft parts of northern berries. *Food Research International*, 44. Doi: 10.1016/j.foodres.2011.02.025

146. Oomah, B.D., Ladet, S., Godfrey, D.V., Liang, J.X., Girard, B. (2000). Characteristics of raspberry (Rubus idaeus L.) seed oil. *Food Chemistry*, 69, 187-193. DOI: 10.1016/S0308-8146(99)00260-5

147. Missouri Botanical Garden. (n.d.). *Rosa rubiginosa*. Retrieved November 2, 2020, from https://www.missouribotanicalgarden.org/PlantFinder/PlantFinderDetails.aspx?taxonid=286363&isprofile=0&

148. Winther, K., Campbell-Tofte, J., & Vinther Hansen, A. S. (2016). Bioactive ingredients of rose hips (Rosa canina L) with special reference to antioxidative and anti-inflammatory properties: In vitro studies. *Botanics: Targets and Therapy*, 11. https://doi.org/10.2147/BTAT.S91385

149. The Editors of Encylopedia Britannica. (2019, October 10). Rose. *Encyclopedia Britannica*. https://www.britannica.com/plant/rose-plant

150. Engels, G., & Brinckmann, J. (2016). Dog rose hip; Rosa canina; Family: Rosaceae. *HerbalGram*, 111, 8-19. http://cms.herbalgram.org/herbalgram/issue111/hg111-herbpro-rosehip.html

151. Dąbrowska, M., Maciejczyk, E., & Kalemba, D. (2019). Rose hip seed oil: Methods of extraction and chemical composition. European *Journal of Lipid Science and Technology, 121*(8), 1800440. https://doi.org/10.1002/ejlt.201800440

152. Nybom, H. & Werlemark, G. (2017). Realizing the potential of health-promoting rosehips from dogroses (Rosa sect. Caninae). *Current Bioactive Compounds*, 13, 3-17. DOI: 10.2174/1573407212666116060709906 35

153. del Valle, J.M., Bello, S., Thiel, J., Allen, A., & Chordia, L. (2000). Comparison of conventional and supercritical CO2-extracted rosehip oil. *Brazilian Journal of Chemical Engineering, 17*(3), 335-348. https://doi.org/10.1590/S0104-66322000000300010

154. Concha, J., Soto, C., Chamy, R., & Zuniga, M.E. (2006). Effect of rosehip extraction process on oil and defatted meal physiochemical properties. *Journal of the American Oil Chemists' Society, 83*(9), 771–775. https://doi.org/10.1007/s11746-006-5013-2

155. Grajzer, M., Szmalcel, K., Kuźmiński, Ł., Witkowski, M., Kulma, A., & Prescha, A. (2020). Characteristics and antioxidant potential of cold-pressed oils—Possible strategies to improve oil stability. *Foods*, 9, 1630. https://doi.org/10.3390/foods9111630

156. Ozcan M. (2002). Nutrient composition of rose (Rosa canina L.) seed and oils. *Journal of Medicinal Food, 5*(3), 137–140. https://doi.org/10.1089/10966200260398161

157. Machmudah, S., Kawahito, Y., Sasaki, M., & Goto, M. (2007). Supercritical CO2 extraction of rosehip seed oil: Fatty acids composition and process optimization. *Journal of Supercritical Fluids*, 41, 421-428. DOI: 10.1016/j.supflu.2006.12.011

158. Eden Botanicals. *Certificate of analysis: rosehip seed co2*. Retrieved March 8, 2022, from https://www.edenbotanicals.com/product_

documents/COA/888_Rosehip_Seed_CO2_Organic_COA_25.pdf

159. Jakovljevic, M., Moslavac, T., Bilic, M., Aladic, K., Bakula, F., & Jokic, S. (2018). Supercritical CO2 extraction of oil from rose hips (Rosa canina L.) and cornelian cherry (Cornus mas L.) seeds. *Croatian Journal of Food Science and Technology, 10*(2), 197-205. DOI: 10.17508/CJFST.2018.10.2.08

160. Timoszuk, M., Bielawska, K., & Skrzydlewska, E. (2018). Evening primrose (Oenothera biennis) biological activity dependent on chemical composition. *Antioxidants, 7*(8), 108. https://doi.org/10.3390/antiox7080108

161. Dąbrowska, M., Maciejczyk, E., & Kalemba, D. (2019), Rose hip seed oil: Methods of extraction and chemical composition. European *Journal of Lipid Science and Technology, 121*(8),1800440. https://doi.org/10.1002/ejlt.201800440

162. Lin, T. K., Zhong, L., & Santiago, J. L. (2018). Anti-inflammatory and skin barrier repair effects of topical application of some plant oils. *International Journal of Molecular Sciences, 19*(1), 70. https://doi.org/10.3390/ijms19010070

163. Kodahl, N., & Sørensen, M. (2021). Sacha inchi (Plukenetia volubilis L.) is an underutilized crop with great potential. *Agronomy, 2021*(11), 1066. https://doi.org/10.3390/agronomy11061066

164. Krivankova, B., Plesny, Z., Lojka, B., Lojkova, J., Banout, J., & Preininger, D. (2007, October 9-11). Sacha inchi (Plukenetia volubilis, Euphorbiaceae): A promising oilseed crop from Peruvian Amazon. In *Utilization of diversity in land systems: Sustainable and organic approaches to meet human needs, Tropentag, Witzenhausen.* Retrieved June 11, 2021, from https://www.tropentag.de/2007/abstracts/links/Krivankova_NnQmCSMU.pdf

165. Avila-Sosa, R., Montero-Rodríguez, A.F., Aguilar-Alonso, P., Vera López, O., Lazcano Hernández, M., Morales-Medina, J.C., & Navarro-Cruz, A.R. (2019). Antioxidant properties of Amazonian fruits: A mini review of in vivo and in vitro studies. *Oxidative Medicine and Cellular Longevity, 2019*, Article 8204129. https://doi.org/10.1155/2019/8204129

166. Liu, Q., Xu, Y.K., Zhang, P., Na, Z., Tang, T., & Shi, Y.X. (2014). Chemical composition and oxidative evolution of sacha inchi (Plukentia [sic] volubilis L.) oil from Xishuangbanna (China). *Grasas Aceites, 65*(1), 1-9. http://dx.doi.org/10.3989/gya.075713

167. Rodríguez, G., Villanueva, E., Glorio, P., & Baquerizo, M. (2015). Estabilidad oxidativa y estimación de la vida útil del aceite de sacha inchi (Plukenetia volubilis L.). *Scientia Agropecuaria, 6*(3), 155-163. DOI: 10.17268/sci.agropecu.2015.03.02

168. Fanali, C., Dugo, L., Cacciola, F., Beccaria, M., Grasso, S., Dacha, M., Dugo, P., & Mondello, L. (2011). Chemical characterization of sacha inchi (Plukenetia volubilis L.) oil. *Journal of Agriculture and Food Chemistry, 59*(24), 13043-13049. https://doi.org/10.1021/jf203184y

169. Ramos-Escudero, F., Muñoz, A.M. Escudero, M.R., Viñas-Ospino, A., Morales, M.R., & Asuero, A.G. (2019). Characterization of commercial sacha inchi oil according to its composition: Tocopherols, fatty acids, sterols, triterpene and aliphatic alcohols. *Journal of Food Science Technology, 56*(10), 4503-4515. https://doi.org/10.1007/s13197-019-03938-9

170. Ramos-Escudero, F., González-Miret, M.L., Viñas-Ospino, & Escudero, M.R. (2019). Quality, stability, carotenoids and chromatic parameters of commercial Sacha inchi oil originating from Peruvian cultivars. *Journal of Food Science Technology, 56*(11), 4901-4910. https://doi.org/10.1007/s13197-019-03960-x

171. Wang, S., Zhu, F., & Kakuda, Y. (2018). Sacha inchi (Plukenetia volubilis L.): Nutritional composition, biological activity, and uses. *Food Chemistry, 265,* 316-328. https://doi.org/10.1016/j.foodchem.2018.05.055

172. Hamaker, B.R., Valles, C., Gilman, R., Hardmeier, R.M., Clark, D., Garcia, H.H., Gonzales, A.E., Kohlstad, I., Castro, M., Valdivia, R., Rodriguez, T., & Lescano, M. (1992). Amino acid and fatty acid profiles of the Inca peanut (Plukenetia volubilis). *Cereal Chemistry, 69*(4), 461-463. Retrieved June 14, 2021, from https://www.cerealsgrains.org/publications/cc/backissues/1992/Documents/69_461.pdf

173. Suppasawat, N., Nuamnaichati, N., Mangmool, S., Srisukh, & Lomarat, P. (2017). Anti-inflammatory activity of sacha inchi (Plukenetia volubilis L.) oil in LPS-stimulated RAW 264.7 cells. *Thai Journal of Pharmaceutical Sciences, 41,* 1-4. Retrieved July 7, 2021, from http://ipnacs2017.weebly.com/uploads/1/5/1/8/15182734/pn-1_narumes_suppasawat_1___1-4__ok.pdf

174. Soimee, W., Nakyai, W., Charoensit, P., Grandmottet, F., Worasakwutiphong, S., Phimnuan, P., & Viyoch, J. (2019). Evaluation of moisturizing and irritation potential of sacha inchi oil. *Journal of Cosmetic Dermatology, 19*(4), 915-924. https://doi.org/10.1111/jocd.13099

175. Saengsorn, K. & Jimtaisong, A. (2017). Determination of hydrophilic-lipophilic balance value and emulsion properties of sacha inchi oil. *Asian Pacific Journal of Tropical Biomedicine, 7* (12), 1092-1096. https://doi.org/10.1016/j.apjtb.2017.10.011

176. Gonzales-Aspajo, G., Belkhelfa, H., Haddioui-Hbabi, L., Bourdy, G., & Deharo, E., (2015). Sacha inchi oil (Plukenetia volubilis L.), effect on adherence of Staphylococcus aureus to human skin explant and keratinocytes in vitro. *Journal of Ethnopharmacology, 171,* 330-334. https://doi.org/10.1016/j.jep.2015.06.009

177. Chadburn, H. & Wilson, B. 2018. *Elaeagnus rhamnoides.* The IUCN Red List of Threatened Species 2018: e.T55686342A119996497. https://dx.doi.org/10.2305/IUCN.UK.2018-1.RLTS.T55686342A119996497.en. Retrieved March 10, 2022, from https://www.iucnredlist.org/species/55686342/119996497

178. Zielińska, A., & Nowak, I. (2017). Abundance of active ingredients in sea-buckthorn oil. *Lipids in Health and Disease, 16,* 95. https://doi.org/10.1186/s12944-017-0469-7

179. Pundir, S., Garg, P., Dviwedi, A., Ali, A., Kapoor, V.K., Kapoor, D., Kulshrestha, S., Lal, U.R., & Negi, P. (2021). Ethnomedicinal uses, phytochemistry and dermatological effects of Hippophae rhamnoides L.: A review. *Journal of Ethnopharmacology, 266,* 113434. 14 pages. https://doi.org/10.1016/j.jep.2020.113434

180. Cenkowski, S., Yakimishen, R., Przybylski, R., & Muir, W.E. (2006). Quality of extracted sea buckthorn seed and pulp oil. *Canadian Biosystems Engineering, 48*(3), 9-16.

181. Nature in Bottle. (2021). *Sea buckthorn oil: Certificate of analysis Batch # 40452108.* Nature in Bottle, Retrieved March 4, 2022, from https://www.natureinbottle.com/product/sea_buckthorn_fruit_pulp_oil

182. Yang, B., Ahotupa, M., Maatta, P., Kallio, H. (2011). Composition and antioxidative activities of supercritical CO2-extracted oils from seeds and soft parts of northern berries. *Food Research International, 44.* DOI: 10.1016/j.foodres.2011.02.025

183. Pavlovic, N., Lendic, K.V., Miskulin, M., Moslavac, T., & Jokic, S. (2016). Supercritical CO2 extraction of sea buckthorn. *Food in Health and*

Disease, 5(2), 55-61.

184. Li, T.S.C., Beveridge T.H.J., Drover, J.C.G. (2007). Phytosterol content of sea buckthorn (Hippophae rhamnoides L.) seed oil: Extraction and identification. *Food chemistry*, 101 (2007), 1633-1639. DOI:10.1016/j.foodchem.2006.04.033

185. Jiang, X., Li, W. Zhou, S. & Jiang, Y. (2020). Changes of physicochemical properties, oxidative stability and cellular anti-inflammatory potentials for sea-buckthorn pulp oils during refining. *RSC Advances*, 10, 36678-36685. DOI: 10.1039/d0ra07095e

186. Zeb, A. (2004). Important therapeutic uses of sea buckthorn (Hippophae): A review. *Journal of Biological Sciences, 4*(5), 687-693.

187. Zielińska, A. & Nowak, I. (2014). Fatty acids in vegetable oils and their importance in cosmetic industry. *Chemik*, 68, 103-110.

188. Koskovac, M., Cupara, S., Kipic, M., Barjaktarevic, A., Milovanovic, O., Kojicic, K., Markovic, M. (2017). Sea Buckthorn Oil—A Valuable Source for Cosmeceuticals. *Cosmetics, 4*(4), 40. https://doi.org/10.3390/cosmetics4040040

189. Marsinach, M.S. & Cuenca, A.P. (2019). The impact of sea buckthorn oil fatty acids on human health. *Lipids in Health and Disease, 18*(1), 145. DOI: 10.1186/s12944-019-1065-9

190. Smida, I. Pentelescu, C., Pentelescu, O., Sweidan, A., Oliviero, N., Meuric, V., Martin, B, Colceriu, L, Bonnaure-Mallet, M., & Tamanai-Shacoori, Z. (2019). Benefits of sea buckthorn (Hippophae rhamnoides) pulp oil-based mouthwash on oral health. *Journal of Applied Microbiology, 126*(5), 1594-1605. DOI: 10.1111/jam.14210

191. Koskovac, M., Cupara, S., Kipic, M., Barjaktarevic, A., Milovanovic, O., Kojicic, K., Markovic, M. (2017). Sea Buckthorn Oil—A Valuable Source for Cosmeceuticals. *Cosmetics, 4*(4), 40. https://doi.org/10.3390/cosmetics4040040

192. Yang, B. & Erkkola, R. (2006). Sea buckthorn oils, mucous membranes and Sjögren's syndrome. *Yksityisääkäri*, 4, 20-21. Retrieved March 8, 2022, from http://www.scicompdf.se/membrasin/yang_erk_2006.pdf

193. Larmo, P.S., Yang, B., Hyssälä, J., Kallio, H.P., Erkkola, R. (2014). Effects of sea buckthorn oil intake on vaginal atrophy in postmenopausal women: A randomized, double-blind, placebo-controlled study. *Maturitas, 79*(3), 316-321. https://doi.org/10.1016/j.maturitas.2014.07.010

194. Barstow, M. (2019). *Calophyllum inophyllum*. The IUCN Red List of Threatened Species 2019: e.T33196A67775081. Retrieved September 6, 2020, from https://dx.doi.org/10.2305/IUCN.UK.2019-1.RLTS.T33196A67775081.en

195. Fern, K. (2019, June 13). Useful Tropical Plants: Calophyllum inophyllum. *Tropical Plants Database*. http://tropical.theferns.info/viewtropical.php?id=Calophyllum+inophyllum

196. Léguillier, T., Lecsö-Bornet, M., Lémus, C., Rousseau-Ralliard, D., Lebouvier, N., Hnawia, E., Nour, M., Aalbersberg, W., Ghazi, K., Raharivelomanana, P., & Rat, P. (2015). The wound healing and antibacterial activity of five ethnomedical Calophyllum inophyllum oils: An alternative therapeutic strategy to treat infected wounds. *PloS One, 10*(9), e0138602. https://doi.org/10.1371/journal.pone.0138602

197. Dweck, A.C. & Meadows, T. (2002). Tamanu (Calophyllum inophyllum) – the African, Asian, Polynesian and Pacific panacea. *International Journal of Cosmetic Science*, 24, 1-8.

198. Raharivelomanana, P., Ansel, J.-L., Lupo, E., Mijouin, L., Guillot, S., Butaud, J.F., Ho, R., Lecellier, G., & Pichon, C. (2018). Tamanu oil and skin active properties: From traditional to modern cosmetic uses. *Oilseeds & Fats, Crops and Lipids, 25*(5). DOI: https://doi.org/10.1051/ocl/2018048

199. Léguillier, T., Lecsö-Bornet, M., Lémus, C., Rousseau-Ralliard, D., Lebouvier, N., Hnawia, E., Nour, M., Aalbersberg, W., Ghazi, K., Raharivelomanana, P., & Rat, P. (2015). The wound healing and antibacterial activity of five ethnomedical Calophyllum inophyllum oils: An alternative therapeutic strategy to treat infected wounds. *PloS One, 10*(9), e0138602. https://doi.org/10.1371/journal.pone.0138602

200. Crane, S., Aurore, G., Joseph, H., Mouloungui, Z., & Bourgeois, P. (2005). Composition of fatty acids triacylglycerols and unsaponifiable matter in Calophyllum calaba L. oil from Guadeloupe. *Phytochemistry, 66*(15), 1825–1831. https://doi.org/10.1016/j.phytochem.2005.06.009

201. Cassien, M. Mercier, A., Thétiot-Laurent, S., Culcasi, M., Ricquebourg, E., Asteian, A., Herbette, G. Bianchini, J.P., Raharivelomanana, P., & Pietri, S. (2021). Improving the antioxidant properties of Calophyllum inophyllum seed oil from French Polynesia: Development and biological applications of resinous ethanol-soluble extracts. *Antioxidants, 10*(199), 23 pages. https://doi.org/10.3390/antiox10020199

202. Leu, T., Raharivelomanana, P., Soulet, S., Bianchini, J.P., Herbette, G., & Faure, R. (2009). New tricyclic and tetracyclic pyranocoumarins with an unprecedented C-4 substituent. Structure elucidation of tamanolide, tamanolide D and tamanolide P from Calophyllum inophyllum of French Polynesia. *Magnetic Resonance in Chemistry, 47*(11), 989–993. https://doi.org/10.1002/mrc.2482

203. Mahmud, S., Rizwani, G., Ahmad, M., Ali, S., Perveen, S., & Ahmad, V. (1998) Antimicrobial studies on fractions and pure compounds of Calophyllum inophyllum Linn. *Pakistan Journal of Pharmacology, 15*(2),13–25.

204. Nguyen, V.L., Truong, C.T., Nguyen, B., Vo, T.V., Dao, T.T., Nguyen, V.D., Trinh, D.T., Huynh, H.K., & Bui, C.B. (2017). Anti-inflammatory and wound healing activities of calophyllolide isolated from Calophyllum inophyllum Linn. *PloS One, 12*(10), e0185674. https://doi.org/10.1371/journal.pone.0185674

205. Yimdjo, M.C., Azebaze, A.G., Nkengfack, A.E., Meyer, A.M., Bodo, B., & Fomum, Z.T. (2004). Antimicrobial and cytotoxic agents from Calophyllum inophyllum. *Phytochemistry, 65*(20), 2789–2795. https://doi.org/10.1016/j.phytochem.2004.08.024

206. Léguillier, T., Lecsö-Bornet, M., Lémus, C., Rousseau-Ralliard, D., Lebouvier, N., Hnawia, E., Nour, M., Aalbersberg, W., Ghazi, K., Raharivelomanana, P., & Rat, P. (2015). The wound healing and antibacterial activity of five ethnomedical Calophyllum inophyllum oils: An alternative therapeutic strategy to treat infected wounds. *PloS One, 10*(9), e0138602. https://doi.org/10.1371/journal.pone.0138602

207. West Coast Institute of Aromatherapy. (2018). *Tamanu Calophyllum inophyllum*. West Coast Aromatherapy. Retrieved March 10, 2022, from https://westcoastaromatherapy.com/article-archives/tamanu/

208. Ansel, J.L., Lupo, E., Mijouin, L., Guillot, S., Butaud, J.F., Ho, R., Lecellier, G., Raharivelomanana, P., & Pichon, C. (2016). Biological activity of Polynesian Calophyllum inophyllum oil extract on human skin cells. *Planta Medica, 82*(11-12), 961–966. https://doi.org/10.1055/s-0042-108205

209. Bhalla, T.N., Saxena, R.C., Nigam, S.K., Misra, G., & Bhargava, K.P. (1980). Calophyllolide--A new non-steroidal anti-inflammatory agent. *The Indian Journal of Medical Research*, 72, 762–765.

210. Pribowo, A., Girish, J., Gustiananda, M., Nandhira, R.G., & Hartrianti, P. (2021). Potential of tamanu (Calophyllum inophyllum) oil for atopic dermatitis treatment. *Evidence-Based Complementary and Alternative Medicine, 2021*(6332867), 9 pages. https://doi.org/10.1155/2021/6332867

211. Kilham, C. (2004) Tamanu oil: A tropical topical remedy. *HerbalGram*, 63, 26-31. Retrieved March 8, 2022, from http://cms.herbalgram.org/herbalgram/issue63/article2709.html

212. Gupta, S. & Gupta, P. (2020). The genus Calophyllum: Review of ethnomedicinal uses, phytochemistry and pharmacology. In J. Singh, V. Meshram, M. Gupta (Eds.). *Bioactive natural products in drug discovery.* Springer. pp. 215-242. https://doi.org/10.1007/978-981-15-1394-7_5

213. Raharivelomanana, P., Ansel, J.-L., Lupo, E., Mijouin, L., Guillot, S., Butaud, J.F., Ho, R., Lecellier, G., & Pichon, C. (2018). Tamanu oil and skin active properties: From traditional to modern cosmetic uses. *Oilseeds & Fats, Crops and Lipids, 25*(5). DOI: https://doi.org/10.1051/ocl/2018048

References
Part Five: The Herbal Oils

1. Ganora, L. (2021). *Herbal Constituents: Foundations of Phytochemistry.*

2. Lavagna, S.M., Secci, D., Chimenti, P., Bonsignore, L., Ottaviani, A., & Bizzarri, B. (2001). Efficacy of Hypericum and Calendula oils in epithelial reconstruction of surgical wounds in childbirth with caesarean section. *Il Farmaco, 56*(2001), 451-453. DOI: 10.1016/s0014-827x(01)01060-6

3. Falniowski, A., Bazos, I., Hodálová, I., Lansdown, R. & Petrova, A. (2011). Arnica montana. The IUCN Red List of Threatened Species 2011: e.T162327A5574104. Retrieved October 1, 2018, from http://dx.doi.org/10.2305/IUCN.UK.2011-1.RLTS.T162327A5574104.en.

4. Arnica - Arnica spp. (2018). United Plant Savers. Retrieved March 14, 2022, from https://unitedplantsavers.org/species-at-risk-list/arnica-arnica-spp/

5. Kriplani, P., Guarve, K., & Baghael, U. S. (2017). Arnica montana L. - a plant of healing: Review. *The Journal of Pharmacy and Pharmacology, 69*(8), 925–945. https://doi.org/10.1111/jphp.12724

6. Barnes, J., Anderson, L.A., & Phillipson, J.D. (2007). *Herbal medicines* (3rd ed.). Pharmaceutical Press. pp. 63-66.

7. Gardner, Z., & McGuffin, M. (Eds.). (2013). *American herbal products associations' botanical safety handbook* 2nd ed. CRC Press. 87-90.

8. Engles, G., & Brinckmann, J. (2015). Arnica. *HerbalGram*,107, 1-6. http://cms.herbalgram.org/herbalgram/issue107/hg107-herbpro-arnica.html

9. van Wyk, B. & Wink, M. (2004) *Medicinal plants of the world.* Timber Press.

10. Perry, N.B., Burgess, E.J., Rodriquez-Guitian, M.A. Franco, R.R., Mosquera, E.L., Smallfield, B., Joyce, N.I., & Littlejohn, R.P. (2009). Sesquiterpene lactones in Arnica montana: helenalin and dihydrohelenalin chemotypes in Spain. *Planta Medica, 75*(6), 660-6. DOI: 10.1055/s-0029-1185362.

11. Knuesel, O., Weber, M., & Suter, A. (2002). Arnica montana gel in osteoarthritis of the knee: An open, multicenter clinical trial. *Advances in Therapy, 19*(5). DOI:10.1007/BF02850361

12. Judzentiene, A. & Budiene, J. (2009). Analysis of the chemical composition of flower essential oils from Arnica montana of Lithuanian origin. *Chemija, 20*(3), 190-194.

13. Ly, G., Knorre, A., Schmidt, T.J., Pahl, H.L. & Merfort, I. (1998). The anti-inflammatory sesquiterpene lactone helenalin inhibits the transcription factor NF-κB by directly targeting. T*he Journal of Biological Chemistry, 273*(50), 33508-33516. DOI: 10.1074/jbc.273.50.33508

14. May, P. (2014, 25 February). *Arnica flower CO_2 extract - Approved efficacy in topical treatment.* Cosmetic Business. Retrieved March 14, 2022, from https://www.cosmeticsbusiness.com/news/article_page/Arnica_Flower_CO2-Extract_Approved_Efficacy_in_Topical_Treatment/95998

15. Flavex. (n.d.). Arnica flower CO2 total extract (organic) information sheet. https://www.flavex.com/en/produkt/arnica-flower-co2-to-extract-4-sesquiterpene-lactones-product-nr-043-002/

16. Mills, S., & Bone, K. (2000). *Principles and practice of phytotherapy.* Churchill Livingstone.

17. Lyss, G., Knorre, A., Schmidt, T. J., Pahl, H. L., & Merfort, I. (1998). The anti-inflammatory sesquiterpene lactone helenalin inhibits the transcription factor NF-kappaB by directly targeting p65. T*he Journal of Biological Chemistry, 273*(50), 33508–33516. https://doi.org/10.1074/jbc.273.50.33508

18. Moore, M. (1993). *Medicinal plants of the Pacific northwest.* Red Crane Books.

19. Petruzzello, M. (2018, May 30). Calendula | description, uses, & facts. Encyclopedia Britannica. https://www.britannica.com/plant/calendula

20. Verma, P. K., Raina, R., Agarwal, S., Kaur, H. (2018). Phytochemical ingredients and pharmacological potential of Calendula officinalis Linn. *Pharmaceutical and Biomedical Research, 4*(2), 1-17. http://pbr.mazums.ac.ir/article-1-199-en.html

21. *Calendula officinalis*. (n.d.). Missouri Botanical Garden. Retrieved July 28, 2020, from http://www.missouribotanicalgarden.org/PlantFinder/PlantFinderDetails.aspx?taxonid=277409

22. Arora, D., Rani, A., & Sharma, A. (2013). A review on phytochemistry and ethnopharmacological aspects of genus Calendula. *Pharmacognosy Reviews, 7*(14), 179–187. https://doi.org/10.4103/0973-7847.120520

23. Andersen, F.A., Bergfeld, W.F., Belsito, D.V., Hill, R.A., Klaasen, C.D., Liebler, D.C., Marks Jr., J.G., Shank, R.C., Slaga, T.J., & Snyder, P.W. (2010). Final report of the cosmetic ingredient review expert panel amended safety assessment of Calendula officinalis–derived cosmetic ingredients. *International Journal of Toxicology 29*(Supplement 4), 221S-243S DOI: 10.1177/1091581810384883

24. Zitterl-Eglseer, K., Reznicek, G., Jurenitsch, J., Novak, J., Zitterl, W., & Franz, C. (2001). Morphogenetic variability of faradiol monoesters in marigold Calendula officinalis L. *Phytochemical Analysis, 12*(3), 199–201. https://doi.org/10.1002/pca.582

25. Hamburger, M., Adler, S., Baumann, D., Förg, A., & Weinreich, B. (2003). Preparative purification of the major anti-inflammatory triterpenoid esters from marigold (Calendula officinalis). *Fitoterapia,74*(4), 328-338. https://doi.org/10.1016/S0367-326X(03)00051-0

26. Nature's Gift, Calendula Total CO2 Certificate of Analysis. Batch #: GE-65114, GE-171001, and GE-58873. https://naturesgift.com/product/calendula-total-co2/

27. Raal, A., Orav, A., Nesterovitsch, J., & Maidla, K. (2016). Analysis of carotenoids, flavonoids and essential oil of Calendula officinalis cultivars growing in Estonia. *Natural Product Communications, 11*(8), 1157–1160.

28. Pintea, A., Bele, C., Andrei, S. & Socaciu, C. (2003). HPLC analysis of carotenoids in four varieties of Calendula officinalis L. flowers. *Acta Biologica Szegediensis, 47*(1-4), 37-40.

29. Zhang, X., Xiong, H., & Liu, L. (2012). Effects of taraxasterol on inflammatory responses in lipopolysaccharide-induced RAW 264.7 macrophages. *Journal of Ethnopharmacology, 141*(1), 206-211. https://doi.org/10.1016/j.jep.2012.02.020

30. Sharma, K., & Zafar, R. (2015). Occurrence of taraxerol and taraxasterol in medicinal plants. *Pharmacognosy Reviews, 9*(17), 19–23. https://doi.org/10.4103/0973-7847.156317

31. Nogueira, A.O., Oliveira, Y.I.S., Adjafre, B.L., de Moraes, M.E.A., & Aragão, G.F. (2019). Pharmacological effects of the isomeric mixture of alpha and beta amyrin from Protium heptaphyllum: A literature review. *Fundamental and Clinical Pharmacology, 33*(1), 4-12. https://doi.org/10.1111/fcp.12402

32. Della Loggia, R., Tubaro, A., Sosa, S., Becker, H., Saar, S., & Isaac, O. (1994). The role of triterpenoids in the topical anti-inflammatory activity of Calendula officinalis flowers. *Planta Medica, 60*(6), 516–520. https://doi.org/10.1055/s-2006-959562

33. Silva, D., Ferreira, M.S., Sousa-Loba, J.M., Cruz, M.T., & Almeida, I.F. (2021). Anti-inflammatory activity of Calendula officinalis L. flower extract. *Cosmetics*, 8, 31. https://doi.org/10.3390/cosmetics8020031

34. Chandran, P. K., & Kuttan, R. (2008). Effect of Calendula officinalis flower extract on acute phase proteins, antioxidant defense mechanism and granuloma formation during thermal burns. *Journal of Clinical Biochemistry and Nutrition, 43*(2), 58–64. https://doi.org/10.3164/jcbn.2008043

35. Martin, D., Navarro Del Hierro, J., Villanueva Bermejo, D., Fernández-Ruiz, R., Fornari, T., & Reglero, G. (2016). Bioaccessibility and antioxidant activity of Calendula officinalis supercritical extract as affected by in vitro codigestion with olive oil. *Journal of Agricultural and Food Chemistry, 64*(46), 8828–8837. https://doi.org/10.1021/acs.jafc.6b04313

36. Givol, O., Kornhaber, R., Visentin, D., Cleary, M., Haik, J., & Harats, M. (2019). A systematic review of Calendula officinalis extract for wound healing. *Wound Repair and Regeneration, 27*(5), 548–561. https://doi.org/10.1111/wrr.12737

37. Parente, L.M., Lino Júnior, R., Tresvenzol, L.M., Vinaud, M.C., de Paula, J.R., & Paulo, N.M. (2012). Wound healing and anti-Inflammatory effect in animal models of Calendula officinalis L. growing in Brazil. *Evidence-based Complementary and Alternative Medicine, 2012*(375671). 7 pages. https://doi.org/10.1155/2012/375671

38. Daucus carota var. sativus. (n.d.). Missouri Botanical Garden. Retrieved December 16, 2020, from https://www.missouribotanicalgarden.org/PlantFinder/PlantFinderDetails.aspx?taxonid=276043&isprofile=0&chr=19

39. Luby, C. H., Maeda, H. A., & Goldman, I. L. (2014). Genetic and phenological variation of tocochromanol (vitamin E) content in wild (Daucus carota L. var. carota) and domesticated carrot (D. carota L. var. sativa). *Horticulture Research*, 1, 14015. https://doi.org/10.1038/hortres.2014.15

40. Bystricka, J., Kavalcova, P., Musilova, J., Vollmannova, A., Toth, T., & Lenkova, M. (2015). Carrot (Daucus carota L. ssp. sativus (Hoffm.) Arcang.) as source of antioxidants. *Acta Agriculturae Slovenica, 105*(2), 303–311. http://dx.doi.org/10.14720/aas.2015.105.2.13

41. Golan, R. (1995). *Optimal wellness*. Ballantine Books.

42. Huang, Z.R., Lin, Y.K., & Fang, J.Y. (2009). Biological and pharmacological activities of squalene and related compounds: potential uses in cosmetic dermatology. *Molecules, 14*(1), 540–554. DOI:10.3390/molecules14010540

43. Pizzorno, J.E. & Murray, T. (1999). *Textbook of natural medicine*. Churchill Livingstone.

44. Oladeji, O. S., & Oyebamiji, A.K. (2020). Stellaria media (L.) Vill. - A plant with immense therapeutic potentials: phytochemistry and pharmacology. *Heliyon*, 6(6). https://doi.org/10.1016/j.heliyon.2020.e04150

45. Ma, L., Song, J., Shi, Y., Wang, C., Chen, B., Xie, D., & Jia, X. (2012). Anti-hepatitis B virus activity of chickweed [Stellaria media (L.) Vill.] extracts in HepG2.2.15 cells. *Molecules, 17*(7), 8633–8646. https://doi.org/10.3390/molecules17078633

46. Blankespoor, J., & Gemma, M. (2021, December 6). The 10 best wild foods and medicinal for beginning foragers and wildcrafters. Chestnut School of Herbal Medicine. https://chestnutherbs.com/best-wild-foods-for-beginning-foragers/

47. Yarnell, E. (2004). *Phytochemistry and pharmacy for practitioners of botanical medicine*. Healing Mountain Publishing.

48. Khela, S. (2012). Symphytum officinale. The IUCN Red List of Threatened Species 2012: e.T202969A2758315. Retrieved March 11, 2022, from https://www.iucnredlist.org/species/202969/2758315

49. Symphytum officinale. (n.d.). Missouri Botanical Garden. Retrieved October 21, 2020, from http://www.missouribotanicalgarden.org/PlantFinder/PlantFinderDetails.aspx?kempercode=b472

50. Comfrey. (2015, March 23). Penn State Hershey. http://pennstatehershey.adam.com/content.aspx?productid=107&pid=33&gid=000234

51. Wiedenfelt, H., Roeder, E., Bourauel, T., & Edgar, J. (2008). *Pyrrolizidine alkaloids: Structure and toxicity*. Bonn University Press.

52. Romm, A. (2018). *Botanical medicine for women's health*. Elsevier. p.356.

53. Stritch, L. 2018. *Populus balsamifera*. The IUCN Red List of Threatened Species. Retrieved on October 02, 2018, from http://dx.doi.org/10.2305/IUCN.UK.2018-1.RLTS.T61959749A61959757.en

54. Populus balsamifera. (2017). Ladybird Johnson Wildflower Center. The University of Texas at Austin. Retrieved April 1, 2022, from https://www.wildflower.org/plants/result.php?id_plant=POBA2

55. *Populus balsamifera*. (n.d.). Plants for a Future. Retrieved October 23, 2020, from https://pfaf.org/user/Plant.aspx?LatinName=Populus+balsamifera

56. Moore, M. (1993). *Medicinal plants of the Pacific northwest*. Red Crane Books.

57. Kis, B., Avram, S., Pavel, I. Z., Lombrea, A., Buda, V., Dehelean, C. A., Soica, C., Yerer, M. B., Bojin, F., Folescu, R., & Danciu, C. (2020). Recent advances regarding the phytochemical and therapeutic uses of Populus nigra L. buds. *Plants, 9*(11), 1464. https://doi.org/10.3390/plants9111464

58. Klemow, K.M., Bartlow, A., Crawford, J., Kocher, N., Shah, J., &

Ritsick, M. (2011). Medical attributes of St. John's wort (Hypericum perforatum). In I. F. F. Benzie & S. Wachtel-Galor (Eds.), Herbal Medicine: Biomolecular and Clinical Aspects (2nd ed.). CRC Press/Taylor & Francis. http://www.ncbi.nlm.nih.gov/books/NBK92750/

59. Maisenbacher, P., & Kovar, K.-A. (1992) Analysis and stability of Hyperici oleum. P*lanta Medica*, 58(4), 351-354. DOI: 10.1055/s-2006-961483

60. Crockett S.L. (2010). Essential oil and volatile components of the genus Hypericum (Hypericaceae). *Natural Product Communications, 5*(9), 1493–1506. https://doi.org/10.1177/1934578X1000500926

61. Miraldi, E., Biagi, M., & Giachetti, D. (2006). Chemical constituents and effect of topical application of Oleum Hyperici on skin sensitivity to simulated sun exposure. *Natural Product Communication, 1*(3), 209-213. https://doi.org/10.1177/1934578X0600100307

62. Sosa, S., Pace, R., Bornancin, A., Morazzoni, P., Riva, A., Tubaro, A., & Della Loggia, R. (2007). Topical anti-inflammatory activity of extracts and compounds from Hypericum perforatum L. T*he Journal of Pharmacy and Pharmacology, 59*(5), 703–709. https://doi.org/10.1211/jpp.59.5.0011

63. Lyles, J. T., Kim, A., Nelson, K., Bullard-Roberts, A. L., Hajdari, A., Mustafa, B., & Quave, C. L. (2017). The chemical and antibacterial evaluation of St. John's wort oil macerates used in Kosovar traditional medicine. *Frontiers in Microbiology*, 8, 1639. https://doi.org/10.3389/fmicb.2017.01639

64. Bertoli, A., Cirak, C., & Teixeira da Silva, J.A. (2011). Hypericum species as sources of valuable essential oils. *Medicinal and Aromatic Plant Science and Biotechnology,* 5 (Special Issue 1), 29-47.

65. Schepetkin, I.A., Özek, G., Özek, T., Kirpotina, L.N., Khlebnikov, A.I., & Quinn, M.T. (2020). Chemical composition and immunomodulatory activity of Hypericum perforatum essential oils. *Biomolecules, 10*(6), 916. https://doi.org/10.3390/biom10060916

66. Saddiqe, Z., Naeem, I., & Maimoona, A. (2010). A review of the antibacterial activity of Hypericum perforatum L. *Journal of Ethnopharmacology, 131*(3), 511–521. https://doi.org/10.1016/j.jep.2010.07.034

67. Schempp, C.M., Hezel, S., & Simon, J. C. (2003). Behandlung der subakuten atopischen Dermatitis mit Johanniskraut-Creme. Eine randomisierte, placebokontrollierte Doppelblindstudie im Halbseitendesign [Topical treatment of atopic dermatitis with Hypericum cream. A randomized, placebo-controlled, double-blind half-side comparison study]. *Der Hautarzt; Zeitschrift fur Dermatologie, Venerologie, und verwandte Gebiete [The Dermatologist; Journal of Dermatology, Venereology, and Related Fields], 54*(3), 248–253.

References
Part Six: The Butters

1. Barker, A. (2021). Attalea speciosa. The IUCN Red List of Threatened Species 2021: e.T111454030A158506703. https://dx.doi.org/10.2305/IUCN.UK.2021-2.RLTS.T111454030A158506703.en

2. Burlando, B., & Cornara, L. (2017). Revisiting Amazonian plants for skin care and disease. *Cosmetics, 4*(3), 25. https://doi.org/10.3390/cosmetics4030025

3. Campos, J.L.A., da Silva, T.L.L., Albuquerque, U.P., Peroni, N., & Araújo, E.L. (2015). Knowledge, use, and management of the babassu palm (Attalea speciosa Mart. ex Spreng) in the Araripe region (Northeastern Brazil). *Economic Botany, 69*(3), 240–250. http://www.jstor.org/stable/24826032

4. Santos, J., da Silva, J.W., dos Santos, S.M., Rodrigues, M.F., Silva, C., da Silva, M.V., Correia, M., Albuquerque, J., Melo, C., Silva, T.G., Martins, R.D., Aguiar Júnior, F., & Ximenes, R.M. (2020). In vitro and in vivo wound healing and anti-inflammatory activities of babassu oil (Attalea speciosa Mart. Ex Spreng., Arecaceae). *Evidence-Based Complementary and Alternative Medicine*, 2020, Article ID 8858291. https://doi.org/10.1155/2020/8858291

5. Souza, M.H., Monteiro, C.A., Figueredo, P.M., Nascimento, F.R., & Guerra, R.N. (2011). Ethnopharmacological use of babassu (Orbignya phalerata Mart) in communities of babassu nut breakers in Maranhão, Brazil. *Journal of Ethnopharmacology, 133*(1), 1–5. https://doi.org/10.1016/j.jep.2010.08.056

6. Araújo, F.R., González-Pérez, S.E., Lopes, M.A., & Viegas, I.dJ.M. (2016). Ethnobotany of babassu palm (Attalea speciosa Mart.) in the Tucuruí Lake protected areas mosaic – Eastern Amazon. *Acta Botanica Brasilica, 30*(2), 193-204. https://doi.org/10.1590/0102-33062015abb0290

7. Codex Alimentarius Commission. (1999). Codex Standard for Named Vegetable Oils. Codex-Stan 210-1999. Food and Agriculture Organization of the United Nations. Retrieved from https://www.fao.org/3/y2774e/y2774e04.htm# TopOfPage

8. Bauer, L.C., Lacerda, E.C.Q, Santos, L.S., Ferrão, S.P.B., Fontan, R.dC.I., Veloso, C.M., & Bonomo, C.F. (2019). Antioxidant activity and bioactive compounds of babassu (Orbignya phalerata) virgin oil obtained by different methods of extraction. *The Open Food Science Journal*,11, 35-43. DOI: 10.2174/1874256401911010035

9. Reis, M., dos Santos, S.M., Silva, D.R., Silva, M.V., Correia, M., Ferraz Navarro, D., Santos, G., Hallwass, F., Bianchi, O., Silva, A.G., Melo, J.V., Mattos, A.B., Ximenes, R.M., Machado, G., & Saraiva, K. (2017). Anti-inflammatory activity of babassu oil and development of a microemulsion system for topical delivery. *Evidence-Based Complementary and Alternative Medicine*, 2017, Article ID 3647801, 14 pages. https://doi.org/10.1155/2017/3647801

10. Nakatsuji, T., Kao, M.C., Fang, J.Y., Zouboulis, C.C., Zhang, L., Gallo, R.L., & Huang, C.M. (2009). Antimicrobial property of lauric acid against Propionibacterium acnes: Its therapeutic potential for inflammatory acne vulgaris. *Journal of Investigative Dermatology, 129*(10), 2480-2488. DOI:10.1038/jid.2009.93

11. Fern, K. (2019, June 13). *Theobroma cacao*. Useful Tropical Plants. http://tropical.theferns.info/viewtropical.php?id=Theobroma+cacao

12. *Theobroma cacao*. (n.d.). Missouri Botanical Garden. Retrieved December 27, 2020, from http://www.missouribotanicalgarden.org/

PlantFinder/PlantFinderDetails.aspx?taxonid=287263

13. Lipp, M., Simoneau, C., Ulberth, F., Anklam, E., Crews, C., Brereton, P., de Greyt, W., Schwack, W., & Wiedmaier, C. (2001). Composition of genuine cocoa butter and cocoa butter equivalents. *Journal of Food Composition and Analysis, 14*, 399-408. DOI:10.006/jfca.2000.0984

14. Jahurul, M.H.A., Zaidul, I.S.M., Norulaini, N.A.N., Sahena, F., Jinap, S., Azmir, J., Sharif, K.M., & Mohd Omar, A.K. (2013). Cocoa butter fats and possibilities of substitution in food products concerning cocoa varieties, alternative sources, extraction methods, composition, and characteristics. *Journal of Food Engineering, 117*(4), 467-476. https://doi.org/10.1016/j.jfoodeng.2012.09.024

15. Naik, B. & Kumar, V. (2014). Cocoa butter and its alternatives: a review. *Journal of Bioresource Engineering and Technology, 1*, 7-17.

16. Roiaini, M., Seyed, H.M., Jinap, S., Norhayati, H. (2016). Effect of extraction methods on yield, oxidative value, phytosterols and antioxidant content of cocoa butter. *International Food Research Journal, 23*(1), 47-54.

17. Missouri Botanical Garden. (n.d.). *Cocos nucifera*. Retrieved 2 April 2021 from http://www.missouribotanicalgarden.org/PlantFinder/PlantFinderDetails.aspx?taxonid=276638

18. Lima, E. B., Sousa, C. N., Meneses, L. N., Ximenes, N. C., Santos Júnior, M. A., Vasconcelos, G. S., Lima, N. B., Patrocínio, M. C., Macedo, D., & Vasconcelos, S. M. (2015). Cocos nucifera (L.) (Arecaceae): A phytochemical and pharmacological review. *Brazilian Journal of Medical and Biological Research = Revista Brasileira de Pesquisas Medicas e Biologicas, 48*(11), 953–964. https://doi.org/10.1590/1414-431X20154773

19. Gooley, T. (2020, February 14). *Why the coconut palm points to the sea*. The Natural Navigator. Retrieved 6 March 2020 from https://www.naturalnavigator.com/news/2020/02/why-the-coconut-palm-points-to-the-sea/

20. Palm Nectar Organics. (n.d.) *How is coconut sugar made?* Retrieved 18 November 2020 from http://palmnectarorganics.com/coconut-sugar/how-is-coconut-sugar-made.php

21. Orsavova, J., Misurcova, L., Ambrozova, J.V., Vicha, R., & Mlcek, J. (2015). Fatty acids composition of vegetable oils and its contribution to dietary energy intake and dependence of cardiovascular mortality on dietary intake of fatty acids. *International Journal of Molecular Sciences, 16*(6), 12871–12890. https://doi.org/10.3390/ijms160612871

22. Eyres, L., Eyres, M. F., Chisholm, A., & Brown, R.C. (2016). Coconut oil consumption and cardiovascular risk factors in humans. *Nutrition Reviews, 74*(4), 267–280. https://doi.org/10.1093/nutrit/nuw002

23. Arlee, R., Suanphairoch, S., & Pakdeechanuan, P. (2013). Differences in chemical components and antioxidant-related substances in virgin coconut oil from coconut hybrids and their parents. *International Food Research Journal, 20*(5), 2103-2109. Retrieved 14 November 2020 from http://www.ifrj.upm.edu.my/20%20(05)%202013/9%20IFRJ%2020%20(05)%202013%20Pakdeechanuan%20182.pdf

24. Nasir, N., Jalaludin, A., Abllah, Z., Shahdan, I., & Manan, W. (2017). Virgin coconut oil and its antimicrobial properties against pathogenic microorganisms: A review. Proceedings of the International Dental Conference of Sumatera Utara 2017. *Advances in Health Science Research, 8*, 192-199. DOI: 10.2991/idcsu-17.2018.51

25. Elmore, L.K., Nance, G., Singleton, S., & Lorenz, L. (2014). Treatment of dermal infections with topical coconut oil: A review of efficacy and safety of Cocos nucifera L. in treating skin infections. *Natural Medicine Journal, 6*(5), 11 pages. Retrieved March 13, 2022, from https://www.naturalmedicinejournal.com/print/632

26. Evangelista, M.T., Abad-Casintahan, F., & Lopez-Villafuerte, L. (2014). The effect of topical virgin coconut oil on SCORAD index, transepidermal water loss, and skin capacitance in mild to moderate pediatric atopic dermatitis: A randomized, double-blind, clinical trial. *Journal of Dermatology, 53*(1), 100–108. https://doi.org/10.1111/ijd.12339

27. Agero, A.L., & Verallo-Rowell, V.M. (2004). A randomized double-blind controlled trial comparing extra virgin coconut oil with mineral oil as a moisturizer for mild to moderate xerosis. *Dermatitis, 15*(3), 109–116. DOI:10.2310/6620.2004.04006

28. Nevin, K. G., & Rajamohan, T. (2010). Effect of topical application of virgin coconut oil on skin components and antioxidant status during dermal wound healing in young rats. *Skin Pharmacology and Physiology, 23*(6), 290–297. https://doi.org/10.1159/000313516

29. Varma, S.R., Sivaprakasam, T.O., Arumugam, I., Dilip, N., Raghuraman, M., Pavan, K.B., Rafiq, M., & Paramesh, R. (2018). In vitro anti-inflammatory and skin protective properties of virgin coconut oil. *Journal of Traditional and Complementary Medicine, 9*(1), 5–14. https://doi.org/10.1016/j.jtcme.2017.06.012

30. Mittal, A., Sara, U.V.S., Asgar, A., & Aqil, M. (2009). Status of fatty acids as skin penetration enhancers – A review. *Current Drug Delivery, 2009*(6), 274-279. DOI: 10.2174/156720109788680877

31. Tsukahara, T. (1961). Fungicidal action of caprylic acid for Candida albicans. *Japanese Journal of Microbiology, 5*(4), 383-394. https://doi.org/10.1111/j.1348-0421.1961.tb00217.x

32. Valipe, S.R. (2011). Investigating the antimicrobial effect of caprylic acid and its derivatives on *Dermatophilus congolensis* and developing a species specific PCR to detect *Dermatophilus congolensis*. [Doctoral dissertation, University of Connecticut.] OpenCommons@UConn. Retrieved from https://www.proquest.com/docview/884826263

33. Thormar, H., Hilmarsson, H., & Bergsson, G. (2006). Stable concentrated emulsions of the 1-monoglyceride of capric acid (monocaprin) and microbial activities against the food-borne bacteria Campylobacter jejuni, Salmonella spp., and Escherichia coli. *Applied and Environmental Microbiology, 72*(1), 522-526. DOI:10.1128/AEM.72.1.522-526.2006

34. Willems, H.M.E., Stultz, J.S., Coltrane, M.E., Fortwendel, J.P., & Peters, B.M. (2019). Disparate Candida albicans biofilm formation in clinical lipid emulsions due to capric acid-mediated inhibition. *Antimicrobial Agents and Chemotherapy, 63*(11), e01394-19. doi:10.1128/AAC.01394-19

35. Rosenblatt, J., Reitzel, R.A., Vargas-Cruz, N., Chaftari, A-M., Hachem, R., & Raad, I. (2017). Caprylic and polygalacturonic acid combinations for eradication of microbial organisms embedded in biofilm. *Frontiers in Microbiology, 8*(1999). doi: 10.3389/fmicb.2017.01999

36. Fernandez, E., Moraes, M., Martinelli, G. & Colli-Silva, M. (2021). *Theobroma grandiflorum*. IUCN Red List of Threatened Species. 2021: e.T191158664A191158666. Retrieved February 2, 2022, from https://dx.doi.org/10.2305/IUCN.UK.2021-1.RLTS.T191158664A191158666.pt

37. Gondim, T.M.S., Thomazini, M.J., Cavalvante, M.J.B., Souza, J.M.L. (2001). *Aspectos da produção de cupuaçu*. Rio Branco: Embrapa Acre.

38. Itriago, C.V., & Filho, A.A.M. & Ribeiro, P.R.E., Melo, A.C., Takahashi, J., Ferraz, V.P., Mozombite, S.M.S., & Santos, R.C. (2017). Inhibition of acetylcholinesterase and fatty acid composition in Theobroma grandiflorum seeds. *Orbital - The Electronic Journal of Chemistry, 9*(3), 127-

130. http://dx.doi.org/10.17807/orbital.v0i0.894

39. Cultural Survival. (2021). *Controversy continues over cupuaçu tree patent.* Cultural Survival. https://www.culturalsurvival.org/news/controversy-continues-over-cupuacu-tree-patent. Retrieved February 3, 2022.

40. Pugliese, A.G., Tomas-Barberan, F.A. Truchado, P., Genovese, M.I. (2013). Flavonoids, proanthocyanidins, vitamin c, and antioxidant activity of Theobroma grandiflorum (cupuassu) pulp and seeds. *Journal of Agricultural and Food Chemistry,* 61, 2720-2828. https://doi.org/10.1021/jf304349u

41. Fleck, C.A. & Newman, M. (2014). Advanced skin care – a novel ingredient. *Journal of the American College of Clinical Wound Specialists,* 4, 92–94.

42. Cultural Survival. (2021). *Controversy continues over cupuaçu tree patent.* Cultural Survival. Retrieved February 3, 2022, from https://www.culturalsurvival.org/news/controversy-continues-over-cupuacu-tree-patent

43. De Oliveira, T.B. & Genovese, M.I. (2013). Chemical composition of cupuassu (Theobroma grandiflorum) and cocoa (Theobroma cacao) liquors and their effects on streptozotocin-induced diabetic rats. *Food Research International,* 51(2), 929-935. http://dx.doi.org/10.1016/j.foodres.2013.02.019

44. Pereira, A.L.F., Abreu, V.K.G., & Rodrigues, S. (2018). Cupuassu – Theobroma grandiflorum. In S. Rodrigues, E.d. Silva, & E.S. de Brito (Eds.), *Fruits reference guide* (pp. 159-162). Elsevier. https://doi.org/10.1016/B978-0-12-803138-4.00021-6

45. Yanes, C.V.I., de Melo Filho, A.A., Ribeiro, P.R.E., Melo, A.C.G.R., Takahashi, J.A., Ferraz, V.P., Mozombite, D.M.S., & dos Santos, R.C. (2017). Inhibition of acetylcholinesterase and fatty acid composition in Theobroma grandiflorum seeds. *Orbital: The Electronic Journal of Chemistry,* 9(3), 127-130. http://dx.doi.org/10.17807/orbital.v0i0.894

46. Krist S. (2020). Cupuacu butter. *In Vegetable fats and oils* (pp. 301-303). Springer, Cham. https://doi.org/10.1007/978-3-030-30314-3_46

47. Barbalho, G.N., Matos, B.N., da Silva Brito, G.F., da Cunha Miranda, T., Alencar-Silva, T., Sodré, F.F., Gelfuso, G.M., Cunha-Filho, M., Carvalho, J.L., da Silva, J.K.d.R., & Gratieri, T. (2022). Skin regenerative potential of cupuaçu seed extract (Theobroma grandiflorum), a native fruit from the Amazon: Development of a topical formulation based on chitosan-coated nanocapsules. *Pharmaceutics,* 14, 207. https://doi.org/10.3390/pharmaceutics14010207

48. Sano, K., Kawanobe, H., & Someya, T. (2018). Effect of cupuassu butter on human skin cells. *Data in Brief,* 21, 516–521. https://doi.org/10.1016/j.dib.2018.10.026

49. Ved, D., Saha, D., Ravikumar, K. & Haridasan, K. 2015. *Garcinia indica.* The IUCN Red List of Threatened Species 2015: e.T50126592A50131340. https://dx.doi.org/10.2305/IUCN.UK.2015-2.RLTS.T50126592A50131340.en.

50. Chate, M.R., Kakade, S.B., & Neeha, V.S. (2019). Kokum (Garcinia indica) fruit: a review. Asian *Journal of Diary and Food Research,* 4, 329-332. Doi: 10.18805/ajdfr.DR-1493

51. Krist S. (2020). Kokum butter. In *Vegetable fats and oils.* (pp. 399-403). Springer, Cham. https://doi.org/10.1007/978-3-030-30314-3_62

52. Swami, S.B., Thakor, N.J., & Patil, S.C. (2014). Kokum (Garcinia Indica) and its many functional components as related to the human health: A review. *Journal of Food Research and Technology,* 2(4), 130-142.

53. Chate, M.R., Kakade, S.B., & Neeha, V.S. (2019). Kokum (Garcinia indica) fruit: a review. *Asian Journal of Diary and Food Research,* 4, 329-332. Doi:10.18805/ajdfr.DR-1493

54. Parthasarathy, U., Nandakishore, O.P., Senthil Kumar, R., & Parthasarathy, V.A. (2014). A comparison on the physico-chemical parameters of seed butters of selected Indian Garcinia spp. *Journal of Global Biosciences,* 3(6), 872-880.

55. IUCN SSC Global Tree Specialist Group & Botanic Gardens Conservation International (BGCI). 2020. *Pycnanthus angolensis.* The IUCN Red List of Threatened Species 2020: e.T61890778A156105592. Retrieved on January 08. 2021, from https://dx.doi.org/10.2305/IUCN.UK.2020-3.RLTS.T61890778A156105592.en

56. Agroforestry Database (2009). *Pycnanthus angolensis.* Retrieved from http://apps.worldagroforestry.org/treedb/AFTPDFS/Pycnanthus_angolensis.PDF

57. Achel, D.G., Alcaraz, M., Kingsford-Adaboh, R., Nyarko, A.K., Gomda, Y. (2012). A review of the medicinal properties and applications of Pycnanthus angolensis (Welw) Warb. *Pharmacology Online,* 2, 1-22.

58. Sofidiya, M.O., & Awolesi, A.O. (2015). Antinociceptive and antiulcer activities of Pycnanthus angolensis. *Revista Brasileira de Farmacognosia,* 25(3), 252-257.

59. Essumang, D.K., Alemawor, J., Abassah-oppong, S., Weremfo, A. (2008). Analysis of fatty acid composition of kombo (Pycnanthus angolensis) butter. *International Journal of Chemical Sciences,* 6(2), 917-925.

60. Gustafson, K., Wu, Q.L., Asate-Dartey, J., and Simon, J.E. (2013). Pycnanthus angolensis: Bioactive Compounds and Medicinal Applications. *African Natural Plant Products Volume II: Discoveries and Challenges in Chemistry, Health, and Nutrition,* 63-78. DOI:10.1021/bk-2013-1127.ch005

61. Akoma International Ltd. (2021). *Kombo butter fairly traded (African nutmeg) K0244. Certificate of analysis. Akoma from the heart.* Retrieved March 13, 2022, from https://cdn.shopify.com/s/files/1/0580/3540/4960/files/COA_-_KOMBO_BUTTER.pdf?v=11321693334405620645

62. Nagre, R.D., Oduro, I., & Ellis, W.O. (2011). Comparative physico-chemical evaluation of kombo kernel fat produced by three different processes. *African Journal of Food Science and Technology,* 2(4), 83-91.

63. Leonard EC, Simonton D: Uses of vegetable butter-based cetyl myristoleate for treating osteoarthritis and other musculoskeletal disease conditions and injuries. InUSA, 2010.

64. Essumang, D.K., Alemawor, J., Abassah-oppong, S., Weremfo, A. (2008). Analysis of fatty acid composition of kombo (Pycnanthus angolensis) butter. *International Journal of Chemical Sciences,* 6(2), 917-925.

65. Gyingiri Achel, D., Alcaraz, M., Kingsford-Adaboh, R., Nyarko, A.K., Gomda, Y. (2012). A review of the medicinal properties and applications of Pycnanthus angolensis (Welw) Warb. *Pharmacology Online,* 2, 1-22.

66. Botanic Gardens Conservation International (BGCI) & IUCN SSC Global Tree Specialist Group. 2019. *Pentadesma butyracea.* The IUCN Red List of Threatened Species 2019: e.T61988986A149003791. Retrieved on January 8, 2021, from https://dx.doi.org/10.2305/IUCN.UK.2019-2.RLTS.T61988986A149003791.en

67. Ayegnon, B.P., Kayode, A.P.P., Nassia, I., Barea, B., Tchobo, F.P., &

Hounhouigan, J.D. (2015). Effects of storage conditions on the fatty acid composition of the butter of tallow tree (Pentadesma butyracea). *Journal of Applied Biosciences*, 92, 8630-8638.

68. Flora Fauna Web (2021, October 14). *Pentadesma butyracea Sabine*. NParks Flora & Fauna Web. Retrieved February 3, 2022, from https://www.nparks.gov.sg/FloraFaunaWeb/Flora/4/5/4532

69. Sinsin, B., & Avocevou, C. (n.d.). *Pentadesma butyracea Sabine*. Prota4U. Retrieved from February 3, 2022, from https://prota4u.org/database/protav8.asp?g=pe&p=Pentadesma+butyracea+Sabine

70. Aissi, M.V., Tchobo, F.P., Natta, A.K, Piobo, G., Villeneuve, P., Sohounhloue, D., & Soumanou, M.M. (2011). Effet des prétraitements post-récolte des amandes de Pentedesma butyracea (Sabine) sur la technologie d'extraction en milieu reel et la qualité du beurre. *OCL, 18*(6), 384-392. http://dx.doi.org/10.1051/ocl.2011.0423

71. Aissi, M.V., Tchobo, F.P., & Soumanou, M.M. (2018). Chemical composition of traditionally processed Pentadesma butyracea Sabine seeds and butter. *Journal of Microbiology, Biotechnology and Food Sciences, 7*(6), 576-579. DOI: 10.15414/jmbfs.2018.7.6.576-579

72. Sinsin, B., & Avocevou, C. (n.d.). *Pentadesma butyracea Sabine*. Prota4U. Retrieved from February 3, 2022, from https://prota4u.org/database/protav8.asp?g=pe&p=Pentadesma+butyracea+Sabine

73. Avocevou-Ayisso, C., Avohou, T.H., Oumorou, M., Dossou, G., & Sinsin, B. (2012). Ethnobotany of Pentadesma butyracea in Benin: A quantitative approach. *Ethnobotany Research and Applications*, 10, 151-166. https://ethnobotanyjournal.org/index.php/era/article/view/447/648

74. Tchobo, F.P., Natta, A.K., Barea, B., Barouh, N., Piombo, G., Pina, M., Villeneuve, P., Soumanou, M.M. & Sohounhloue, D.C.K. (2007), Characterization of Pentadesma butyracea sabine butters of different production regions in Benin. *Journal of American Oil Chemists' Society, 84*(8), 755-760. https://doi.org/10.1007/s11746-007-1102-0

75. Sinsin, B., & Avocevou, C. (n.d.). *Pentadesma butyracea Sabine*. Prota4U. Retrieved from February 3, 2022, from https://prota4u.org/database/protav8.asp?g=pe&p=Pentadesma+butyracea+Sabine

76. Ayegnon, B.P., Kayodé, A.P., Tchobo, F.P., Azokpota, P., Soumanou, M.M., & Hounhouigan, D.J. (2015). Profiling the quality characteristics of the butter of Pentadesma butyracea with reference to shea butter. *Journal of the Science of Food and Agriculture, 95*(15), 3137–3143. https://doi.org/10.1002/jsfa.7052

78. Tchobo, F.P., Alain, A.G., Jean-Pierre, N., Mickael, L., Bruno, B., Piombo, G., Armand, N.K., Pierre, V., Mansourou, S.M., & Dominique, S.K.C. (2013). Evaluation of the chemical composition of Pentadesma butyracea butter and defatted kernels. *International Journal of Biosciences, 3*(1), 101-108.

79. Ganesan, S.K. (2021). *Mangifera indica*. The IUCN Red List of Threatened Species 2021: e.T31389A67735735. Retrieved February 3, 2022, from https://dx.doi.org/10.2305/IUCN.UK.2021-2.RLTS.T31389A67735735.en

80. Wu, S., Tokuda, M., Kashiwagi, A., Henmi, A., Okada, Y., Tachibana, S., & Nomura, M. (2015). Evaluation of the fatty acid composition of the seeds of Mangifera indica L. and their application. *Journal of Oleo Science, 64*(5), 479–484. https://doi.org/10.5650/jos.ess14238

81. Shah, K.A., Patel, M.B., Patel, R.J., & Parmar, P.K. (2010). Mangifera indica (mango). *Pharmacognosy reviews, 4*(7), 42–48. https://doi.org/10.4103/0973-7847.65325

82. Ediriweera, M.K., Tennekoon, K.H., & Samarakoon, S.R. (2017). A review on ethnopharmacological applications, pharmacological activities, and bioactive compounds of Mangifera indica (Mango). *Evidence-Based Complementary and Alternative Medicine*, Article ID 6949835, 24 pages. https://doi.org/10.1155/2017/6949835

83. Shah, K. A., Patel, M. B., Patel, R. J., & Parmar, P. K. (2010). Mangifera indica (mango). *Pharmacognosy reviews, 4*(7), 42–48. https://doi.org/10.4103/0973-7847.65325

84. Wu, S., Tokuda, M., Kashiwagi, A., Henmi, A., Okada, Y., Tachibana, S., & Nomura, M. (2015). Evaluation of the fatty acid composition of the seeds of Mangifera indica L. and their application. *Journal of Oleo Science, 64*(5), 479–484. https://doi.org/10.5650/jos.ess14238

85. Mwaurah, P.W., Kumar, S., Kumar, N., Panghal, A., Attkan, A.K., Singh, V.K., & Garg, M.K. (2020). Physicochemical characteristics, bioactive compounds and industrial application of mango kernel and its products: A review. *Comprehensive Reviews in Food Science and Food Safety, 19*(5), 2421– 2446. https://doi.org/10.1111/1541-4337.12598

86. Nadeem, M., Imran, M., & Khalique, A. (2016). Promising features of mango (Mangifera indica L.) kernel oil: A review. *Journal of Food Science and Technology, 53*(5), 2185–2195. https://doi.org/10.1007/s13197-015-2166-8

87. Jin, J., Wang, Y., Su, H., Warda, P., Xie, D., Liu, Y., Wang, X., Huang, J., Jin, Q. & Wang, X. (2017) Oxidative stabilities of mango kernel fat fractions produced by three-stage fractionation. *International Journal of Food Properties, 20*(11), 2817-2829, DOI: 10.1080/10942912.2016.1253096

88. Kassi, A.B.B., Soro, Y., Koffi, E.N., & Sorho, S. (2019). Physicochemical study of kernel oils from ten varieties of Mangifera indica (Anacardiaceae) cultivated in Cote d'Ivoire. *African Journal of Food Science, 13*(7), 135-142. DOI:10.5897/AJFS2019.1827

89. Cosiaux, A., Gardiner, L.M. & Couvreur, T.L.P. 2016. *Elaeis guineensis*. The IUCN Red List of Threatened Species 2016: e.T13416970A13416973. Retrieved January 8, 2021, from https://dx.doi.org/10.2305/IUCN.UK.2016-3.RLTS.T13416970A13416973.en

90. *Elaeis guineensis (African oil palm)*. (2019, November 22). Invasive Species Compendium; CABI. https://www.cabi.org/isc/datasheet/20295

91. *Oil palm*. (2016, January 11). Encyclopedia Britannica. https://www.britannica.com/plant/oil-palm

92. Cernansky, R. (2019, March 26). *As palm oil production ramps up in Africa, communities work to avoid problems plaguing other regions*. Ensia. Retrieved March 14, 2022, from https://ensia.com/features/sustainable-palm-oil-production-west-central-africa/

93. *Oil palm*. (2016, January 11). Encyclopedia Britannica. https://www.britannica.com/plant/oil-palm

94. *Palm oil*. (n.d.). World Wildlife Fund. Retrieved March 14, 2022, from https://wwf.panda.org/discover/our_focus/food_practice/sustainable_production/palm_oil/

95. Reddy, M. T., Kalpana, M., Sivaraj, N., Kamala, V., Pandravada, S. R., & Sunil, N. (2019). Indigenous traditional knowledge on health and equitable benefits of oil palm (Elaeis spp.). *OALib, 06*(01), 1–25. https://doi.org/10.4236/oalib.1105103

96. Makerere University Institute of Environment and Natural Resources. 1998. *Vitellaria paradoxa*. The IUCN Red List of Threatened Species 1998: e.T37083A10029534. https://dx.doi.org/10.2305/IUCN.UK.1998.

RLTS.T37083A10029534.en

97. Burnett, C.L., Fiume, M.M., Bergfelt, W.F., Belsito, D.V., Hill, R.A., Klaassen, C.D., Liebler, D., Marks, Jr., J.G., Shank, R.C., Slaga, T.J., Snyder, P.W., & Andersen, F.A. (2017). Safety assessment of plant-derived fatty acid oils. *International Journal of Toxicology*, 36 (Supplement 3), 51S-129S. doi:10.1177/1091581817740569

98. *Vitellaria paradoxa*. (n.d.). Plants for a Future. Retrieved March 13, 2022, from https://pfaf.org/user/Plant.aspx?LatinName=Vitellaria+paradoxa

99. Teketay, D., Gurmu, D., & Bekelem, T. (2003). Vitellaria paradoxa: A multipurpose industrial oilseed tree. *Walia*, 23, 3-23.

100. Akihisa, T., Kojima, N., Katoh, N., Kikuchi, T., Fukatsu, M., Shimizu, N., & Masters, E.T. (2011). Triaglycerol and triterpene ester composition of shea nuts from seven African countries. *Journal of Oleo Science, 60*(8), 385-391. Retrieved March 12, 2022, from https://www.jstage.jst.go.jp/article/jos/60/8/60_8_385/_pdf/-char/en

101. Codex Standard CXS 325R-2-17. 2017. Fatty acid composition of unrefined shea butter.

102. Maranz, S., & Wiesman, Z. (2004). Influence of climate on the tocopherol content of shea butter. *Journal of Agricultural and Food Chemistry, 52*(10), 2934-2937. https://doi.org/10.1021/jf035194r

103. Aremu, M.O., Andrew, C., Salau, R.B, Atolaiye, B.O., Yebpella, G.G., & Enemali, M.O. (2019). Comparative studies on the lipid profile of shea (Vitallaria paradoxa C.F. Gaertn.) fruit kernel and pulp. *Journal of Applied Sciences*, 19, 480-486. DOI: 10.3923/jas.2019.480.486

104. Hofo, F.G., Akissoe, N., Linnemann, A.R., Soumanou, M., Van Boekel, M.A.J.S. (2014). Nutritional composition of shea products and chemical properties of shea butter: A review. *Critical Reviews in Food Science and Nutrition*, 54, 673-686.

Image Credits

Part One: About Carrier Oils

- Pg. 6, 24, 32, 69, 122, 142, 175, 186, 198 Watercolor orange sunflower Frame / ID 125660363 © Andrey Yanushkov | Dreamstime.com
- Pg. 8 Woman dropping oil I bottle / By polinaloves AdobeStock_434436718
- Pg. 8 Balms with pottery / By Jade Shutes
- Pg. 10 Oil drop splash / By Corona Borealis AdobeStock_263779210
- Pg. 13 Oil pouring lab 2 / By ARTFULLY-79 AdobeStock_147499053
- Pg. 21 Oil pouring lab 3 / By ARTFULLY-79 AdobeStock_147499100
- Pg. 23 Jojoba seeds and oil / By liga cerina/EyeEm AdobeStock_248176254

Part Two: Lipids and the Skin

- Pg. 25 Skin Anatomy / ID 52370573 © Designua | Dreamstime.com
- Pg. 26 Woman / ID 177092229 © Fizkes | Dreamstime.com
- Pg. 26 Layers of Protection / By Jade Shutes
- Pg. 27 Relationship between Skin Barrier and Dermal microbiota / By Camille Charlier
- Pg. 28 pH scale / ID 113123203 © Dijarm | Dreamstime.com
- Pg. 30 Cream in hand / ID 190445671 © Prostockstudio | Dreamstime.com
- Pg. 31 Woman with oil / ID 192845928 © Puhhha | Dreamstime.com

Part Three: The Core Carrier Oils

- Pg 35 Sweet Almond / ID 161435333 © Barmalini | Dreamstime.com
- Pg. 37 Apricot tree / ID 14775564 © Xue Haifeng | Dreamstime.com
- Pg. 39 Apricot oil / By mescioglu AdobeStock_277439394
- Pg. 40 Argan / By paolo airenti | shutterstock_33693988
- Pg. 42 Woman making argan oil / By primipil AdobeStock_269768817.jpeg
- Pg. 43 Baobab / ID 95039690 © Yuliia Yurasova | Dreamstime.com
- Pg 44 Baobab / ID 22743713 © Maniec | Dreamstime.com
- Pg. 46 Baobab fruit / By wasanajai AdobeStock_459869347
- Pg. 47 Camelina Sativa plants with ripe seeds / By Inga AdobeStock_265687440
- Pg. 49 Camelina seeds and oil / By Dionisvera AdobeStock_283907623
- Pg. 50 By Kenneth Bosma - Seeds on a Female Jojoba Bush, (https://en.wikipedia.org/wiki/Jojoba#/media/File:Jojoba.jpg)
- Pg. 53 Jojoba oil and seeds / ID 161386904 © Chernetskaya | Dreamstime.com
- Pg. 54 Bernard DUPONT from FRANCE Wikimedia (https://commons.wikimedia.org/wiki/File:Marula_(Sclerocarya_birrea)_fruits_and_leaves_(12907256475).jpg
- Pg. 56 Olive tree / ID 11541034 © Tomo Jesenicnik | Dreamstime.com
- Pg. 57 Olive tree / By Michel AdobeStock_292875296
- Pg. 59 Olive oil / By Dušan Zidar AdobeStock_78245730

- Pg. 60 Safflower / By Singha Songsak AdobeStock_58770079
- Pg. 63 Sesame seeds and oil / By mirzamlk AdobeStock_213082495
- Pg. 65 Sesame oil and seeds / By mescioglu AdobeStock_267679432
- Pg. 66 Sunflower / Jade Shutes
- Pg. 67 Sunflower oil with seeds / By airborne77 AdobeStock_63480300

Part Four: The Enhancer Carrier Oils

- Pg. 72 Oil with glass pipette / By MelissaAdobeStock_228202680
- Pg. 73 Avocado / ID 31340108 © Rozenn Leard | Dreamstime.com
- Pg. 76 Black cumin / By Madeleine Steinbach AdobeStock_178806429
- Pg. 78 Black cumin / ID 164694217 © Halil Ibrahim Mescioglu | Dreamstime.com
- Pg. 79 Borage / Jade Shutes
- Pg. 81 Borage plant / ID 95790165 © Jurate Buiviene | Dreamstime.com
- Pg. 82 Castor seeds / ID 174838567 © (null) (null) | Dreamstime.com
- Pg. 83 Castor plant / ID 157656557 © Rumxde1 | Dreamstime.com
- Pg. 84 Castor oil with seeds / By Alexander Ruiz AdobeStock_348691342
- Pg. 85 Evening Primrose / ID 72364161 © Km271170kav | Dreamstime.com
- Pg. 87 Evening primrose oil / ID 187513061 © Madeleinesteinbach | Dreamstime.com
- Pg. 88 Hemp / ID 154389547 © Maksym Dragunov | Dreamstime.com
- Pg. 89 Hemp seeds / ID 153810235 © Volodymyr Pishchanyi | Dreamstime.com
- Pg. 91 Hemp oil / By vladk213 AdobeStock_433299187
- Pg. 92 Meadowfoam / ID 184750805 © Chernetskaya | Dreamstime.com
- Pg. 94 Meadowfoam field / By Jennifer L Morrow AdobeStock_352691792
- Pg. 95 Neem / ID 39132461 © Kurapy11 | Dreamstime.com
- Pg. 87 Neem oil / By wasanajai AdobeStock_459866950
- Pg. 98 Pomegranate #1 / ID 16704567 © Natallia Yaumenenka | Dreamstime.com
- Pg. 101 Pumpkin and oil / Jade Shutes
- Pg. 102 Pumpkin / Stocksy_txpf0577b66Jze000_Small_420136
- Pg. 103 Pumpkin seeds and oil / AdobeStock_210528609
- Pg. 104 Raspberry / ID 22517816 © Bbbrrn | Dreamstime.com
- Pg. 106 Raspberry / Jade Shutes
- Pg. 107 Rose / ID 77757742 © Alima007 | Dreamstime.com
- Pg. 108 Rose / ID 76861330 © Btwcapture | Dreamstime.com
- Pg. 110 Rosehip seed oil / ID 127828846 © Madeleinesteinbach | Dreamstime.com
- Pg. 111 Sacha inchi / ID 92812630 © Kanasatra Kaewsaenthip | Dreamstime.com
- Pg. 113 Sacha inchi oil / By Luis Echeverri Urrea AdobeStock_276817845
- Pg. 114 Sea buckthorn / ID 153536690 © Pisotckii | Dreamstime.com
- Pg. 115 Sea buckthorn / ID 95494176 © Zeninaasya | Dreamstime.com
- Pg. 115 Sea buckthorn oils / Jade Shutes
- Pg. 117 Sea buckthorn berries / By Elena AdobeStock_377057143
- Pg. 120 Tamanu / By youli AdobeStock_439452659

Part Five: The Herbal Oils

- Pg. 125 Herbs in jar / Jade Shutes
- Pg. 125 Jade Shutes
- Pg. 127 Arnica Hans Hillewaert / https://commons.wikimedia.org/wiki/File:Arnica_montana_(flower_head).jpg
- Pg. 129 Arnica flowers / ID 100931839 © Jeremy Christensen | Dreamstime.com
- Pg. 130 Calendula / Jade Shutes
- Pg. 132 Drying Calendula / Jade Shutes
- Pg. 133 Carrots / Jade Shutes
- Pg. 134 Carrots dehydrator / Jade Shutes
- Pg. 135 Chickweed / ID 121611430 © Stefan Rotter | Dreamstime.com
- Pg. 136 Chickweed / ID 87316538 © Macsstock | Dreamstime.com
- Pg. 137 Comfrey / Jade Shutes
- Pg. 139 Cottonwood / Jade Shutes
- Pg. 140 Cottonwood bud / Jade Shutes
- Pg. 141 St John's wort / ID 12128248 © Vitaly Ilyasov | Dreamstime.com
- Pg 142 St. John's wort oil / Jade Shutes

Part Six: The Butters

- Pg. 146 Blueberry butter / Jade Shutes
- Pg. 147 Babassu / ID 186617648 © Wirestock | Dreamstime.com
- Pg. 150 Cocoa#1 / ID 20241573 © Saiko3p | Dreamstime.com
- Pg. 151 Cocoa #2 / Jade Shutes
- Pg. 153 Coconut / Jade Shutes
- Pg. 157 Cupuacu / Jade Shutes
- Pg. 159 Cupuaca / By guentermanaus AdobeStock_95988628
- Pg. 160 Kokum / ID 125575544 © EPhotocorp | Dreamstime.com
- Pg. 162 Kombo / Jade Shutes
- Pg. 164 Kpangnan / Jade Shutes
- Pg. 167 Mango / Jade Shutes
- Pg. 169 Palm / ID 162096900 © Shuttersyndicate | Dreamstime.com
- Pg. 172 Palm fruit / By dolphfyn AdobeStock_56330217
- Pg. 173 shea butter / ID 26961199 © Hlphoto | Dreamstime.com
- Pg. 175 Unrefined and refined shea butter / Jade Shutes

Appendices

- Pg. 189 Save the Earth / By Denys Holovatiuk AdobeStock_481697688
- Pg. 191 Oil drop splash / By Corona Borealis AdobeStock_263779210

Index

A

Abrasions 59, 63, 122, 142, 180, 187
Acid Mantle 28
Acne 16, 18, 26, 27, 28, 42, 49, 53, 62, 63, 69, 78, 91, 94, 97, 98, 100, 103, 106, 113, 120, 122, 149, 155, 178, 179, 182, 183, 184, 185, 186, 187, 200, 205, 208, 212, 217
Acne blemishes 103, 185
Acne-prone skin 62, 69, 94, 149, 155
Acne scars 122, 187
Adansonia digitata **43**
After-sun care 78, 182
Aging skin 59, 62, 69, 78, 134, 159, 180, 182, 187
Alleviate pain from burns 46, 178
All skin types 36, 53, 62, 69, 75, 94, 113, 178, 179, 180, 181, 182, 184, 186
Almond, Sweet **35**, See Sweet Almond
Alpha-linolenic acid 15, 17, 38, 45, 48, 55, 74, 83, 90, 102, 105, 109, 112, 116, 118, 158, 168, 192, 193
Amyrin 131
Analgesic 84, 122, 131, 140, 183
Anti-aging 91, 113, 115, 117, 119, 186, 201, 207
Antibacterial 16, 17, 19, 28, 75, 91, 96, 97, 113, 122, 129, 132, 182, 201, 205, 214, 217
Anti-inflammatory 8, 16, 17, 18, 19, 20, 21, 30, 31, 62, 69, 78, 81, 84, 86, 87, 91, 96, 97, 100, 103, 106, 110, 119, 122, 131, 132, 135, 140, 142, 159, 172, 179, 180, 181, 183, 184, 185, 187, 200, 201, 204, 208, 212, 214, 215, 216, 217, 218
Anti-irritant 175
Antimicrobial 16, 29, 78, 122, 129, 132, 156, 200, 203, 206, 218
Antinociceptive 16, 78, 84, 183
Antioxidant 8, 19, 20, 21, 22, 28, 31, 33, 34, 49, 59, 64, 65, **71**, 74, 75, 78, 81, 87, 91, 94, 100, 103, 105, 106, 110, 113, 116, 117, 118, 119, 122, 128, 132, 142, 163, 180, 182, 184, 185, 186, 187, 190, 201, 204, 205, 208, 209, 211, 212, 214, 216, 218, 219
Appendices 187
Apricot 3, 9, 15, **37**, 178, 191, 192, 193, 196, 198, 204, 221
   Formulating with 39
   Nutrient Profile 38
Argan 3, 15, **40**, 41, 42, 178, 191, 192, 198, 204, 221
   Formulating with 42
   Nutrient Profile 41
Argania spinosa **40**

Arnica 4, **127**, 215, 222
   Arnica CO2 Extract 128
   Chemistry 128
   Formulating with 129
   Phytochemistry 128
   Safety Information 128
Arnica montana **127**
Arthritic joints 140
Arthritis 129
Atopic dermatitis 18, 26, 27, 28, 30, 62, 69, 81, 87, 119, 122, 144, 155, 161, 180, 181, 182, 183, 202, 208, 215, 217, 218
Attalea speciosa **147**
Avocado 4, 15, **73**, 182, 191, 193, 196, 198, 207, 222
   Formulating with 75
   Nutrient Profile 74
Ayurvedic Doshas 197
Azadirachta indica **95**

B

Babassu 4, 15, 145, **147**, 194, 195, 197, 198, 222
   Formulating with 149
   Nutrient Profile 148
Baobab 3, 15, **43**, 178, 191, 192, 197, 198, 205, 221
   Formulating with 46
   Nutrient Profile 45
Barrier Function 28
Bedsores 117, 119
Beta-carotene 22, 112, 134
Black Cumin **76**, 182, 191, 192, 193, 195, 196, 197, 198
   Formulating with 78
   Nutrient Profile 77
Blackheads 17, 117, 186, 187
Borage 4, 15, **79**, 182, 191, 192, 193, 195, 196, 198, 201, 208, 209, 222
   Formulating with 81
   Nutrient Profile 80
Borago officinalis **79**
Botanical Families 198
Bruises 129, 138, 142
Burns 21, 40, 46, 48, 103, 106, 110, 115, 117, 119, 120, 122, 129, 132, 142, 151, 154, 178, 185, 186, 187, 216
Bursitis 129
Butters 144
   Benefits of 144
   Classification of 145
   Melting points of 145

Storage of 144

C

Calendula 4, 129, **130**, 215, 216, 222
    Calendula CO2 Extract 131
    Formulating with 129, 132
    Phytochemistry 131
    Safety Information 132
Calendula officinalis **130**
Calophyllum inophyllum **120**
Camelina 3, 15, **47**, 179, 191, 192, 193, 195, 197, 198, 205, 221
    Formulating with 49
    Nutrient Profile 48
Camelina sativa **47**
Cannabis sativa **88**
Capric acid 15, 16, 148, 154, 171
Caprylic acid 15, 16, 148, 154, 171, 194
Carotenoids 5, 22, 72, 102, 112, 116, 118, 131, 182, 183, 185, 186, 187, 195
    Significant Sources 195
Carrot 4, **133**, 216
    Formulating with 134
    Phytochemistry 134
Carrot infused oil 134
Carthamus tinctorius **60**
Castor 4, 15, **82**, 183, 191, 194, 198, 208, 209, 222
    Formulating with 84
    Nutrient Profile 83
Cellular regeneration 17, 46, 75, 100, 110, 184
Ceramides 29
Chapped lips 110, 152, 159, 175, 185
Cheilitis 110, 185
Chemistry of Carrier Oils 10
Chickweed 4, **135**, 222
    Formulating with 136
    Phytochemistry 136
Chlorophyll 74, 75, 102
Cholesterol 29
Chronic skin conditions 105
Cocoa 4, 15, 16, 145, **150**, 191, 194, 196, 198, 200, 218, 222
    Formulating with 152
    Nutrient Profile 151
Coconut 4, 15, 145, **153**, 191, 194, 195, 197, 198, 209, 218, 222
    Formulating with 155
    Nutrient Profile 154
Cocos nucifera **153**
Comfrey 4, **137**, 216, 222
    Formulating with 138
    Phytochemistry 138
    Safety Information 138
Contusions 127, 129, 132

Cooling 9, 87, 149, 152, 155, 175
Core Carrier Oils 33
Core Carrier Oils Chart 178
Cottonwood 4, 125, **139**, 222
    Formulating with 140
    Phytochemistry 140
Cracked nipples 132
Cucurbita maxima **101**
Cupuaçu 15, 144, 145, **157**, 194, 198
    Formulating with 159
    Nutrient Profile 158

D

Damaged skin 20, 42, 100, 119, 159, 178, 184, 185
Damaged tissue 132, 142
Dandruff 49, 51, 53, 62, 69, 74, 97, 179, 184
Daucus carota var. *sativus* **133**
Decrease inflammation 103
Dehydrated 30, 75, 133, 134, 182, 190
Dermal Microbiome 26
Dermatitis 18, 26, 27, 28, 30, 31, 55, 62, 69, 81, 87, 91, 97, 98, 119, 122, 132, 135, 142, 144, 149, 154, 155, 160, 161, 174, 175, 179, 180, 181, 182, 183, 184, 202, 203, 208, 215, 217, 218
Docosahexaenoic acid 17, 18, 193
Dry, damaged hair 97, 184
Dryness 28, 30, 36, 152, 159, 161, 172, 175, 178
Dry skin 17, 28, 30, 35, 36, 39, 49, 54, 59, 78, 106, 115, 155, 159, 168, 172, 175, 178, 180, 182, 185

E

Eczema 18, 20, 22, 26, 27, 31, 35, 36, 40, 46, 49, 53, 55, 59, 62, 75, 78, 81, 86, 87, 91, 97, 110, 117, 119, 120, 122, 128, 134, 144, 149, 155, 159, 166, 168, 178, 179, 180, 181, 182, 183, 184, 185, 186, 187, 202
    Dry eczema 46, 55, 75, 168, 178, 179, 182
EFA deficiency 30, 31, 49, 62, 69, 91, 110, 113, 179, 183
Eicosapentaenoic acid 17, 18, 193, 201
Elaeis guineensis **169**
Emollient 16, 18, 21, 30, 35, 36, 40, 43, 49, 50, 65, 75, 78, 79, 81, 84, 85, 87, 91, 93, 94, 95, 97, 100, 101, 103, 108, 110, 117, 119, 149, 150, 155, 156, 159, 162, 164, 169, 173, 178, 180, 181, 182, 183, 184
Emulsifier 159
Enhancer Carrier Oils 71
Enhancer Carrier Oils Chart 182
Epidermal barrier 30, 87, 183
Epidermal regeneration 117, 186
Evening Primrose 4, **85**, 183, 191, 192, 193, 196, 222
    Formulating with 87
    Nutrient Profile 86

F

Fat-soluble Vitamins and Nutrients 20
Fats vs. Oils 23
Fatty Acid Chart 15
Fatty Acid Naming Conventions 14
Fatty Acids 12
Fatty Acids and the Skin 29
Flaking 117, 119, 186, 187
Flea 97
Foot fungus 97, 184
Fractionated Coconut Oil 156
Fragile 55, 75, 179, 182
Fungal skin infections 69, 78

G

Gamma-linolenic acid 15, 17, 18, 80, 86, 90, 193
Garcinia indica **160**
Glossary of Terms 190

H

Hair 17, 25, 27, 40, 41, 46, 49, 50, 51, 53, 54, 55, 57, 59, 62, 65, 69, 78, 97, 113, 127, 149, 154, 155, 161, 165, 166, 178, 179, 180, 182, 184, 186, 190
   Care 49, 94, 168
   Loss 17, 40, 57, 78, 113, 154, 182, 186
Helianthus annuus **66**
Hematomas 129
Hemp 4, 15, 18, **88**, 183, 191, 192, 193, 195, 196, 197, 198, 209, 222
   Formulating with 91
   Nutrient Profile 90
Herbal Oils 124
   Dilution 124
   How to make 125
   Shelf life 126
   Storage 124
Herpes lesions 142
Hippophaë rhamnoides **114**
Hives 120, 149
How to make an herbal oil 125
   Double-boiler method 125
   Folk method 125
Humectants 31
Hydration 28, 30, 42, 75, 106, 155, 178, 185, 203, 204
Hyperextensions 140
Hypericum perforatum **141**
Hyperpigmentation 16, 17, 78, 110, 119, 185, 201, 210

I

Improves elasticity 175
Inflamed skin conditions 46, 55, 69, 106, 110, 179, 185
Inflammation 12, 17, 18, 20, 27, 30, 31, 36, 39, 57, 74, 75, 78, 79, 103, 110, 114, 117, 119, 126, 127, 129, 130, 135, 140, 142, 147, 154, 161, 162, 163, 178, 182, 185, 186, 187, 200, 201, 203, 209, 211, 212
Inflammatory conditions 18, 49, 119
Injured skin 78, 182
Insect bites or stings 122, 187
Irritation 28, 30, 78, 113, 136, 138, 182, 186, 200, 202, 213
Itch 36, 39, 75, 134, 136, 155, 178, 182

J

Joint pain 40, 163, 174
Joint stiffness 129
Jojoba 3, 15, 19, **50**, 179, 191, 194, 195, 197, 198, 205, 221
   Fatty Acid and Unsaponifiable Fractions 51
   Formulating with 53
   Nutrient Profile 51
   Wax Esters 52

K

Kapha 53, 97, 122, 179, 184, 187, 197
Kokum 5, 15, 145, **160**, 194, 198, 219, 222
   Formulating with 161
   Nutrient Profile 161
Kombo 5, 15, 145, **162**, 191, 194, 198, 219, 222
   Formulating with 163
   Nutrient Profile 163
Kpangnan 5, 15, 145, **164**, 193, 194, 198, 222
   Formulating with 166
   Nutrient Profile 165

L

Lauric acid 15, 16, 148, 154, 163, 171, 194
Lecithin 22
Lice 64, 96, 97, 184, 211
Limnanthes alba **92**
Linoleic acid 14, 15, 17, 36, 38, 41, 45, 48, 51, 55, 58, 60, 61, 62, 64, 66, 68, 69, 74, 77, 80, 83, 86, 90, 91, 96, 99, 102, 105, 109, 110, 112, 116, 118, 121, 148, 151, 154, 158, 161, 163, 165, 168, 171, 174, 180, 181, 193, 201, 210
Lipids of the Stratum Corneum 29
Lubricates joints 163

M

Major Components of Carrier Oils 12
Mangifera indica **167**
Mango 5, 15, 145, **167**, 194, 198, 220, 222
   Formulating with 168
   Nutrient Profile 168
Marula 3, 15, **54**, 179, 191, 193, 197, 198, 221

Formulating with 55
Nutrient Profile 55
Mature 39, 42, 43, 47, 49, 75, 94, 96, 101, 113, 120, 150, 152, 153, 159, 174, 178, 179, 182, 186
Mature skin 39
Meadowfoam 4, 15, 19, **92**, 184, 188, 191, 194, 195, 197, 198, 210, 222
Formulating with 94
Nutrient Profile 93
Medium Chain (C8-C12) Fatty Acids 195
Methods of Extraction 9
Cold Pressing 9
Solvent Extraction 9
Supercritical Fluid CO2 9
Minor Components Chart 19
Minor Components of Carrier Oils 18
Mixed Tocopherols 71
Moisturizers and Skin Barrier Repair 30
Monounsaturated fatty acids 16
Myalgia 129
Myristic acid 15, 16, 45, 51, 148, 151, 154, 163, 171, 194, 200

N

Nasal decongestant 175
Natural Moisturizing Factor 3, 29
Neem 4, 15, **95**, 184, 191, 193, 194, 195, 196, 197, 198, 210, 222
Formulating with 97
Nutrient Profile 96
Nigella sativa **76**
Nonsaponifiable lipids 10
Nourishing 42, 65, 78, 178, 180, 182
Nutrient-deficient 91, 183

O

Occlusive 8, 28, **31**, 155
Oenothera biennis **85**
Olea europaea **56**
Oleic acid 14, 15, **16**, 36, 38, 41, 45, 48, 51, 55, 58, 60, 61, 62, 64, 66, 68, 69, 74, 77, 80, 83, 86, 90, 93, 96, 99, 102, 105, 109, 112, 116, 118, 121, 148, 151, 154, 158, 161, 163, 165, 168, 171, 174, 180, 181, 193, 200
Olive 3, 15, **56**, 127, 130, 133, 135, 137, 139, 141, 180, 191, 193, 194, 195, 197, 198, 206, 221
Formulating with 59
Nutrient Profile 58
Omega-3 5, 17, 18, 193
Omega-3 Fatty Acids 5, 193
Omega-6 5, 17, 18, 193
Omega-6 Fatty Acids 5, 193
Omega-9 5, 16, 193

P

Pain and swelling 140
Pain due to inflammation 163
Palm 5, 15, 22, 145, 147, **169**, 189, 194, 195, 198, 218, 220, 222
Formulating with 172
Nutrient Profile 171
Palmitic acid 15, 16, 36, 38, 41, 45, 48, 51, 55, 58, 61, 64, 68, 74, 77, 80, 83, 86, 90, 96, 99, 102, 105, 109, 112, 116, 118, 121, 148, 151, 154, 158, 161, 163, 165, 168, 171, 174, 194
Palmitoleic acid 14, 15, 16, 41, 45, 51, 58, 74, 118, 151, 163
Pathogenic bacterial 53
Penetration enhancer 16, 59, 62, 69, 78, 180
Pentadesma butyracea **164**
Persea americana **73**
pH 28
Photodamage 30, 91, 94, 122, 184
Phytosterols 19, 20, 209
Pitta 53, 87, 97, 122, 149, 155, 179, 183, 184, 187, 197
Plukenetia volubilis **111**
Polyphenols 58, 90, 194
Polyunsaturated fatty acids 17
Pomegranate 4, 15, **98**, 184, 191, 194, 195, 196, 198, 211, 222
Formulating with 100
Nutrient Profile 99
Populus balsamifera **139**
Post-menopausal women 42, 178
Pregnancy and breastfeeding 138
Preventative aging care 53, 106, 178, 184, 186
Problematic skin 17, 42, 117, 178, 186, 187
Prunus amygdalis var. *dulcis* **35**
Prunus armeniaca **37**
Psoriasis 18, 22, 26, 27, 30, 31, 35, 40, 46, 51, 53, 55, 75, 78, 81, 87, 91, 100, 119, 120, 122, 132, 144, 149, 159, 161, 168, 175, 178, 179, 182, 183, 184, 187
Pumpkin 4, 15, **101**, 185, 191, 192, 193, 195, 196, 198, 211, 222
Formulating with 103
Nutrient Profile 102
Punica granatum **98**
Pycnanthus angolensis **162**
Pyrrolizidine alkaloids 81

R

Rashes 134, 136
Raspberry 4, **104**, 185, 191, 193, 198, 212, 222
Formulating with 106
Nutrient Profile 105
Refining 9
Bleaching 9

Deodorizing 9
Winterizing 9
Refrigeration **34**, 74
   Borage seed 79
   Evening primrose 85
   Hemp seed 88
   Pomegranate 98
   Raspberry seed 104
   Rosehip seed 108
Regeneration 8, 16, 17, 46, 87, 91, 100, 106, 110, 115, 117, 138, 159, 184, 185, 186
Regenerative skincare 53, 119, 172, 183
Restore a damaged skin barrier 42, 178
Rheumatism 57, 76, 95, 112, 122, 127, 129, 139, 170, 174, 187
Ricinus communis **82**
Rosacea 26, 27, 91, 100, 132, 183, 184, 202
Rosa spp. 107
Rose **107**, 198, 207, 212, 213, 222
   Formulating with 110
   Nutrient Profile 109
Rosemary CO2 Extract Antioxidant 71
   Borage seed 81
   Evening primrose 87
   Hemp seed 91
   Pomegranate 100
   Raspberry seed 106
   Rosehip seed 110
   Sea buckthorn pulp 119
Rough skin 152, 159
Rubus idaeus **104**

S

Sacha Inchi **111**, 186, 191, 192
   Formulating with 113
   Nutrient Profile 112
Safflower 4, 15, 60, 61, 62, 180, 191, 193, 196, 198, 206, 222
   Formulating with 62
   Linoleic acid-rich 62
   Nutrient Profile 61
   Oleic acid-rich 62
Saponifiable fraction 10
Saponifiable lipid 10
Saturated fatty acids 16
Scabies 40, 60, 97, 170, 184
Scalp 27, 49, 53, 62, 65, 69, 78, 97, 127, 155, 179, 180, 182
   dry scalp 53
   itchy scalp 49
Scaly skin 17, 22, 122, 187
Scars 40, 46, 74, 106, 110, 119, 122, 178, 185, 187
Sclerocarya birrea **54**
Sea Buckthorn **114**, 186, 187, 191, 192, 193, 194, 195, 196, 198, 214
Sea Buckthorn Pulp Oil **118**
   Formulating with 119
   Nutrient Profile 118
Sea Buckthorn Seed Oil **116**
   Formulating with 117
   Nutrient Profile 116
Sebaceous glands 27
Seborrheic dermatitis 97, 149, 184
Sebum 3, 27, 28
Sensitive 25, 39, 44, 47, 49, 81, 156, 163, 175, 178, 182
Sesame 4, 15, **63**, 180, 191, 192, 194, 196, 197, 198, 206, 222
   Formulating with 65
   Nutrient Profile 64
Sesamum indicum **63**
Shea 5, 15, 145, **173**, 194, 196, 198
   Formulating with 175
   Nutrient Profile 174
Shelf Lives 191
   Extend the Shelf Life of Other Oils 197
Shingles 122, 187
Simmondsia chinensis **50**
Skin 25
   Anatomy & Physiology 25
   Barrier disruption 17, 62, 69
   Barrier repair 42, 117
   Ecology 26
   Elasticity 19, 42, 49, 87, 100, 168, 178, 179, 184, 204
   Hydration 28, 30, 42, 155, 178, 203
   Itching 36, 178
   Skin-soothing 62, 180, 181
Softens and soothes the skin 46
Spoilage 33
Sprains and strains 129
Squalene 7, 18, 19, 21, 28, 36, 38, 41, 48, 58, 74, 80, 90, 99, 102, 105, 109, 118, 184, 185, 195, 201, 202, 204, 208, 212, 216
Stearic acid 15, 16, 36, 38, 41, 45, 48, 55, 58, 61, 64, 68, 74, 77, 80, 83, 86, 90, 96, 99, 102, 105, 109, 112, 116, 118, 121, 148, 151, 154, 158, 161, 163, 165, 168, 171, 174, 194, 200
Stellaria media **135**
Stiffness and swelling 129
St. John's wort 4, **141**
   Formulating with 142
   Phytochemistry 142
   Safety Information 142
Storage 33
Stratum corneum 8, 12, 17, 20, 22, 25, 26, 27, 28, 29, 30, 31, 117, 119, 186, 187, 200, 206, 207
Stretch marks 25, 42, 46, 53, 55, 168, 178, 179
Sunburn 30, 100, 117, 122, 144, 168, 184, 187
Sun-damaged skin 100, 119, 159, 184

Sunflower 4, 15, 17, **66**, 127, 133, 135, 139, 181, 191, 193, 195, 196, 197, 198, 202, 206, 222
    Formulating with 69
    Linoleic acid-rich 69
    Nutrient Profile 68
    Oleic acid-rich 69
Suppleness 21, 49, 59, 168, 179, 180
Suppositories 119, 152, 161
Sustainability 188
Sweet Almond **35**, 178, 191, 192, 193, 198, 221
    Formulating with 36
    Nutrient Profile 36
Swimmer's itch 97, 184
Symphytum officinale **137**

T

Tamanu 4, 15, **120**, 187, 191, 192, 194, 195, 197, 198, 214, 215, 222
    Formulating with 122
    Nutrient Profile 121
Taraxasterol 131
Tattoo aftercare 53, 179
Tension 84, 183
Theobroma cacao **150**
Theobroma grandiflorum **157**
TEWL (see Transepidermal Water Loss)
Tissue regeneration 46, 106, 110, 117, 185
Tissue repair 132
Tocopherols 18, 19, 21, 36, 38, 41, 48, 51, 55, 61, 64, 68, 71, 74, 77, 83, 86, 90, 93, 96, 99, 102, 105, 109, 112, 116, 118, 121, 148, 151, 154, 158, 161, 165, 168, 171, 174, 201, 208, 213
Transepidermal Water Loss 3, 8, 12, 16, 17, 19, 27, **29**, 30, 31, 42, 62, 69, 81, 106, 110, 117, 119, 144, 155, 177, 181, 182, 184, 185, 186, 190
Traumatic injuries 129
Trophic ulcers of the skin 110, 185

U

Ulcers 48, 95, 99, 110, 119, 130, 132, 135, 137, 142, 162, 185
Unsaponifiable fraction 10
UV blocking 117
UV-damage 17, 18
UV-hyperpigmented skin 17, 91, 183
UV-protective 122
UV radiation 19, 33, 78, 182, 185

V

Varicose veins 129
Vata 49, 53, 55, 65, 87, 179, 180, 183, 197
Vitamin A 22, 109, 202
Vitamin D 22
Vitamin E 21, 22, 48, 71
Vitellaria paradoxa **173**
Vitiligo 78, 132, 182, 208

W

Wax esters 52
Wound healing 16, 17, 21, 27, 31, 39, 53, 63, 69, 75, 103, 110, 117, 119, 120, 122, 135, 141, 142, 149, 161, 170, 178, 179, 185, 186, 200, 203, 204, 207, 212, 214, 216, 217, 218
Wound Healing or Skin Regeneration Carrier Oils **197**
Wrinkles 31, 40, 42, 62, 69, 91, 152, 159, 178, 183

X

Xerosis 28, 29, 30, 155, 218

Y

Yeast infections 97, 184

Z

Zero Waste 188